Clinical Obsessive-Compulsive Disorders in Adults and Children

Clinical Obsessive-Compulsive Disorders in Adults and Children

Edited by

Robert Hudak
University of Pittsburgh School of Medicine

and

Darin D. Dougherty
Harvard Medical School

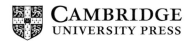

CAMBRIDGE
UNIVERSITY PRESS

CAMBRIDGE UNIVERSITY PRESS
Cambridge, New York, Melbourne, Madrid, Cape Town,
Singapore, São Paulo, Delhi, Tokyo, Mexico City

Cambridge University Press
The Edinburgh Building, Cambridge CB2 8RU, UK

Published in the USA of America by Cambridge University Press, New York

www.cambridge.org
Information on this title: www.cambridge.org/9780521515696

First published 2011

Printed in the United Kingdom at the University Press, Cambridge

A catalog record for this publication is available from the British Library

Library of Congress Cataloging in Publication data
Clinical obsessive-compulsive disorders in adults and children / edited
by Robert Hudak, Darin D. Dougherty.
p. ; cm.
Includes bibliographical references and index.
ISBN 978-0-521-51569-6 (hardback)
1. Obsessive-compulsive disorder.   I. Hudak, Robert, 1966–
II. Dougherty, Darin D.   III. Title.
[DNLM: 1. Obsessive-Compulsive Disorder. WM 176]
RC533.C6335   2011
616.85′227–dc22
2010038772

ISBN 978-0-521-51569-6 Hardback

Contents

Contributors

Andrea Allen
Mount Sinai School of Medicine, New York, USA

Jonathan S. Abramowitz
Department of Psychology, University of
North Carolina at Chapel Hill, Chapel Hill,
NC, USA

Michael H. Bloch
Yale Child Study Center, New Haven, CT, USA

Elaine Davis
Obsessive Compulsive Foundation of Western PA,
Pittsburgh, PA, USA

Darin D. Dougherty
Harvard Medical School and Department of
Psychiatry of Massachusetts General Hospital, Boston,
MA, USA

Beth Forhman
Adjunct Faculty, Graduate School of Social Work,
Adelphi University, Garden City, NY, USA

Andrew R. Gilbert
Department of Psychiatry, University of
Pittsburgh School of Medicine, Pittsburgh,
PA, USA

Christina M. Gilliam
The Institute of Living, Hartford, CT, USA

Andrew Goddard
Indiana University, Indianapolis, IN, USA

Benjamin D. Greenberg
Butler Hospital, Warren Alpert Medical School of
Brown University, Providence, RI, USA

Robert Hudak
University of Pittsburgh School of Medicine,
Pittsburgh, PA, USA

Sony Khemlani-Patel
Psychiatry Department, North Shore University
Hospital, Great Neck, NY, USA

Terri Laterza
Adult OCD Intensive Outpatient Program, Western
Psychiatric Institute and Clinic, Pittsburgh, PA, USA

Fugen Neziroglu
Hofstra University, Hempstead, New York, USA

Signi A. Page
UPMC Medical Education Program Pittsburgh,
Pittsburgh, PA, USA

Stefano Pallanti
Mount Sinai Medical Centre, New York, USA

Katharine A. Phillips
Butler Hospital and the Department of Psychiatry and
Human Behavior, Alpert Medical School of Brown
University, Providence, RI, USA

Kalie D. Pierce
Adult OCD Intensive Outpatient Program, Western
Psychiatric Institute and Clinic, Pittsburgh, PA, USA

Michael Poyurovsky
Rappaport Faculty of Medicine, Technion, Israel
Institute of Psychiatry, Haifa, Israel

Yong-Wook Shin
Clinical Cognitive Neuroscience Center, SNU-MRC,
Seoul, Korea

David F. Tolin
The Institute of Living, Hartford and Yale University
School of Medicine, New Haven, CT, USA

Aureen P. Wagner
The OCD and Anxiety Consultancy, Rochester,
NY, USA

Preface

While obsessive-compulsive disorder (OCD) is one of the most common psychiatric disorders, accurate diagnosis and treatment are still too often lacking. Past studies have suggested that 17.5 years elapse, on average, between the onset of OCD symptoms and adequate diagnosis and treatment. Recently, greater attention is being paid to OCD in lay media outlets, which has resulted in a greater public awareness of OCD. Also, clinicians are receiving more training regarding the diagnosis and treatment of OCD than in the past. Hopefully, these factors will shorten the gap between symptom onset and adequate treatment. However, even with this growing knowledge base, clinicians are often required to seek out expert knowledge regarding OCD in order to optimize their diagnostic and treatment strategies. While no textbook can be a substitute for individual teaching and supervision, a review of contemporary diagnostic and treatment strategies should enhance the clinical acumen of readers and help to ensure that readers provide their patients with optimal care. The goal of this volume is to describe the current state of knowledge concerning the diagnosis and treatment of OCD and to describe how it is appropriately applied in a clinical treatment setting.

The clinical presentation, the underlying etiology, and pharmacotherapy treatment of OCD are all addressed in this text. The first chapter covers basic information concerning OCD, including epidemiology and phenomenology. Hudak also provides case examples to illustrate certain diagnostic challenges in OCD. Dougherty and Greenberg discuss the latest findings regarding the neurobiology of OCD in Ch. 2. In addition, they review surgical treatments for intractable OCD. First-line medication treatments are reviewed in Ch. 3, by Page and Hudak, while pharmacological augmentation strategies are described by Goddard and Shin in Ch. 4.

Comorbidity is the rule rather than the exception in OCD. Therefore, multiple chapters deal with treatment concerns in patients with comorbid disorders. In Ch. 5, Abramovitz discusses OCD treatment in patients with comorbid mood disorders including a discussion of postpartum OCD, while in Ch. 6 Poyurovsky covers the important topic of the relationship between psychosis and OCD. Finally, Gilbert, in Ch. 7, reviews medication strategies in the treatment of another special population, children and adolescents.

Psychotherapy plays a critical role in treatment and management, and Neziroglu and colleagues (Ch. 8) discuss the principles behind exposure with response prevention therapy. Hoarding represents a specific type of OCD symptoms requiring its own individual therapies, and a review is provided by Gilliam and Tolin in Ch. 9. Psychotherapy in children and adolescents can require different strategies than in adults, and Wagner in Ch. 10 provides detailed clinical information regarding the use of psychotherapy in this population. The perception of OCD in the community at large can have effects on access to OCD treatment. This issue, as well as strategies to mitigate this problem, is reviewed by Davis in Ch. 11. Family members are greatly affected by OCD and this issue almost always needs to be addressed in treatment. Allen and Pallanti, in Ch. 12, provide an invaluable discussion regarding the inclusion of family in treatment. Laterza, Pierce, and Hudak in Ch. 13 review the different levels of treatment (outpatient, day programs, residential programs, etc.) available to OCD patients, and provide case examples of how differing intensities of therapy impacts outcome.

Finally, OCD is often considered a spectrum disorder. Therefore, other putative spectrum disorders are reviewed in chapters by Phillips (Ch. 14: body dysmorphic disorder) and Bloch (Ch. 15: trichotillomania).

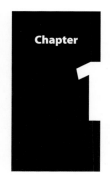

Chapter

1

Introduction to obsessive-compulsive disorder

Robert Hudak

History and diagnosis

There is probably no other psychiatric illness that has gone through a more fascinating evolution in its conceptualization during contemporary times than obsessive-compulsive disorder (OCD). Just in the last 30 years the change in the perception and treatment of OCD has been dramatic. In fact, this process is still ongoing as psychiatry increasingly moves towards a multidimensional model of OCD. This work-in-progress will be interesting to follow. At the turn of the twentieth century, Freud wrote about obsessions as defensive psychological responses to unconscious impulses. He also talked about the underlying role of childhood sexual experiences. Pierre Janet first provided clinical descriptions of OCD in 1903 in *Les Obsessions et la Psychasthenie*. As a result, through most of the following decades, OCD was thought to result from unresolved unconscious conflicts. For years, parents were thought to be the root cause of this disorder through "excessively harsh toilet training" (Adams 1973). It is important to note, however, that a disease model should not simply present a theory that on the surface appears to explain an illness but should also predict a related treatment. Significantly, no treatment based on the resolution of unconscious impulses was ever shown to work for OCD.

With psychoanalytic models clearly not valid in explaining the pathology of OCD, cognitive models were then explored. The cognitive models postulated that individuals with OCD may possess dysfunctional beliefs including over-inflated personal responsibility, overestimation of threat, the need to control thoughts, and perfectionism (Freeston *et al.* 1996; Boucard *et al.* 1999). Interestingly, it was not until the latter part of the twentieth century that a model for OCD based on

biological underpinnings became widely accepted. Because of the heterogeneous nature of the symptoms of OCD, it is unlikely that a single factor will be identified as the biological origin for OCD. Consequently, multiple avenues of research are being explored. Genetic, neuroanatomical, and infectious causes for OCD are the focus of current research and the underlying cause of OCD is likely multifactorial.

As defined by the *Diagnostic and Statistical Manual of Mental Disorders,* 4th edition (DSM-IV; American Psychiatric Association 1994), OCD has fairly straightforward criteria. The DSM simply asks that a person has either obsessions (Box 1.1) or compulsions (Box 1.2), that at some point during the disorder the person has recognized that the symptoms were excessive or unreasonable, and that they cause marked distress, are time consuming, or significantly interfere with the patients functioning. The DSM-IV does allow that the person can have poor insight (i.e., not recognize that the symptoms are unreasonable or excessive). Because of the intrusive nature of an obsession, a person may describe it as an alien thought, or as a feeling as if the thought is not their thought. However, the person will state that they know that the thought is coming from their own mind: just that it feels as if it is not. Careful interviewing by the practitioner should easily distinguish this from thought insertion, a symptom of schizophrenia that is not seen in OCD.

The differential diagnosis of OCD can be difficult enough that the illness has been termed chameleon-like (Attiullah *et al.* 2000). A contributing factor in this difficulty is that obsessions can focus on virtually any thought content. While OCD is sometimes portrayed as the illness in which people have a fear of germs or a need to check things, the content of obsessions can include virtually anything. It is the nature of the

Clinical Obsessive-Compulsive Disorders in Adults and Children, ed. Robert Hudak and Darin D. Dougherty.
Published by Cambridge University Press. Copyright © Cambridge University Press 2011.

Box 1.1   Required diagnostic criteria of obsessions

1. Recurrent and persistent thoughts, impulses, or images that are experienced, at some time during the disturbance, as intrusive and inappropriate and caused marked anxiety or distress.
2. The thoughts, impulses, or images are not simply excessive worries about real-life problems.
3. The person attempts to ignore or suppress such thoughts, impulses, or images, or to neutralize them with some other thought or action.
4. The person recognizes that the obsessional thoughts, impulses, or images are a product of his or her own mind (not imposed from without as in thought insertion).

Box 1.2   Required diagnostic criteria of compulsions

1. Repetitive behaviors (e.g., hand washing, ordering, checking) or mental acts (e.g., praying, counting, repeating words silently) that the person feels driven to perform in response to an obsession, or according to rules that must be applied rigidly.
2. The behaviors or mental acts are aimed at preventing or reducing distress or preventing some dreaded event or situation; however, these behaviors or mental acts either are not connected in a realistic way with what they are designed to neutralize or prevent or are clearly excessive.

Table 1.1 Content of the primary obsession

Content	Percentage
Contamination	38
Fear of harming self or others	24
Symmetry concerns	10
Somatic	7
Religious	6
Sexual	6
Hoarding	5
Unacceptable urges	4
Miscellaneous	1

thought (i.e., its intrusive nature) that determines the obsession, not the content of the thought. People may also describe experiences in which their thoughts are "sticky" and seem to repeat or skip like a record album that has a scratch. Some obsessions occur more commonly than others. Table 1.1 contains a list of the most common obsessions as reported by the DSM-IV Field Trial, which examined the primary presenting symptom (Foa *et al.* 1995).

It should be noted that obsessions are defined as thoughts, impulses, or images; some clinicians forget that obsessions can present in forms other than thoughts. This can be a factor in the misdiagnosis of OCD. A patient with an obsessional image may describe their symptoms in such a way that it can be confused with a visual hallucination. For example, obsessions of aggression towards their children are recognized phenomena of OCD in the postpartum period (Abramowitz *et al.* 2003). Obsessional images can coexist as well. One woman presented to our clinic with an obsessional image that involved her ripping out her baby's cornea and seeing the baby covered in blood. Such a vivid obsessional image is often described as a hallucination by the patient. Careful questioning should help in distinguishing between the two. It is important to note that the mothers with postpartum obsessions find these thoughts morally repugnant and they represent no increase in the risk of harm to the child.

Many patients report that their primary obsession is not a well-defined thought, such as "I wonder if I really locked the door." Instead, they report a difficulty performing a certain task until it feels "just right." They may be unable to stop an action such as hand washing not because they are worried about germs but because they get a feeling that it has not yet been done correctly. They may have a difficult time making decisions or initiating actions until they feel that it is the "correct" or "proper" time to do so. In some patients, the inability to

Table 1.2 Content of the primary compulsion

Content	Percentage
Checking	28
Cleaning/washing	27
Miscellaneous	12
Repeating	11
Mental rituals	11
Ordering	6
Hoarding	4
Counting	2

make decisions can be so severe that it is termed obsessional slowness.

Table 1.2 contains the most common compulsions as reported by the DSM-IV Field Trial, which examined the primary presenting symptom (Foa *et al.* 1995). The authors found that up to 80% of OCD patients had mental compulsions, a significant fact because mental compulsions were not recognized by DSM-III. Among the potential negative outcomes by DSM-III would be that designing behavioral therapy targeting rituals could suffer as a result. Many patients also incorrectly identified themselves as being in a "pure obsessional" subcategory as a result of this diagnostic neglect. The current criteria state much more clearly that compulsions may exist as mental and not just as physical acts. Compulsive rituals such as counting, praying, and mental reviewing are now considered compulsions under the criteria. DSM-IV trials suggested that approximately 10% of OCD patients have mental rituals as their primary compulsion.

Other studies have noted that most people have multiple obsessions and compulsions (Rasmussen and Tsuang 1986; Pinto *et al.* 2006). Various OCD symptoms can occur simultaneously in individual patients. For example, at the same time as a person is engaging in a hand washing ritual, they may also be performing a counting ritual. An examination of the most common obsessions and compulsions show that the rates of obsessions and their expected compulsions are not always identical. For example, the rate of contamination obsessions in the study was 38% while the rate of cleaning as a ritual was only 27%. This disparity can be explained by the fact that obsessions and compulsions do not necessarily follow what a non-OCD sufferer

may believe is a realistic or logical correlate. For example, the person who believes their hands are contaminated may not compulsively wash their hands in response but instead respond to that obsession by repeating phrases (e.g., "I am clean, I am clean, I am clean"). Since the compulsion is not inherently goal-directed or rewarding, it is not necessarily recognized as any more logical than the obsession (Cameron 2007).

Another significant category in the DSM-IV is the qualifier for "poor insight." Prior editions stated that the person must have recognized the absurdity of their symptoms at least during one point in the course of their illness. The DSM-IV Field trials showed that 8% of current OCD patients did not recognize their obsessions as being unreasonable, and that 5% never did (Foa *et al.* 1995).

The diagnosis of OCD is essentially the same whether the patient is a child or adult, and clinically the disease appears the same in both groups (Swedo *et al.* 1989), with the possible exception of a higher rate of poor insight in children (Goodman 1999). Interestingly, this makes OCD fairly unusual compared with other psychiatric disorders, where symptoms usually appear differently in children as opposed to adults.

Epidemiology

At one time, OCD was thought to be a rare condition. While the illness has been written about for more than 100 years, it was believed to be a uncommon disorder that would be seldom seen or diagnosed. This changed with the publication of the Epidemiological Catchment Area (ECA) study (Karno *et al.* 1988). This study was based on a large household sample of US residents and it determined that the lifetime prevalence of OCD was between 1.9% and 3.3% (Goodman 1999). This was initially a surprise because these numbers were much higher than expected. However, data from other studies subsequently performed at multiple sites worldwide generally agree with the ECA, the data being fairly consistent in most nations; the sole exception being Taiwan, which tends to have rates differing from other countries for all psychiatric disorders studied (Horwath and Weissman 2000). These studies, therefore, indicate that OCD is the fourth most common psychiatric disorder behind specific phobias, substance disorders, and major depression (Rasmussen and Eisen 1994).

Because of the potential for severe impairment, the World Health Organization has listed OCD among the 10 medical and psychiatric conditions most likely to cause disability (Murray *et al.* 1996). The ECA study further showed that approximately 36% of patients with OCD had occupational difficulties. One estimate showed that someone with OCD may lose three years of wages because of the illness during the course of their lives. Approximately one quarter of OCD patients experience problems with marital relationships, and patients with OCD are less likely to marry than people without OCD (Goodman 1999).

The age of onset has been examined in epidemiological studies. There are some difficulties with comparing numbers from these studies because of the disparity of the definition of age of onset. Authors have looked at the age when symptoms first began, when the symptoms first caused distress, or when the person first met DSM criteria. This is not an insignificant concern, as many patients with OCD will report the presence of subclinical symptoms for many years before they became severe enough to cause distress or to seek treatment. According to the ECA study, the age of onset of OCD is in the mid-20s for people in the USA. In the other countries studied, the range of age of onset can vary from early to mid-20s to early 30s. Data indicates an average age of onset of 21, with an earlier average age of onset for men at 19 years compared with women at 22 years of age (Rasmussen and Eisen 1994). It is not at all unusual for OCD to present earlier than these ages: 21% of patients report symptoms before puberty. A positive family history of OCD, as well as a personal or family history of tics was also associated with an earlier age of onset (Attiullah *et al.* 2000). A person with comorbid obsessive-compulsive personality disorder (OCPD) may have a somewhat earlier age of onset when compared with OCD patients without OCPD (Coles *et al.* 2008).

There is also a phenomenon of late-onset OCD. It has been reported that 11% of OCD patients will have onset of symptoms after the age of 30 years (Grant 2007). As is often the case, many of these patients also reported the presence of minor or subclinical obsessions prior to the onset of OCD. This group of patients is more likely to be married than OCD patients with a younger age of onset, but no further difference demographically has been noted between the groups. The late-onset group was less likely to have checking as a primary symptom (checkers tend to have an earlier age of onset) and are less likely to have comorbid personality disorders. Significantly, these individuals tend to have a lower severity of symptoms and a corresponding improved response to cognitive-behavioral therapy. One should note some studies have not shown a difference in severity level between early- and late-onset OCD, and no difference in level of insight or functional impairment. People with late-onset OCD did have a lower rate of psychiatric comorbidity (Pinto *et al.* 2006). The phenomenon of late-onset OCD is an ongoing area of study.

Case example 1

Ms. L is a 31-year-old white woman who presented to an OCD intensive treatment program precisely one year and three days after the onset of her OCD. She is able to specify the exact day and minute her symptoms started, as she was typing an e-mail at the time. She started having severe hand tremors that she described as "hand-flapping" and became quite concerned that she had multiple sclerosis or Lyme disease. She had a complete neurological work-up that failed to identify any abnormalities, yet she continued to have intrusive thoughts about being ill and compulsions involving body scans to ensure she was not sick. At her initial evaluation, she stated that she had intrusive thoughts her entire life. These included concerns about getting AIDS from mosquitoes or fears that she might be gay. She did not consider these thoughts to be troublesome; since they did not interfere with her life she did not seek treatment.

Ms. L illustrates some of the difficulties in performing epidemiological studies. While her clear recollection of the specific day of onset of symptoms is not typical, it is not a unique clinical experience either. Her onset can be defined at age 30 when she first had obsessions severe enough to seek treatment. Alternatively, her onset can be said to have started with her early life history of intrusive thoughts. Like many people with such as history, Ms. L was not able to say exactly when those started, except to say it was her "entire life." Because OCD has been known to have its onset as early as the first two or three years of life (do Rosario-Campos *et al.* 2005), these subclinical obsessions may not be considered unusual by the person as they have always been present. It should also be noted that many OCD patients will give a clear history that some of their earliest memories consist of obsessions. These factors can make determining the age of onset problematic.

The information on gender distribution in OCD has also changed over the years. What was once considered to be conventional wisdom has changed somewhat. This is because the ECA study engendered a dramatic change in how OCD was regarded by the mental health community. It had been believed that OCD had an equal gender distribution: that men and women suffered from the disorder in equal proportions. The ECA studies were carried out at cross-national sites (which included the USA, Edmonton Canada, Puerto Rico, Munich, Taiwan, Korea, and New Zealand) and showed a picture that did not necessarily agree with this earlier hypothesis. Most of the studies showed that women seem to have a slight increase in the rate of OCD, except for the Munich site, which showed a small preponderance of men. The ratio of women to men in all of the studies was less than 2 to 1. So, if indeed OCD does tend to occur more often in women, the difference is not as great as in disorders such as major depression, which women suffer in rates twice that of men.

Evolution towards a multidimensional model

In DSM-IV, OCD is classified as an anxiety disorder, although strictly speaking it is not a disorder of anxiety. While obsessions may indeed provoke anxiety in the affected individual, the anxiety is a consequence of the intrusive thought itself. In the instance of an obsession that involved spreading contamination to others, it would be natural for someone to experience anxiety and fear for the safety of others, even though the thought itself is recognized as irrational. The anxiety is a result of the overestimation of threat that can occur in OCD (Rachman 1993) and is not the underlying cause of the obsession itself. Additionally, obsessions do not always provoke anxiety in the patient.

Disgust is also a common emotional response to obsessional content, particularly when related to contamination or religious obsessions (Husted *et al.* 2006; Olatunji *et al.* 2007). There are suggestions of neuroanatomical differences between people who experience disgust instead of anxiety-related obsessions (Berle and Phillips 2006). Other OCD patients may experience a feeling of incompleteness or of things "just not feeling right" (Ecker and Gonner 2008). Sometimes, the obsessions can provoke guilt, irritability, shame, or just a general feeling of discomfort.

Because of these facts, it has been proposed that an Obsessive-Compulsive Spectrum Disorders category should be created (Castle and Phillips 2006; Stein and Lochner 2006; Matsunaga and Seedat 2007). Such a classification would likely necessitate the removal of OCD from the Anxiety Disorders category. Some authors have argued that OCD is better served by being placed in a category of Obsessive-Compulsive Spectrum Disorders, as greater overlap exists with illnesses such as body dysmorphic disorder, hypochondriasis, trichotillomania, pathological excoriations or skin picking, and Tourette's syndrome, among others, than is seen between OCD and other illnesses listed under Anxiety Disorders (Hollander *et al.* 2007; Pallanti and Hollander 2008). This question may ultimately be resolved as the consideration of OCD evolves towards the multidimensional model.

Symptom dimensions

From the time of the earliest descriptions of OCD, authors have tried to divide OCD into different subcategories, including Falret's "*folie du doute*" (madness of doubt) and "*delire du toucher*" (delusion of touch) in 1869 (de Mathis *et al.* 2006). In more recent times, authors have divided symptoms into various categories, including washers, checkers, symmetry, aggressive thoughts, and hoarders. An additional classification proposes OCD symptoms be segregated based on the origin of the obsessions. They would either be classified as autogenous, where obsessions tend to come into conscious thought spontaneously, or as reactive, such as where obsessions are evoked by external stimuli (Lee *et al.* 2005). In 1980, the DSM-III simply defined OCD without addressing specific symptoms or subtypes. As more research has been carried out – including observational studies, factor and cluster analytical studies, and various biologic investigations including genetic and neuroimaging studies – newer multidimensional models for OCD are being developed. The different dimensions of OCD (which regard OCD as comprising different sets of OCD symptoms) may indicate different treatment responses and different comorbidities depending upon the specific obsessional dimension. Research in the fields of the genetics, neurobiology, and treatment of OCD may find these dimensional phenotypes of value in more clearly defining parameters of subject selection for studies as well as determining more

Table 1.3 The association between obsessive-compulsive disorder factors and comorbid diagnosis

Disorder	Factor			
	I	II	III	IV
Tic disorders	+		−	
Depressive disorders	+			
Bipolar disorder		+		
Generalized anxiety disorder	+			
Social phobia	+			
Panic disorder agoraphobia and alcohol/substance abuse	+	+		
Eating disorders			+	

closely related correlates of their findings (Leckman *et al.* 2007; Stein *et al.* 2010).

As the dimensional approach has been studied more extensively, various dimensions appear to be associated with their own distinctive traits. Using factor analytic methods, many studies have shown that OCD can be viewed as having four factors (Hasler *et al.* 2005; Mataix-Cols *et al.* 2005). The studies have been fairly consistent but occasionally show anywhere between three and six factors (Leckman *et al.* 2007). Some of the disparity occurs because some studies differ on whether or not aggressive–sexual–religious symptoms form a unique factor. Additionally, somatic obsessions have occasionally been loaded on to differing factors. Nonetheless, the most common factors identified are as follows.

> *Factor I.* Associated with aggressive, sexual, religious obsessions and related checking compulsions. Somatic obsessions generally fall into the factor I group as well.
> *Factor II.* Associated with obsessions of symmetry and compulsions of repeating, counting, ordering, and arranging.
> *Factor III.* Associated with contamination obsessions and cleaning compulsions.
> *Factor IV.* Associated with hoarding and collecting.

The various studies from Leckman (2007) and Mataix-Cols and colleagues (Mataix-Cols *et al.* 2005, Mataix-Cols 2006) have demonstrated that comorbidities can be associated with these factors. Table 1.3 outlines some of the pertinent information from these studies.

Analyses have shown that tic disorders, including Tourette's syndrome, are positively associated with factor I and negatively associated with factor III. Depressive disorders are found to be associated with factor I while bipolar disorder is more strongly associated with factor II. Generalized anxiety and social phobia are associated with factor I, while symptoms of panic, agoraphobia, and alcohol and substance abuse are associated with both factors I and II. Interestingly, there does not appear to be an association between other anxiety disorders, or substance abuse, and factor III. One can hypothesize that this may be because of the fact that people with contamination obsessions are more likely to experience disgust in response to their obsessions (as opposed to anxiety) and, therefore, may not feel an increased need to self-medicate with alcohol. Factor III is associated with eating disorders. There are some epidemiological associations with these factors as well. Men are more likely to have factor I obsessions while women are more likely to fall into factor III. Factors I and II are associated with an earlier age of onset than the other factors.

While OCD symptoms are known to fluctuate during the course of someone's life, preliminary longitudinal studies seem to indicate that patients maintain symptoms within their respective dimension (Mataix-Cols 2002). Further studies are needed to confirm this finding. When symptoms are classified by the autogenous and reactive model, a preliminary study has also shown that those patients do not fluctuate between subtypes (Besiroglu *et al.* 2006). Reviewing the above information, it does appear that a dimensional approach to OCD can help to integrate prior studies and classifications based on age of onset, gender, or presence of comorbid and obsessive compulsive spectrum conditions. This will likely have an influence on the development of the DSM-V (Leckman *et al.* 2007) and contribute towards a better understanding of the phenomenology of OCD (Mataix-Cols 2006).

Potential genetic and autoimmune causative factors

Research to elucidate the potential genetic origins of OCD is extensive and ongoing (Pauls 2008). Analyses of the incidence of OCD in twins show that monozygotic twins have a higher rate of OCD than dizygotic twins, serving as a good indication of the genetic nature of the illness. While case studies were published as early as 1929, it was with the advent of the DSM-III in the 1980s that such studies recruited enough subjects to have adequate authority. Subsequent family studies helped to confirm that the transmission of OCD did indeed occur on a familial basis.

Current research has been focused on determining if a genetic linkage of certain loci and the expression of OCD can be identified. Recent additional work is investigating the correlation between specific symptoms such as compulsive hoarding and an association with a specific susceptibility locus. Future work is likely to focus on genome-wide association studies in an attempt to help to identify potentially problematic genes (Hemmings and Stein 2006). Since OCD likely has a multifactoral etiology, it is improbable that a single gene will be found to be the cause of the illness. However, as further genetic studies are carried out containing large enough sample sizes, people with a common genetic etiology are more likely to be identified as dimensional subgroups within the larger sample (Kim and Kim 2006). Such a large study would of course necessitate a significant funding commitment.

Another potential causative factor for OCD under investigation is a fascinating area involving sequelae from group A beta-hemolytic streptococcal (GAS) infection (Snider and Swedo 2004). It has long been recognized that a neurological disorder called Sydenham's chorea could follow such an infection, and that obsessive compulsive symptoms can be associated with the chorea. In the late 1980s and early 1990s, it was discovered that some children would develop OCD and/or tic disorders following a GAS infection and in the absence of Sydenham's chorea. This syndrome is known as PANDAS (pediatric autoimmune neuropsychiatric disorders associated with streptococcal infections). While a controversy still exists as to whether PANDAS is a true causative factor of OCD, the hypothesis that cross-reactive antineuronal antibodies may play a role in the etiology of OCD in these children is gaining evidence (Murphy *et al.* 2006). These anti-GAS antibodies appear to react in the neurons in the caudate, putamen, and globus pallidus. Antibiotic prophylaxis as well as intravenous immunoglobulin and plasma exchange have been shown to improve OCD symptoms in preliminary studies, but currently there are no formal recommendations for general treatment.

While PANDAS is likely to be responsible for only a minority of OCD cases, the criteria set up by Snider and Swedo (2004) and currently used to recognize this subgroup are:

- the presence of a tic disorder and/or OCD
- prepubertal age at onset, usually between 3 and 12 years of age
- abrupt symptom onset and/or episodic course of symptom severity: often parents can pinpoint the date of onset, which is unusual in OCD, and the OCD symptoms may completely remit between episodes in PANDAS but are unlikely to do so in OCD in the absence of PANDAS
- temporal association between symptom exacerbations and streptococcal infections, with the OCD symptoms usually occurring after the infection
- presence of neurological abnormalities during periods of symptom exacerbation, including tics and choreiform movements.

Further research is being carried out to help to elucidate epidemiological issues such as symptoms and course, and potential treatment of PANDAS in addition to the specific cellular basis of the illness.

Comorbidity of psychiatric disorders in OCD

It is well known that patients with OCD will commonly have other psychiatric disorders. The ECA study reported that two thirds of OCD patients met the criteria for another psychiatric disorder at some point in their lives (Karno *et al.* 1988). Other studies have tended to show similar incidences (Tükel *et al.* 2002). In a study performed in an OCD specialty treatment center, it was found that 31% of OCD patients met the criteria for major depressive disorder (MDD) during the period of their treatment at the center, as well as 67% of the study participants indicating a lifetime history of MDD. Additionally, incidence of patients meeting a clinical criteria at some point in their lives was reported as 18% for social phobia, 17% for eating disorders, 14% for alcohol dependence, and 12% for panic disorder; the incidence of these diagnoses presenting at the time of the study were 11%, 8%, 8%, and 6%, respectively (Attiullah *et al.* 2000).

Depression may be secondary and reactive to the OCD symptoms or a primary diagnosis; distinguishing between the two can be difficult. Regardless, the finding that MDD occurs in approximately two thirds of OCD patients is an important consideration for the clinician. Since MDD is an illness that is associated with suicidality, it follows that the potential for suicide exists in patients with OCD. Unfortunately, suicide in OCD has only had limited research. One study reported that up to 70% of people with OCD had thoughts that life was not worth living, about half of their sample had either suicidal thoughts or passive death wishes, and 10% of their sample reported a history of suicide attempts (Torres *et al.* 2007). Another study found that the rate of suicide attempts in patients with OCD was as high as 27% (Kamath *et al.* 2007). While it appears that suicidality is a potential area of concern for clinicians who treat OCD, any risk factors for suicide unique to OCD are not well delineated at this time. Whether there is a relationship between the severity of OCD symptoms and suicidality is not clear because of some conflicting data. Larger studies will need to be carried out to clarify this point. The type of OCD symptoms from which a person suffers has been suggested as a risk factor but has not been well studied. The presence of depression and hopelessness are correlated to a higher degree with suicidal ideation (Kamath *et al.* 2007), although insight into obsessional symptoms has a less clear association with suicidal thoughts. It is clear that there is an under-recognized potential for suicide in OCD; this should be screened for and addressed in a rigorous manner.

Bipolar disorder and OCD are known to occur together. Various authors have stated that up to a third of patients with bipolar disorder also meet the criteria for OCD. Interestingly, it has been noted that obsessive and compulsive symptoms rarely occur during a manic episode (Attiullah *et al.* 2000). Most patients with bipolar disorder and OCD will report that their OCD symptoms get better as they become manic. In a case study reported by Gordon and Rasmussen (1988), a patient's OCD became worse in direct proportion to his depression and remitted during manic episodes. This is a fairly typical pattern clinically, and it is not unusual for bipolar patients to report this phenomenon as a motivating factor for their decision to discontinue use of mood stabilizers. In addition to the euphoria associated with mania, they enjoy the absence of their OCD.

Other anxiety disorders commonly occur with OCD as indicated above, and it is becoming increasingly recognized that generalized anxiety disorder (GAD) is found frequently in OCD patients. As many as 20% of OCD patients have comorbid GAD (Abramowitz and Foa 1998). It can be difficult clinically to distinguish obsessions and the worries displayed in GAD in individuals presenting with both disorders as they have shared clinical characteristics. The intense preoccupation with worry over occurrences of potentially low probability is often seen in both illnesses and, therefore, this high comorbidity is not entirely unexpected.

As noted above, eating disorders can occur in approximately 17% of patients with OCD. When patients with eating disorder are properly screened, it has been found that 41% of them may also suffer from OCD (Kaye *et al.* 2004). It has long been recognized that the two disorders share some clinical characteristics. Patients with eating disorders can display perfectionism; rigidity, especially in matters concerning their dietary habits; and harm avoidance (Attiullah *et al.* 2000). These symptoms can be heightened in someone suffering from both illnesses. It should be noted that a common obsession involves a fear of food being contaminated; people with this symptom will often experience weight loss. Such pathology would not warrant the diagnosis of an eating disorder. Because eating disorders are potentially lethal, screening for this condition is highly warranted while examining patients with OCD.

The association between tic disorders and OCD has long been recognized. It has been found that between 5 and 10% of patients with OCD will have met the criteria for Tourette's syndrome at some point in their lifetime, and up to 20% will have had multiple tics at some point (Swedo *et al.* 1989). Patients with Tourette's syndrome are more likely to have OCD symptoms related to symmetry and ordering, and compulsions of touching and counting (Hasler *et al.* 2005). Among patients with tics disorders, approximately one quarter are diagnosed with comorbid OCD, and as many as half report obsessional-like symptoms. Because of the high rate of comorbidity, this has led to speculation that these disorders may share a genetic relationship.

The comorbidity of OCD and schizophrenia is an area that is receiving much interest in the literature but is still in flux because of significant differences in findings from different studies. Most clinicians and researchers agree that OCD occurs at a higher rate in people with schizophrenia than it does in the general population, but the exact rate varies greatly between studies. The rates of OCD in schizophrenia have been reported to be anywhere from 7.8% to 41% (Attiullah *et al.* 2000). Discrepancies may be attributed to differing methods of screening for obsessive compulsive symptoms as well as inconsistent criteria in defining OCD or obsessive compulsive symptoms. See Ch. 6 for more details.

Obsessive-compulsive personality disorder

A controversy still exists concerning any potential relationship between OCPD and OCD. It is common in day-to-day practice to hear a clinician mention the relationship between OCPD and OCD, or to hear talk about OCD and OCPD being on a continuum. There is little evidence to support these notions. The concept of OCPD is based in psychoanalytic theory and was written about in the early 1900s. Freud talked about anal character types who were preoccupied with notions of orderliness, parsimony, and obstinacy (Fineberg *et al.* 2007). While early writings suggested that OCPD traits sometimes preceded the development of OCD, it was noted as early as the 1930s that OCPD traits also occurred without subsequent development of OCD. Modern studies have also not shown any definitive relationship between the two disorders (Attiullah *et al.* 2000). The fact that both disorders share very similar sounding names has likely contributed to the confusion. The first edition of the DSM mentioned a "compulsive personality," and in the DSM-II, the name was changed to "obsessive compulsive personality." In the same edition, an alternative name was also introduced – "anankastic personality"–

to help to decrease confusion with OCD. However, the term anankastic was dropped from DSM-III and OCPD is the only official designation at present. Interestingly, the anankastic term was kept in the *International Statistical Classification of Diseases and Related Health Problems* (ICD) classification, and is still in use in ICD-10 (World Health Organization 1994) coding and terminology.

The DSM-IV describes OCPD as a disorder characterized by "a preoccupation with orderliness, perfectionism, and mental and interpersonal control, at the expense of flexibility, openness, and efficiency." In other words, people with OCPD are very rigid individuals with a low tolerance for changes and spontaneity. The full criteria appear in Box 1.3.

Studies have shown that criteria 1, 2, 6, and 8 to be the most consistent and useful criteria in the diagnosis of OCPD whereas 3 and 7 have little predictive value (Grillo *et al.* 2001). Criterion 5 deals with hoarding and can easily be confused with the hoarding subtype of OCD. The diagnostic criterion of OCPD is, therefore, in flux, likely to change over time, and gives pause to the hypothesis of connecting it to OCD.

Various studies have shown different rates of comorbidity of OCD and OCPD. While the numbers differ depending on which study is read, most data show that OCD is more likely to occur in the absence of OCPD than with it (Torres and Del Porto 1995; Attiullah *et al.* 2000; Crino and Andrews 1996). Recent data have suggested that only approximately 25% of OCD patients have comorbid OCPD (Pinto *et al.* 2006). Personality disorders are considered to be stable disorders, yet in an OCD specialty treatment center,

---

Box 1.3 Diagnostic criteria for obsessive-compulsive personality disorder

1. Is preoccupied with details, lists, order, organization, or schedules to the extent that the major point of the activity is lost.
2. Shows perfectionism that interferes with task completion (e.g., is unable to complete a project because his or her own overly strict standards are not met).
3. Is excessively devoted to work and productivity to the exclusion of leisure activities and friendships (not accounted for by obvious economic necessity).
4. Is overconscientious, scrupulous, and inflexible about matters of morality, ethics, or values (not accounted for by cultural or religious identification).
5. Is unable to discard worn-out or worthless objects even when they have no sentimental value.
6. Is reluctant to delegate tasks or to work with others unless they submit to exactly his or her way of doing things.
7. Adopts a miserly spending style toward both self and others; money is viewed as something to be hoarded for future catastrophes.
8. Shows rigidity and stubbornness.

approximately 80% of patients who had a diagnosis of a personality disorder upon admission for OCD treatment failed to meet the criteria for the personality disorder after appropriate OCD treatment (Baer and Jenike 1992). This finding further supports the hypothesis that a significant relationship between OCD and OCPD is unlikely to exist.

The driving force behind the respective pathologies of OCD and OCPD is different. The person with OCPD has no obsessions: no intrusive thoughts exist which trouble the individual. Rather than being compelled to perform what an OCD sufferer usually recognizes as silly, repetitive, and useless tasks, the individual with OCPD feels that their actions are correct and necessary. The person with OCPD shows little discomfort with their symptoms while the person with OCD will show anxiety or anguish over their illness. Some of the confusion may result because the symptoms can look similar on the surface. For example, a person with obsessions regarding order and symmetry may appear to have OCPD-like perfectionism. However, that is only a superficial similarity; confusion would only occur if the clinician focuses on the behavior (i.e., arranging and ordering) that the person was exhibiting and not assessing whether it is ego-syntonic or not (Grant and Odlaug 2008). The underlying reason for the behaviors is very different, and with careful questioning the clinician can usually determine the nature of the behavior.

Another potential area for confusion of OCD and OCPD may occur through ritual avoidance in OCD. When OCD symptoms are more severe, the resultant elaborate and time-consuming rituals can be very exhausting to perform. As a result, their compulsions can take the form of avoidance; in other words, rather than performing a ritual, they will avoid the situation that will trigger the obsession. They may develop rigid rules to follow in order to avoid a feared situation. As an example, a person with contamination obsessions may require that family or visitors remove shoes or clothing worn outside, or even insist that people shower and change before entering the house. These rules are the result of their desire not to have to perform extensive cleaning rituals. While this person would be considered rigid and orderly, these problems are not stemming from an underlying OCPD diagnosis but are a result of the OCD. Understanding that the OCD precedes the rigidity is an important determination in clarifying the diagnosis (Baer and Jenike 1992). If the rigidity responds to OCD treatment, resulting in

a lessening or elimination of this trait, a diagnosis of OCPD would not be warranted.

Course of OCD

The course of OCD is chronic and lifelong. Symptoms will fluctuate over the lifetime of the individual, exhibiting a waxing and waning in severity of symptoms (DSM-IV). The likelihood of full remission among adult sufferers is low (Eisen *et al.* 1999). However, differing definitions of the following categories has tended to obfuscate the data. The course of OCD has classically been divided into three categories (Goodwin *et al.* 1969):

1. Episodic course with periods of incomplete remission
2. Phasic course with periods of complete remission between exacerbations
3. Continuous and unremitting course but most patients experiencing fluctuations in the level of symptoms, and a minority experiencing a chronic and deteriorative course.

Studies showed differing rates of the categories, with estimates of the continuous course at approximately 50–80%, with a minority (approximately 10%) experiencing a deteriorating course (Attiullah *et al.* 2000). One potential problem with the categories can be how to differentiate the episodic course from the continuous course owing to the typical waxing and waning of symptoms. The definition between an incomplete remission and someone with continuous OCD experiencing a good period may not always be clear, and it may differ depending on the criteria set for a particular study.

For the most part, these studies were carried out before the advent of serotonin reuptake inhibitors (SRIs) and exposure with response prevention therapy (ERP). Modern treatments may change the way the course of the illness is viewed (Steketee *et al.* 1999). With treatment, one third of patients have been known to experience a 75% reduction in symptoms (Orloff *et al.* 1994). While many patients will report improvement in OCD after treatment, the majority will still be sick enough to meet full criteria for OCD. However, these patients can report significant improvement in the reduction of the strength of the obsessions and in their degree of impairment. Only a minority of patients, approximately 12%, will experience complete remission (Eisen *et al.* 1999).

In women, the possibility exists for onset of OCD during pregnancy and/or during the postpartum period. Most of the studies performed in this area have methodological problems because of their retrospective nature, making firm conclusions difficult. Wisner *et al.* (1999) reported that 57% of women in the postpartum period with depression will experience obsessional thoughts. Women experiencing postpartum depression are also more likely to experience intrusive, obsessional thoughts than women with major depression unrelated to pregnancy. Pregnancy seems to be associated with onset of OCD in a small number of women, with estimates from various studies ranging anywhere from 10% to 66% of women with a diagnosis of OCD reporting onset or worsening of symptoms with pregnancy (Abramowitz *et al.* 2003). Most patients retrospectively report no change in OCD during pregnancy, with approximately 17% reporting worsening of symptoms, and 14% describing improvement. Additional work is required to fully explore the relationship between pregnancy and OCD.

Insight in OCD

Some individuals with OCD are known to have poor insight into their symptoms. Children especially appear to be more likely to describe obsessions as senseless and, therefore, may have poorer insight (Volz and Heyman 2007). For the first time, the DSM-IV has recognized this aspect of OCD, and added a qualifier of "poor insight." It states that the qualifier of "poor insight" may be given if the obsession is exaggerated in intensity but not quite to the level of a delusion. Clinically, patients may exhibit poor insight globally (i.e., the person has poor insight into their OCD during the entire course of their illness) or it may occur only after they have been sick for a period of time. However, even people with otherwise good insight into their symptoms will often report impaired insight during the time period that they are engaged in a compulsion and are experiencing severe anxiety. In addition to poor insight, the DSM-IV states that an OCD patient may be given an additional diagnosis of "delusional disorder" or "psychotic disorder not otherwise specified" if the patient has lost the ability to do reality testing and when the belief in the obsessions reaches delusional proportions.

Discussing insight and OCD is fraught with difficulties as this is still an area that is not completely settled. Measuring insight has been problematic; until the publication of the Brown Assessment of Beliefs Scale (BABS), there was no accepted scale to measure insight (Eisen *et al.* 1998). The term "overvalued idea" (OVI) appears in the DSM-IV yet does not appear in the diagnostic criteria for OCD. The relationship between OVI and obsessions, as well as delusions, has not yet been clearly delineated (Kozak and Foa 1994). The DSM glossary defines overvalued ideation as "an unreasonable and sustained belief that is maintained with less than delusional intensity (i.e., the person is able to acknowledge the possibility that the belief may not be true)." The issue of whether or not obsessions evolve into OVI and then into delusions, and, therefore, can be considered to be on a continuum is not settled. There has been little research carried out to examine the difference, if any, between an obsession and OVI. It has been argued that the strength of the belief in obsessions is broadly distributed and that a continuum of insight, rather than categories of obsessions/OVI/delusions, is more accurate (Kozak and Foa 1994). These authors noted that delusions have the same range of insight. Since insight tends to be a state-dependent phenomenon (i.e., insight is poor in the midst of an obsessional crisis and better when the person is less anxious) the idea that obsessions, OVI, and delusions are on a continuum ultimately may not be valid. Unfortunately, the DSM-IV inappropriately clouds the issue of insight in the descriptive text of OCD. It gives the example of poor insight as a person with the obsession that they have willed the death of another person and stating this has reached "delusional proportions." The example of someone with good insight is given as having a fear of germs. The reason given for good insight in the text is that germs are "ubiquitous." This example is based upon the content of the obsession and not on the strength of the conviction, which is truly the determining factor for insight.

Whether people with poor insight respond differently to treatment is still controversial. One difficulty in studying these patients is getting them to agree to therapy, especially behavioral therapy. Some clinicians have noted that OCD patients with poor insight do indeed respond to ERP as long as they are willing to engage in treatment (Eisen *et al.* 2001), and there is little difference in the response to pharmacotherapy or behavioral therapy (Kozak and Foa 1994). Since this has not been studied extensively, it should be considered to be an ongoing issue. However, there is no evidence at this time that patients with poor insight should not be offered therapy. If they agree to participate, the same therapy and protocol as other patients should be offered.

Misdiagnosis of OCD

Mental health evaluations tend to miss OCD (Grant and Odlaug 2008). While it is recognized as a serious mental illness, it is common for patients to be under psychiatric treatment for some time before a diagnosis of OCD is finally made. On average, people with OCD see three to four doctors and spend nine years seeking treatment before they receive a correct diagnosis. This delayed diagnosis, combined with the fact that individuals suffering with OCD often put off seeking treatment when the disorder manifests, results in an average of 17 years from the onset of OCD symptoms until the patient start receiving appropriate treatment (Hollander and Wong 1998). A study from a health maintenance organization demonstrated that the clinically recognized rate of OCD was less than 10% of the estimated population prevalence (Fireman *et al.* 2001). Even when patients do receive a correct diagnosis of OCD, less than 10% of the patients will be offered a medication regimen that is consistent with the current standards of care (Hankin *et al.* 2009). As few as one in five adolescents with OCD receive treatment for their illness (Valleni-Basile *et al.* 1994). There are numerous reasons why OCD is potentially subject to underdiagnosis: (1) reluctance of patients to divulge their symptoms; (2) lack of recognition of the diversity of presenting symptoms in OCD by professionals, leading to a subsequent misdiagnosis; and (3) failure to ask OCD screening questions in the routine mental status examination (Rasmussen and Eisen 1990).

Obsessions are quite commonly accompanied by shame and embarrassment, resulting in patients often failing to reveal symptoms to their loved ones, primary care physician, or psychiatrist. The patient may not initially present their symptoms to a mental health professional but may present them in a medical setting where it is unlikely that OCD would be considered in a differential. Often people voice other complaints such as depression, anxiety, or panic attacks. Only with direct questioning are obsessional symptoms shared with the clinician. Failure to recognize the varied forms of OCD is another contributor to the underdiagnosis of OCD. While compulsive cleaning and checking rituals are commonly recognized as OCD, it actually can involve virtually any feature imaginable: obsessions can concern almost any topic. Occasionally, people who report staying up all night ritualizing or who describe their anxiety or obsessions as "racing thought" can be misdiagnosed as bipolar. Symptoms

such as "just right" OCD and obsessional slowness are not routinely taught to mental health clinicians and are, therefore, poorly recognized. Patients with OCD and obsessional slowness have been misdiagnosed as having catatonic schizophrenia when the inability to initiate actions becomes severe enough. Obsessions are often mistakenly called delusions. As a result, OCD can be thought of as a "the great imitator" with its ability to mimic many other psychiatric illnesses.

Mental health professionals often do not routinely screen for OCD symptoms during mental status examinations. Most psychiatrists and psychologists receive minimal specific training in OCD and consequently do not have enough knowledge about this disorder. Clinical psychologists do not learn ERP as part of their training; psychiatrists rarely rotate through specialized OCD programs. Training for social workers, mental health counselors, and nurses is even less comprehensive in addressing OCD and treatment protocols for this disorder.

To facilitate the diagnosis of OCD in the clinical setting, routine screening questions should be given to patients, particularly those with anxiety or depressive complaints. Questions that may be asked as part of the mental status examination would include:

Do you wash your hands excessively, or do you have to check things over and over?
Do you have thoughts that make you anxious, or that you consider to be bothersome or that do not make sense?
Do you have thoughts that you try to get rid of but cannot?
Do you have behaviors or rituals that you have to do repeatedly, and that you feel compelled to do even though it seems silly?

A key point in those screening questions is that while the first question regarding hand washing and checking will capture most OCD, it will still miss a significant percentage of patients. Therefore, a complete screening should continue with the additional questions to increase the likelihood of identifying additional cases of OCD.

Obsessions versus delusions

One of the more difficult challenges facing a clinician is trying to distinguish between obsessions and delusions. It is a clinical distinction that appears straightforward, yet in practice is one of the more vexing problems in the mental health field. Clinical experience in an OCD specialty clinic has shown that OCD is often misdiagnosed as a psychotic disorder. A case series involving what the authors termed "transformation obsessions" illustrates how this misdiagnosis may occur (Volz and Heyman 2007). Nine patients presented to their clinic with obsessions that involved the fear of turning into someone or something else, or assuming unwanted characteristics. Several of these patients were initially given a diagnosis of a psychotic disorder. Prior to a specialty OCD clinic referral, the treating physicians deemed these symptoms to be bizarre in nature in spite of the fact that there is no basis in psychiatric literature to make the differentiation between obsessions and delusions based upon their bizarre nature of the content of the thought (e.g., the thought consisting of a physical impossibility).

The importance of making the correct differential diagnosis between obsessions and delusions cannot be overstated: an incorrect diagnosis will negatively affect the patient's treatment and outcome. Patients report feeling hopeless and stigmatized when they are given an incorrect psychotic diagnosis.

Obsessions are defined as "recurrent and persistent unwanted thoughts, images, or impulses that are inappropriate or intrusive and cause marked anxiety" (DSM-IV). A delusion is defined as "a false belief based on incorrect inference about external reality that is firmly sustained despite what almost everyone else believes" (DSM-IV). The terms ego-dystonic and ego-syntonic were de-emphasized in the DSM-IV; however, they are useful in distinguishing between obsessions and delusions. Ego-dystonic is defined as anything that is unacceptable to the part of the psyche that mediates reality testing, impulse control, and thought content (Ayd 1995). This term describes an obsession. The presence of an ego-dystonic thought is distressing to the individual. In contrast, ego-syntonic can be defined as any thought that is acceptable to the part of the psyche that mediates reality testing, impulse control, and thought content (Ayd 1995). This term describes a delusion. The presence of a delusion is not distressing to the person who has it. While it has been argued that the strength of the conviction differentiates between obsessions and delusions, people with both obsessions and delusions may have a range of insight into their symptoms (Kozak and Foa 1994). (See above in the discussion of insight in OCD.) While people suffering from obsessions with poor insight

may not always be able to describe their thoughts as irrational, the description of a thought as irrational and/or intrusive is indicative of an obsession, or if the individual knows that what they are worried about is silly or bizarre. By contrast, a delusional person has total belief in their delusion and does not question its presence in their mind.

Along with confusion regarding the role of insight into the differentiation between obsessions and delusions, clinical experience indicates that it is common practice for mental health practitioners to attempt to distinguish between delusions and obsessions based upon the concept of bizarreness (i.e., whether the thought is physically impossible). It should be noted that no systemic surveys have studied this issue, yet evidence of this practice has been widely observed. Practitioners have also been noted to classify obsessions into subcategories based on whether they think a particular thought is "non-bizarre" or "bizarre." There has never been a suggestion that obsessions should be viewed differently based upon their "bizarreness;" treatment protocols are the same in either instance and there is no indications that treatment response will differ. Therefore, there is no reason to subcategorize obsessions based on bizarreness. The case studies below illustrate that if the approach to making a clinical diagnosis is not based upon accepted protocols, patients may receive incorrect diagnoses and/or incorrect treatment leading to poor outcomes.

Case example 2

Mrs. A was referred to an OCD intensive outpatient program by her private psychiatrist because of non-response. She had been given a diagnosis of OCD with delusions. She was employed as an administrative assistant and was performing well at her job. Mrs. A had not been responding well to outpatient treatment consisting solely of pharmacological treatment. She was on a moderate dose of a selective SRI (SSRI) as well as a second-generation antipsychotic and had some side effects to these, mostly complaining of daytime fatigue. Her primary symptoms involved checking her surroundings for lint that may have fallen from her clothing. She stated that she felt that if the lint was away from the main body of clothing, it would "get lonely because it had no one to talk to." She said that she was less worried if two pieces of lint fell off her clothes: they would be able to talk to each other and would not be as unhappy. She was able to express to staff at the clinic that she knew full well that lint was not sentient and did not get lonely. She fully recognized the absurdity of these thoughts, and in fact much of her anxiety stemmed from the fact that she was so preoccupied with a thought that she herself found ridiculous. There was no evidence of a psychotic disorder (no delusions, hallucinations, or thought disorder). She received intensive ERP. Her antipsychotic medication was discontinued, and she was switched to a different SSRI. Her daytime somnolence resolved at that time. She had a very good response to treatment; after eight weeks she was discharged and resumed her full-time employment.

In the case of Mrs. A, the incorrect thought by the psychiatrist that the obsessions were delusional in nature because of their bizarre content led to morbidity in this patient; the attempt to tailor her treatment based upon that faulty assumption was certain to fail. Initial treatment with ERP therapy was delayed because of the mistaken belief that therapy might not work in someone with so-called "bizarre" obsessions. In addition, SSRIs were not fully utilized: the dose was not sufficient to produce an antiobsessional response because of the psychiatrist's focus on the nature of the obsessions and the mistaken diagnosis. She also was placed on antipsychotic medication, which is not a first-line treatment for OCD. This led to significant side effects, including daytime sedation, leading to work difficulties, weight gain, and exposed her to the possibility of extrapyramidal side effects.

Mrs. A had significant morbidity as a result of an incorrect diagnosis. She was told she had OCD with delusions. This was based upon what was considered to be the bizarre nature of her obsessions: the fear that lint can talk and get lonely. Yet, the DSM makes no mention of a delusions qualifier for OCD. Once a patient is diagnosed as having an obsession, no qualifier should be made based on the content of the obsession. Whether an obsession is physically possible or not is irrelevant. The DSM-IV does allow for the qualifier for poor insight, but that was not an issue here. A representation of a thought algorithm that the referring psychiatrist was using is shown in Fig. 1.1. When the problematic thought was identified (lint will get lonely), the determination was made regarding whether the thought was obsessional or delusional. The psychiatrist did indeed make a correct determination: seeing that the thought was ego-dystonic (i.e., that the patient herself recognized the intrusive and silly nature of the thought) it was termed an obsession.

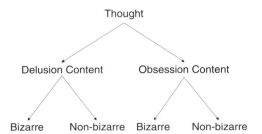

Fig. 1.1 Incorrect diagnostic algorithm for classifying obsessional content.

However, an incorrect assumption quickly followed. In the case of delusions, one does need to determine whether or not they are bizarre, as this has clinical significance. In the case of Mrs. A, the psychiatrist incorrectly assumed that same standard applied to her obsessions and erroneously termed her OCD as delusional in nature. Obsessions with atypical content are actually fairly common. In addition to the transformation obsessions noted by Volz and Heyman (2007), other examples include unwillingness to touch a computer screen for fear of getting contaminated with a computer virus; fears that a certain song playing on the radio would cause "song germs" to contaminate any food in the room; and a man who feared that his daughter would be trapped and suffocate in the envelope when he paid his bills.

In addition to the incorrect thought by clinicians that obsessions should be classified as bizarre or non-bizarre, a similar mistake is sometimes made when trying to distinguish between delusions and obsessions. Occasionally, a mental health clinician will incorrectly ascribe a bizarre thought to be a delusion simply based on the bizarre nature of the thought. A phrase that is often heard is that the thought "sounds delusional." If the problematic thought is taken to be non-bizarre, it is more likely to be ascribed as obsessional. This incorrect belief again can lead to significant morbidity in psychiatric patients.

Case example 3

Miss B was a 26-year-old woman admitted to the inpatient unit for an electroconvulsive therapy consult after being transferred from a state psychiatric hospital during a nine month hospital stay. She was currently suffering from severe depression and had a diagnosis of treatment-resistant schizophrenia lasting seven years. She had been tried on many first-generation and second-generation antipsychotic drugs including high-dose clozapine with no response at all in her schizophrenia symptoms. She related that she had concerns that she was being watched or spied upon by cameras. She had rituals that involved checking her closet and clothes to ensure that no cameras were present. She had torn apart her bedroom door piece by piece to reassure herself that no camera was present, and only felt comfortable with her door when she accompanied her father to the lumber yard and watched a new door being cut. She stated this act assured her that no cameras could have been hidden in the wood. Because checking rituals for cameras or spy devices is extremely unusual behavior in delusional individuals, she was questioned further. She admitted that she never actually had the belief that she was being spied upon. She only had the worry that she may be observed. She was able to describe the thought as intrusive and unrealistic. The checking rituals were an attempt to reassure herself that "everything was OK." She also had a long history of fear of photographs: she had thoughts that people in pictures could see her undress. When she dressed in her room, she would set down any pictures face down so that they could not see her. She described this as upsetting and bizarre, as she knew such a thing was impossible. She was screened for other OCD symptoms, and it was discovered that she had significant symmetry concerns, specifically the desire to have all of the individual carpet fibers in her room lying in the same direction. This included a ritual that involved the straightening out her carpet, which could last up to two days. No history of delusions, hallucinations, or thought disorder past or present was discovered. Her affect was full and appropriate with none of the blunting that is often seen in schizophrenia. The patient had never been screened for OCD symptoms by her psychiatrists in her seven-year mental health history and she had never been placed on SSRIs. During her electroconvulsive therapy course, she was taken off her clozapine and placed on high-dose SSRIs for antiobsessional effect. She responded extremely well to the electroconvulsive therapy and her depression remitted. With SSRI use, she related that her OCD symptoms were greatly reduced in severity for the first time in her life. Miss B was then transferred back to the state hospital in order to arrange for discharge. Immediately upon transfer to the state hospital, she was taken off of her antiobsessional medications and placed back on clozapine in spite of recommendations

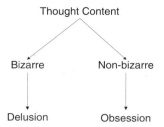

Fig. 1.2 Incorrect diagnostic algorithm for classifying bizarre thought content.

to the contrary. She decompensated rapidly and remained in the state hospital unable to be discharged.

In this example, the intrusive nature of Miss B's thoughts was not taken into consideration and as a result she was diagnosed schizophrenic despite the absence of hallucinations, thought disorder, or blunting of her affect. Her rituals involving checking for spying devices were overlooked in spite of the fact that delusional patients do not typically exhibit such rituals seeking reassurance. Because OCD was never considered and was not screened for on a routine basis, the presence of other, easily recognizable OCD symptoms were never uncovered. Unfortunately, this misdiagnosis was a source of significant morbidity for this patient. She endured a lengthy state hospital admission as well as significant side effects from antipsychotic medications. She had continued symptoms (except during the brief period of time she was placed on antiobsessional drugs) and decompensated even further when OCD treatment was discontinued.

In this instance, the treating psychiatrists made a common error involving the differential diagnosis between obsessions and delusions: because the thoughts were initially deemed bizarre (i.e., being spied upon by cameras) they were considered to be delusions. A representation of the incorrect diagnostic algorithm used in this case can be seen in Fig. 1.2. A thought that is considered to be bizarre or physically impossible, or one that simply "sounds psychotic" to the clinician, is then assumed to be a delusion. Only if the problematic thought is noted to be non-bizarre is the possibility of an obsession considered.

Distinguishing obsessions and delusions in diagnosis

The two cases above demonstrate that significant morbidity can result when the diagnostic criteria for

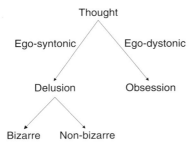

Fig. 1.3 Correct diagnostic algorithm for classifying obsessions and delusions.

obsessions and delusions are obfuscated in the mind of the clinician. An understanding the proper algorithm is vital in making this distinction (Fig. 1.3). Once the problematic thought is identified, the mental health clinician needs to determine if that thought is ego-dystonic or ego-syntonic. This determination is made on the basis of the nature of the thought (i.e., the way the person experiences the thought) and not on the content of the thought (i.e., what the thought is about). If the thought is ego-syntonic and, therefore, seen to be realistic and appropriate to the patient, it is appropriate to label it as a delusion. At that point, the delusion can be classified as either bizarre or non-bizarre. In contrast, if the presenting problematic thought it determined to be ego-dystonic and, therefore, seen to be intrusive and inappropriate to the patient, then the thought should be labeled obsessional. No further subtyping or classification based on whether the concern is something that is physically possible is necessary.

It can be difficult to determine if a thought is ego-syntonic or ego-dystonic when the OCD patient lacks insight. Because both delusions and obsessions can have virtually any content, a specific thought that is not commonly seen can create confusion (Volz and Heyman 2007). Thought insertion and thought withdrawal are classic, well-known delusions; fears of germs are one of the most common obsessions. However, clinicians should be prepared to see either delusions or obsessions manifest in virtually any form. There are some additional clinical clues that can be helpful in this clinical differentiation. A delusional patient has no doubt about what they are experiencing. To them, this thought is very natural. They have no concerns about the presence of the thought in their mind and no doubt that the thought is real. By contrast, the obsessional person is not convinced that their

fear is real and will seek reassurance. Reassurance seeking may manifest by the patient asking questions such as, "Are you sure that the germs will not make me sick?" or "How can I be sure that I will not kill my children?" Questions such as these illustrate their lack of certainty, a symptom seen in OCD. Magical thinking should be noted: if present it is indicative of OCD. Magical thinking is defined as the belief that one's thoughts, words, or actions might or will somehow cause or prevent a specific outcome in a way that defies the normal laws of cause and effect (Ayd 1995). This belief that one's thoughts can affect the outside world (e.g., as in a superstition) can be confused for psychosis if not carefully assessed. An example of magical thinking in OCD would be someone who compulsively taps a desk to prevent a family member from being killed in a car accident. Paranoia, which may be seen in delusional individuals, can be considered to be the exact opposite phenomena: it is the belief that outside events are influencing that person. An example of this would be someone who believes they are being controlled by a television personality with the same first name.

Careful questioning of patients' symptoms and keeping in mind the principles of diagnosing obsessions and delusions can minimize clinical errors and help to improve patient outcomes.

Summary

This chapter was designed to provide an introduction to OCD and to explain many of its clinical features to the reader. Many of the topics eluded to in this discussion will be explored in depth in later chapters. It is hoped that the reader will have gained an understanding of the history of the recognition and classification of OCD, as well as understanding some of the potential changes regarding classification in future editions of the DSM. Diagnostic criteria as well as some of the major areas contributing to under- and misdiagnosis have been outlined. The scope of this chapter only allowed for a brief overview of many of the facets of the multidisciplinary investigations that will influence how the medical profession ultimately views this disorder. It is hoped that knowledge gained through these investigations into the etiology of OCD will also lead to more effective and refined treatment protocols.

The misdiagnosis and underdiagnosis of OCD is a looming problem for individuals facing this disorder. Better education of both the professional community and the general population about OCD may help to alleviate some of the marked distress these people unnecessarily experience as they negotiate the mental health process in search of help for a disorder that often take years to diagnose. Challenges do face the medical community in the proper diagnosis of OCD; only through a greater recognition and understanding of OCD can this situation begin to resolve.

References

Abramowitz JS, Foa EB (1998). Worries and obsessions in individuals with obsessive-compulsive disorder with and without comorbid generalized anxiety disorder. *Behav Res Ther* **36**: 695–700.

Abramowitz JS, Schwartz SA, Moore KM, Luenzmann KR (2003). Obsessive-compulsive symptoms in pregnancy and the puerperium: a review of the literature. *Anxiety Disord* **17**: 461–478.

Adams P (1973). *Obsessive Children* (p. 193). New York: Brummer/Mazel.

American Psychiatric Association (1994). *Diagnostic and Statistical Manual of Mental Disorders*, 4th edn. Washington, DC: American Psychiatric Press.

Attiullah N, Eisen JL, Rassmussen SA (2000). Clinical features of obsessive-compulsive disorder. *Psych Clin N Am* **23**: 469–491.

Ayd FJ (1995). *Lexicon of Psychiatry, Neurology, and the Neurosciences*. Baltimore, MD: Williams & Wilkins.

Baer L, Jenike MA (1992). Personality disorders in obsessive-compulsive disorder. *Psychiatr Clin N Am* **15**: 803–812.

Berle D, Phillips ES (2006). Disgust and obsessive-compulsive disorder: an update. *Psychiatry* **69**: 288–238.

Besiroglu L, Uguz F, Ozbebit O, *et al.* (2006). Longitudinal assessment of subtype categories in obsessive-compulsive disorder. *Depress Anxiety* **113**: 440–446.

Boucard C, Rheaume J, Ladouceur R (1999). Responsibility and perfectionism in OCD: an experimental study. *Behav Res Ther* **37**: 293–248.

Cameron CL (2007). Obsessive-compulsive disorder in children and adolescents. *J Psychiatr Ment Health Nurs* **14**: 696–704.

Castle DJ, Phillips KA (2006). Obsessive-compulsive spectrum of disorders: a defensible construct? *Aust N Z J Psychiatry* **40**: 114–120.

Crino RD, Andrews G (1996). Personality disorder in obsessive-compulsive disorder: a controlled study. *J Psychiat Res* **30**: 29–38.

Coles ME, Pinto A, Mancebo MC, Rasmussen SA, Eisen JL (2008). OCD with comorbid OCPD: a subtype of OCD? *J Psychiatry Res* **42**: 289–296.

de Mathis MA, Diniz JB, do Rosario MC, *et al.* (2006). What is the optimal way to subdivide obsessive-compulsive disorder? CNS *Spectr* **11**: 762–768, 771–774, 776–779.

do Rosario-Campos MC, Leckman JF, Curi M, *et al.* (2005). A family study of early-onset obsessive-compulsive disorder. *Am J Med Genet B Neuropsychiatr Genet* **136B**: 92–97.

Ecker W, Gonner S (2008). Incompleteness and harm avoidance in OCD symptom dimensions. *Behav Res Ther* **46**: 895–904.

Eisen JL, Phillips KA, Rasmussen SA, *et al.* (1998). The Brown Assessment of Beliefs Scale (BABS): reliability and validity. *Am J Psychiatry* **155**: 102–8.

Eisen JL, Goodman WK, Keller MB, *et al.* (1999). Patterns of remission and relapse in obsessive-compulsive disorder: a 2-year prospective study. *J Clin Psychiatry*. **60**: 346–351.

Eisen JL, Rasmussen SA, Phillips KA, *et al.* (2001). Insight and treatment outcome in obsessive-compulsive disorder. *Compr Psychiatry* **42**: 494–497.

Fireman B, Koran LM, Leventhal JL, Jacobson A (2001). The prevalence of clinically recognized obsessive-compulsive disorder in a large health maintenance organization. *Am J Psychiatry* **158**: 1904–1910.

Fineberg NA, Sharma P, Sivakumaran T, Sahakian B, Chamberlain S (2007). Does obsessive-compulsive personality disorder belong within the obsessive-compulsive spectrum? CNS *Spectr* **12**: 467–482.

Foa EB, Kozak MJ, Goodman WK, *et al.* (1995). DSM-IV field trial: obsessive-compulsive disorder. *Am J Psychiatry* **152**: 90–96.

Freeston MH, Rheaume J, Ladouceur R (1996). Correcting faulty appraisals of obsessional thoughts. *Behav Res Ther* **34**: 433–446.

Goodman WK (1999). Obsessive-compulsive disorder: diagnosis and treatment. *J Clin Psychiatry* **60**(Suppl 18): 18: 27–32.

Goodwin DW, Guze SB, Robbins E (1969). Follow-up studies in obsessional neurosis. *Arch Gen Psychiatry* **20**: 182–187.

Gordon A, Rasmussen SA (1988). Mood related obsessive compulsive symptoms in a patient with bipolar affective disorder. *J Clin Psychiatry* **49**: 27–28.

Grant JE, Odlaug BL (2008). Challenges in diagnosing and treating obsessive-compulsive disorder. *Psychiatric Times* **25**(Suppl 2): 25–30.

Grant JE, Mancebo MC, Pinto A, *et al.* (2007). Late-onset obsessive compulsive disorder: clinical characteristics and psychiatric comorbidity. *Psychiatry Res 30* **152**: 21–27.

Grillo CM, McGlashan TH, Morey LC, *et al.* Internal consistency, intercriterion overlap and diagnostic efficiency of criteria sets for dsm-iv schizotypal, borderline, avoidant, and obsessive-compulsive personality disorders. *Acta Psychiatr Scand* **104**: 264–272.

Hankin CS, Koran LM, Bronstone A, *et al.* (2009). Adequacy of pharmacotherapy among medicaid-enrolled patients newly diagnosed with obsessive-compulsive disorder. *CNS Spectr* **14**: 695–703.

Hasler G, LaSalle-Ricci VH, Ronquillo JG, *et al.* (2005). Obsessive-compulsive disorder symptom dimensions show specific relationships to psychiatric comorbidity. *Psychiatry Res* **135** 121–132.

Hemmings S, Stein DJ (2006). The current state of association studies in obsessive-compulsive disorder. *Psychiatr Clin N Am* **29** 411–444.

Hollander E, Wong C (1998). Psychosocial function and economic cost of obsessive-compulsive disorder. *CNS Spectr* **3**: 48–58.

Hollander E, Kim S, Khanna S, Pallanti S (2007). Obsessive-compulsive disorder and obsessive-compulsive spectrum disorders: diagnostic and dimensional issues. *CNS Spectr* **12**(Suppl 3): 5–13.

Horwath E, Weissman MM (2000). The epidemiology and cross-national presentation of obsessive-compulsive disorder. *Psychiatr Clin N Am* **23**: 493–507.

Husted DS, Shapira NA, Goodman WK (2006). The neurocircuitry of obsessive-compulsive disorder and disgust. *Prog Neuropsychopharmacol Biol Psychiatry* **30**: 389–399.

Janet P (1903). *Les Obsessions et la Psychasthenie*. Paris: Felix Alcan.

Kamath P, Janardhan Reddy YC, Kandavel T (2007). Suicidal behavior in obsessive-compulsive disorder. *J Clin Psychiatry* **68**: 1741–1750.

Karno M, Golding JM, Sorenson SB, *et al.* (1988). The epidemiology of obsessive-compulsive disorder in five US communities. *Arch Gen Psychiatry* **45**: 1094–1099.

Kaye WH, Bulik CM, Thornton L, Barbarich N, Masters K (2004). Comorbidity of anxiety disorders with anorexia and bulimia nervosa. *Am J Psychiatry* **161**: 2215–2221.

Kim SJ, Kim C (2006). The genetic studies of obsessive-compulsive disorder and its future directions. *Yonsei Med J* **47**: 443–454.

Kozak MJ, Foa EB (1994). Obsessions, overvalued ideas, and delusions in obsessive-compulsive disorder. *Behav Res Ther* **12**: 343–353.

Leckman JF, Rauch SL, Mataix-Cols D (2007). Symptom dimensions in obsessive-compulsive disorder: implications for the DSM-V. *CNS Spectr* **12**: 376–387, 400.

Lee HJ, Kwon SM, Kwon JS, Telch MJ (2005). Testing the autogenous-reactive model of obsessions. *Depress Anxiety* **21**: 118–129.

Mataix-Cols D (2006). Deconstructing obsessive-compulsive disorder: a multidimensional perspective. *Curr Opin Psychiatry* **19**: 84–89.

Mataix-Cols D, Rauch S, Baer L, *et al.* (2002). Symptom stability in adult obsessive-compulsive disorder: data from a naturalistic two-year follow-up study. *Am J Psychiatry* **159**: 263–268.

Mataix-Cols D, Rosario-Campos MC, Leckman JF (2005). A multidimensional model of obsessive-compulsive disorder. *Am J Psychiatry* **162**: 228–238.

Matsunaga H, Seedat S (2007). Obsessive-compulsive spectrum disorders: cross-national and ethnic issues. *CNS Spectr* **12**: 392–400.

Murphy TK, Sajid MW, Goodman WK (2006). Immunology of obsessive-compulsive disorder. *Psychiatr Clin N Am* **29** 445–469.

Murray CJ, Lopez AD (1996). *The Global Burden of Disease*. Boston, MA: Harvard University Press;.

Olatunji BO, Abramowitz JS, Williams NL, Connoly KM, Lohr JM (2007). Scrupulosity and obsessive-compulsive symptoms: confirmatory factor analysis and validity of the Penn Inventory of Scrupulosity. *J Anxiety Disord* **21**: 771–787.

Orloff LM, Battle MA, Baer L, *et al.* (1994). Long-term follow-up of 85 patients with obsessive-compulsive disorder. *Am J Psychiatry* **51**: 441–442.

Pallanti S, Hollander E (2008). Obsessive compulsive disorder spectrum as a scientific "metaphor". *CNS Spectr* **13**(Suppl 14): 6–15.

Pauls D (2008). The genetics of obsessive-compulsive disorder: a review of the evidence. *Am J Med Genet* **148C**: 133–139.

Pinto A, Mancebo MC, Eisen JL, Pagano ME, Rasmussen SA (2006). The Brown Longitudinal Obsessive-Compulsive Study: clinical features and symptoms of the sample at intake. *J Clin Psychiatry* **67**: 703–711.

Rachman S (1993). Obsessions, responsibilities, and guilt. *Behav Res Ther* **31**: 149–154.

Rasmussen SA, Eisen JL (1990). Epidemiology of obsessive compulsive disorder. *J Clin Psychiatry* **51**(Suppl): 10–13.

Rasmussen SA, Eisen JL (1994). Epidemiology and differential diagnosis of obsessive-compulsive disorder. *J Clin Psychiatry* **55**(Suppl): 5–14.

Rasmussen SA, Tsuang MT (1986). Clinical characteristics and family history in DSM-III obsessive-compulsive disorder. *Am J Psychiatry* **143**: 317–322.

Rodrigues Torres A, Del Porto JA (1995). Comorbidity of obsessive-compulsive disorder and personality disorders. a Brazilian controlled study. *Psychopathology* **28**: 322–329.

Snider LA, Swedo SE (2004). PANDAS: current status and directions for research. *Mol Psychiatry* **9**: 900–907.

Stein DJ, Lochner C (2006). Obsessive-compulsive spectrum disorders: a multidimensional approach. *Psychiatr Clin N Am* **29** 343–351.

Stein DJ, Fineberg NA, Bienvenu OJ, *et al.* (2010). Should OCD be classified as an anxiety disorder in DSM-V? *Depress Anxiety* **27**: 495–506.

Steketee G, Eisen J, Dyck I, Warshaw M, Rasmussen S (1999). Predictors of course in obsessive-compulsive disorder. *Psychiatry Res* **89**: 299–238.

Swedo SE, Rapoport JL, Leonard H, Lenane M, Cheslow D (1989). Obsessive compulsive disorder in children and adolescents: clinical phenomenology of 70 consecutive cases. *Arch Gen Psychiatry* **46**: 335–341.

Torres AR, Ramos-Cerqueira AT, Torresan RC, *et al.* (2007). Prevalence and associated factors for suicidal ideation and behaviors in obsessive-compulsive disorder. *CNS Spectr* **12**: 711–718.

Tükel R, Polat A, Ozdemir O, Aksut D, Turksoy N (2002). Comorbid conditions in obsessive-compulsive disorder. *Compr Psychiatry* **43**: 204–209.

Valleni-Basile LA, Garrison CZ, Jackson KL, *et al.* (1994). Frequency of obsessive-compulsive disorder in a community sample of young adolescents. *J Am Acad Child Adolesc Psychiatry* **33**: 782–791.

Volz C, Heyman I (2007). Case series: transformation obsession in young people with obsessive-compuslive disorder (OCD). *J Am Acad Child Adolesc Psychiatry* **46**: 766–772.

Wisner, Peindl, Gigliotti, Hanusa. (1999). Obsessions and compulsions in women with post-partum depression. *J Clin Psych* **60**: 176–180.

World Health Organization (1994). *International Statistical Classification of Diseases and Related Health Problems*, 10th revision. Geneva: World Health Organization.

Chapter

2

Neurobiology and neurocircuitry of obsessive-compulsive disorder and relevance to its surgical treatment

Darin D. Dougherty and Benjamin D. Greenberg

Introduction

This chapter reviews current neurobiological models of obsessive-compulsive disorder (OCD) and their relevance to surgical treatments for OCD. First, the cortico-striato-thalamo-cortical (CSTC) circuitry implicated in the pathophysiology of OCD is described and the supporting data (mostly neuroimaging) is reviewed. The chapter concludes with a review of neurosurgical treatments for OCD that are believed to impact this circuitry.

Neurobiology and neurocircuitry

Neuroanatomical models of OCD and related disorders emphasize the CSTC circuitry. In classic articles, Alexander and colleagues introduced and reviewed the organization of multiple, parallel, segregated CSTC circuits (Alexander *et al.* 1986, 1990). Each CSTC circuit involves projections from a variety of cortical zones to specific corresponding subterritories of striatum, which, in turn, send projections via other intermediate basal ganglia targets to ramify within the thalamus. These circuits are ultimately closed via reciprocal projections from thalamus back to the same prefrontal cortical regions from which the cortico-striatal projections originated. Multiple CSTC circuits run in parallel and subserve separate functions. These have been designated the affective circuit, the sensorimotor circuit, the ventral cognitive circuit, and the dorsal cognitive circuit. Neuroimaging supports a central role for a specific CSTC circuit, the ventral cognitive circuit, in OCD pathophysiology. Nodes within this circuitry include the orbital frontal cortex (OFC) and anterior cingulate cortex (ACC) as well as basal ganglia and thalamus. Multiple lines of neuroimaging evidence support the role of dysfunction within this circuitry in the pathophysiology of OCD.

Structural neuroimaging

Structural neuroimaging studies have found subtle differences in OFC, striatal, and thalamic volumes in subjects with OCD compared with controls (Robinson *et al.* 1995; Jenike *et al.* 1996). In a preliminary study that addressed the potential confound of chronic medication exposure, voxel-based morphometry revealed greater gray matter density within the hypothesized circuitry in children with OCD than in healthy controls or their unaffected siblings (Gilbert *et al.* 2008). This may be viewed as consistent with functional neuroimaging reporting hypermetabolism and increased resting-state perfusion in striatum, anterior cingulate, and orbital cortex (Szeszko *et al.* 2008). Magnetic resonance spectroscopy studies also suggest neurochemical abnormalities in this circuitry, including reductions in *N*-acetylaspartate (a purported marker of healthy neurons) within the striatum and medial thalamus in OCD (Ebert *et al.* 1997; Bartha *et al.* 1998).

Connections within circuitry implicated in OCD may also be abnormal in the illness. A diffusion tensor magnetic resonance imaging study found increased fractional anisotropy (a measure of white matter structure) in the cingulum bundle bilaterally and in the left anterior limb of the internal capsule in patients compared with healthy controls (Cannistraro *et al.* 2007). This is early evidence of abnormal connections between nodes within putative OCD circuitry. It is also consistent with observations that ablating or modulating these white matter pathways (as in

Clinical Obsessive-Compulsive Disorders in Adults and Children, ed. Robert Hudak and Darin D. Dougherty.
Published by Cambridge University Press. Copyright © Cambridge University Press 2011.

anterior cingluotomy, anterior capsulotomy, or deep brain stimulation (DBS) of the ventral anterior limb of the internal capsule/ventral striatum) is associated with therapeutic improvement (discussed further below).

Functional neuroimaging

Functional imaging has been used extensively in OCD research. It has consistently documented hyperactivity (increased metabolism or perfusion) in CSTC circuits in OCD subjects at rest compared with healthy volunteers. Specifically, neutral state paradigms utilizing positron emission tomography and single photon emission computed tomography have consistently found increased regional brain activity within OFC and ACC in patients with OCD compared with healthy volunteers (Baxter et al. 1988, 1992; Nordahl et al. 1989; Machlin et al. 1991; Swedo et al. 1989; Rubin et al. 1992). However, differences in the striatum and thalamus (other, albeit smaller, structures within the ventral cognitive circuit) have been inconsistent with these findings (Baxter et al. 1988; Machlin et al. 1991; Rauch et al. 1997). Further, hyperactivity within OFC, ACC, and caudate nucleus is accentuated during provocation of OCD symptoms (McGuire et al. 1994; Rauch et al. 1994, 1997; Breiter et al. 1996). Conversely, studies have consistently found reduced activity in these same regions after successful OCD treatment. It is especially interesting that this can be observed regardless of the mode of treatment, including pharmacological (Benkelfat et al. 1990; Hoehn-Saric et al. 1991; Baxter et al. 1992; Swedo et al. 1992; Perani et al. 1995), behavioral (Baxter et al. 1992; Schwartz et al. 1996), and neurosurgical (Mindus et al. 1986) therapies. Imaging also suggests that activity in this circuitry before treatment might predict responses to therapies. Activity within OFC predicts subsequent response to medication or behavior therapy (Baxter et al. 1992; Swedo et al. 1992; McGuire et al. 1994; Brody et al. 1998; Saxena et al. 1999; Rauch et al. 2002) while baseline activity in the posterior cingulate cortex predicts subsequent response to fluvoxamine (Rauch et al. 2002) and anterior cingulotomy (Rauch et al. 2001). Response prediction, using neuroimaging and other physiological or clinical features of individual patients, would be an especially important advance for neurosurgical treatments, where the risks and expense of procedures are quite significant (discussed further below).

Surgery

History

Lobotomy emerged before the current era of empirical psychiatry. Therapeutic nihilism for severe disorders was pervasive, and current ethical and regulatory contexts had yet to emerge. Among those who first received lobotomies in the 1930s were patients with severe obsessions. Reported successful outcomes were greeted with much publicity (Anon. 1937). Lobotomy's use accelerated (Valenstein 1986; Pressman 1998) until effective alternatives appeared and its heavy adverse effect burden was recognized (El-Hai 2005). There was vocal skepticism from the beginning (Fins 2003), but it was only decades later, when wide use of lobotomy had essentially ended (replaced by dramatically more limited use of stereotactic procedures), that opposition rose to the level of national governments in the USA and elsewhere (US National Commission 1977). Ironically, even Walter Freeman, who later became an "evangelist" for lobotomy, actually began by emphasizing care in patient selection and outcomes measurement (Freeman et al. 1942).

Surgical techniques: stereotactic ablation

Four lesion procedures remain in use for OCD: anterior capsulotomy, anterior cingulotomy, subcaudate tractotomy, and limbic leucotomy. In each, bilateral lesions are made under magnetic resonance imaging guidance. In addition to OCD, all have been used for highly refractory depression. Some (e.g., anterior capsulotomy) have also been applied to non-OCD anxiety disorders or medically intractable chronic pain (anterior cingulotomy).

Outcomes cannot be fairly assessed until six months to two years after surgery. Direct comparison of procedures is rare; there is one published example (Kullberg 1977). Early reports used global improvement measures (e.g., from "much improved" to "worse" after surgery). Usually ratings of "improved" or better were considered satisfactory. Newer studies have been prospective, using validated measures. Prospective studies of anterior cingulotomy and gamma ventral capsulotomy for OCD are continuing at major centers.

Anterior capsulotomy

Anterior capsulotomy, originated by Tailarach, was developed further by Leksell. The target is the anterior limb of the internal capsule, impinging on the underlying ventral striatum. It is intended to interrupt fibers connecting prefrontal cortex and subcortical nuclei including the dorsomedial thalamus. The original anterior capsulotomy procedure used thermocoagulation via burr holes in the skull. Since lesions can include most of the anterior capsule in the coronal plane, the resulting ablation volumes can be large. Lesions have been repeated in patients judged to have poor responses, and some case series have reported combined results of single procedures, repeated procedures, and radiosurgery (Ruck *et al.* 2008). It would be expected that adverse effect burdens would generally be greatest for the largest total lesion volumes. Beginning in the 1980s, the Leksell Gamma Knife (Elekta, Stockholm) has been used to lesion the anterior limb of the internal capsule without craniotomy. In the early 1990s, a more discrete gamma knife procedure was developed, which resulted in ablations that were typically smaller than thermocapsulotomy lesions. The more recent gamma procedure is called "gamma ventral capsulotomy," since the lesions are within the ventral half of the anterior capsule. A sham surgery-controlled, double-blind study of gamma ventral capsulotomy for OCD is underway at the University of Sao Paulo, Brazil (Lopes *et al.* 2009). This is the first controlled trial of a lesion procedure in psychiatry.

Outcomes

All the reports reviewed below used open-label ablation. Early work suggested favorable responses in approximately half of OCD patients or those with major affective disorders ($n = 116$) (Herner 1961). Poor results were seen in schizophrenia (14% favorable) or non-OCD anxiety disorders (20% favorable). Later, satisfactory outcomes were described in 71% of OCD patients after capsulotomy (Bingley *et al.* 1977). In a review, 170 (67%) of 253 OCD patients were significantly improved (Waziri 1990). A literature review found "satisfactory" outcomes in 64% (137 of 213) of all patients; the OCD patients improved most (Mindus *et al.* 1994). Follow-up data, however, were inadequate in 149, a major limitation. Therapeutic response (35% improvement on the Yale–Brown Obsessive Compulsive Scale [Y-BOCS]) has been reported at 60% for patients with OCD who underwent gamma ventral capsulotomy. A recent comparison of patients who received several different types of capsulotomy within a relatively small sample (25 in total) revealed lasting improvement (35% Y-BOCS reduction at 4–17 years after surgery) in 48% of OCD patients. No significant difference in benefit between the thermocapsulotomy and gamma knife capsulotomy was seen in the modest subsets receiving these different procedures (Ruck *et al.* 2008). Interestingly, in that study, effectiveness seemed greater when lesion volumes were smaller.

Adverse effects

Short-term adverse effects of thermocapsulotomy include headache, confusion, and incontinence, especially for capsulotomies performed via thermocoagulation. Weight gain, fatigue, memory loss, incontinence, and seizure have been reported as infrequent but in some cases permanent side effects (Feldman *et al.* 2001). In contrast to thermocapsulotomy, discussed above, gamma ventral capsulotomy radiosurgery typically has a short postoperative recovery period and can be an outpatient procedure. Similar to the course of therapeutic change, adverse effects usually develop slowly after gamma ventral capsulotomy.

Studying a population of 26 patients with various, typically non-OCD, anxiety disorders, Ruck *et al.* (2008) found that capsulotomy alleviated severe symptoms; however, seven patients suffered from significant apathy and decline in executive function on retrospective examination. The risk for cognitive complications, including frontal lobe dysfunction, was confirmed in a subsequent study. The elevated cognitive risk associated with capsulotomies was verified in the OCD population by the same group of investigators, reporting data from 25 OCD patients followed for a mean of 10.9 years after surgery. While thermocapsulotomy and gamma knife anterior capsultomy (an earlier version of the procedure) were found to be effective for alleviating OCD symptoms, 10 of 25 patients presented with apathy and significant deterioration of executive function. The authors suggested that smaller lesions with less medial and posterior extension, particularly in the right hemisphere, were less prone to cause these adverse effects. It is also important to note that apathy and executive dysfunction was overwhelmingly seen in patients who underwent repeated procedures (resulting in larger total lesion volumes) or gamma knife lesions at high radiation doses (up to 200 Gy). As noted above, there may be less risk, and possibly better outcomes, with relatively smaller total lesion volumes.

Serious adverse effects of the gamma knife radio-surgical procedure include radiation-induced edema and delayed cyst formation (which may or may not be symptomatic). Development of clinically significant edema appears to reflect individual differences in sensitivity to radiation that remain poorly understood. Late cyst formation (from two to greater than five years after surgery) has occurred in from 1.6% to 3.6% of patients after surgery for arteriovenous malformations and may in part be related to the extent of postoperative radiation-induced edema (Pan *et al.* 2005).

Anterior cingulotomy

Anterior cingulotomy was first used for intractable pain; however, it was noticed that patients with comorbid anxiety or depressive conditions had the best results after cingulotomy. Ballantine and colleagues (1987) later studied its safety and effectiveness for several psychiatric indications. The Massachusetts General Hospital group has performed over 1000 cingulotomies since 1962. The target is within the dorsal anterior cingulate cortex at the margin of the cingulum bundle white matter. Two or three lesions of approximately 1.0 cm^3 are made on each side by thermocoagulation through burr holes, under local anesthesia. Making the smallest possible lesion is the goal, so depending on their response patients may return months after the first operation for a second procedure to extend the lesions.

Outcomes

In 1987, Ballantine and colleagues reviewed the long-term results of 198 patients who underwent the procedure for major affective disorder, OCD, or anxiety disorder. Significant improvement, determined using a subjective functional/symptomatic rating scale, occurred for patients with severe affective disorders (62%), OCD (56%), and anxiety disorders (79%) (Ballantine *et al.* 1987). When these data were analyzed using more rigid outcome criteria, only 33% showed substantial benefit from the cingulotomy (Cosgrove 2000). A 2002 review of 44 patients who had undergone cingulotomies since 1991 reported that, 32% of patients with OCD were full responders and another 14% were partial responders (Dougherty *et al.* 2002). It should be noted that it may take as long as three to six months for the beneficial effects of cingulotomies to emerge (Cosgrove 2000).

Because of the relatively good success and clearly low morbidity and mortality rates, cingulotomy has been the most widely used psychiatric neurosurgical procedure in North America over the last several decades. A more recent study (Kim *et al.* 2003) of stereotactic bilateral anterior cingulotomy as a treatment for refractory OCD found a mean Y-BOCS severity reduction of 36% after 12 months, 6 of the 14 patients met responder criteria (35% Y-BOCS reduction plus a Clinical Global Impression score of much or very much improved) at 12 months. There was no significant cognitive dysfunction after cingulotomy.

Adverse effects

Cingulotomies have a relatively low rate of side effects. Of the more than 1000 cingulotomies performed at Massachusetts General Hospital, there had been no deaths, no infections, and only two subdural hematomas (Greenberg *et al.* 2009). Short-term postoperative side effects include headache, nausea, or difficulty with urination, which usually resolve within a few days. The most common serious side effect is seizure (rates ranging from 1% to 9%) (Binder and Iskandar 2000).

Subcaudate tractotomy

Subcaudate tractotomy, introduced in 1964, was intended to limit adverse effects by restricting lesion size. By targeting the substantia innominata (white matter just inferior to the head of the caudate nucleus), the goal was to interrupt nerve fibers connecting OFC to subcortical structures.

Outcomes

By 1973, this procedure had been performed in over 650 patients with major depression, OCD, or anxiety, with reported success rates around 50% (Knight 1973). In 1994, Bridges and colleagues reviewed 1300 cases of subcaudate tractotomy used for treatment of anxiety, phobic anxiety, OCD, major depressive disorder, or bipolar disorder. They concluded that 40–60% of patients benefited from the procedure to the point of living normal or near-normal lives. Suicide rates were reduced from 15% (in a similarly affected control group) to 1%.

Adverse effects

Short-term side effects include somnolence lasting up to a few days postoperatively, confusion lasting up to one month postoperatively, and possibly temporary decreases in certain cognitive functions. The most common major adverse effect is seizure (at least 1.6% of cases), although mild personality changes have been noted (Greenberg *et al.* 2009). Only one surgery-related death was reported.

Limbic leucotomy

Limbic leucotomy was introduced by Kelly and colleagues in the UK in 1973. It combines subcaudate tractotomy and anterior cingulotomy. The lesions have typically been made via thermocoagulation or with a cryoprobe. Historically, the precise placement of the lesions was guided by intraoperative stimulation; pronounced autonomic responses were believed to designate the optimal lesion site.

Outcomes

In an early study, Kelly *et al.*(1973) reported significant improvement (using a five-point global rating scale) in 89% of patients with OCD. In 1993, Hay and colleagues reported a moderate to marked improvement in 10 (38%) of their 26 OCD patients treated with limbic leucotomy. Most recently, Cho and colleagues (2008) reported a marked response (in the top three categories of the Clinical Global Personality Social Status Rating Scale) in 12 (69%) of their 18 patients with intractable affective disorders who underwent limbic leucotomy. They showed significant improvement in depression (Hamilton Depression Rating Scale averages reduced from 42 to 20), anxiety (average Hamilton Anxiety Rating Scale scores decreased approximately 50%). Negative symptoms also improved. These results were sustained over a seven-year follow-up period. In a different clinical population, Price and colleagues have reported that limbic leucotomy may benefit patients with severe self-mutilation from repetitive, tic-like behaviors (Price *et al.* 2001).

Adverse effects

The most significant complications reported for this procedure are seizure and enduring lethargy. Overall, short-term side effects for limbic leucotomy include headache, confusion, lethargy, perseveration, and lack of sphincter control. While most of these effects are transient, it is common for confusion to last several days; as a result, patients often have a longer postoperative hospital stay with this procedure than with either cingulotomy or subcaudate tractotomy (Greenberg *et al.* 2009). A more recent study of limbic leucotomy for OCD reported that mean Y-BOCS scores decreased from 34 to 3, which is a large decrease compared with that seen in other studies of the effects of neurosurgery in OCD. In 10 of the 12 patients, there was long-term follow-up (for a mean of 45 months), during which they were described as having returned to a previous (improved) level of psychosocial functioning (Kim *et al.* 2002).

Deep brain stimulation

Use of DBS occurred as early as 1948, when J. L. Pool used an electrode in the caudate nucleus in a woman with depression and anorexia (Pool 1954). Modern psychiatric DBS began fifty years later, when Nuttin and colleagues (1999) treated otherwise intractable OCD by DBS of a site based initially on an anterior capsulotomy target. The procedure is essentially the same as for movement disorders. Leads with multiple electrode contacts are implanted via skull burr holes. Patients are typically sedated but awake. Lead placement (typically bilateral) is guided by multimodal imaging and dedicated computer targeting platforms. In contrast to DBS for Parkinson's disease, microelectrode recording is not routinely used for target identification in OCD, although it may be used for research purposes in the operating room. Intraoperative "macrostimulation" (i.e., using the lead just implanted, which is very large compared with neurons) is used to determine if adverse effects (Shapira *et al.* 2006) or physiological (Okun *et al.* 2004) or behavioral effects of acute stimulation suggest that the lead location should be modified. In a separate surgical phase (on the same or a different day), the neurostimulator is implanted subdermally (e.g., in the upper chest wall). It is connected to the brain leads via wires tunneled under the skin. This phase of surgery is carried out under general anesthesia.

Adjusting DBS is an outpatient procedure typically performed by a specially trained psychiatrist. Various combinations of electrodes can be activated, at different polarities, intensities, and frequencies. This parameter "survey" and optimization is time consuming and requires attentive, long-term follow-up. If no beneficial settings can be identified despite extensive efforts, the electrodes can be inactivated and the devices may be removed, fully or partially. Sometimes the brain electrodes are left in place given the (apparently small) risk of hemorrhage upon removal. In our experience, complete device explantation is relatively rare.

Outcomes

For OCD, benefit has been reported after application of DBS to the ventral anterior limb of the internal capsule/ventral striatum (Greenberg et al. 2010), in more anterior locations in the internal capsule (Abelson et al. 2005), the ventral caudate (Aouizerate et al. 2004), or the subthalamic nucleus (Mallet et al. 2008). The OCD targets have been most influenced by the more focal stereotactic ablation procedures that have continued in use since the 1940s, by anatomical considerations derived from neuroimaging, and by direct clinical observations of patients receiving DBS for other indications who had comorbid OCD symptoms (Mallet et al. 2008). Modification of the ventral anterior limb of the internal capsule/ventral striatum target led to improved effectiveness for OCD with lower current drain (Greenberg et al. 2010).

Adverse effects

Safety profiles have been variable in these small-scale reports on DBS for OCD. Adverse effects have ranged from transient psychiatric symptom exacerbations (Greenberg et al. 2010) to permanent neurological sequelae (Mallet et al. 2008) or, on longer-term follow-up, suicide in the context of psychosocial stress (Abelson et al. 2005). But, as for efficacy, only quite tentative conclusions about safety can be drawn given the data available. Comparisons of outcomes from DBS at one target with those for another are especially difficult given the small samples and variability in entry criteria and other techniques. A "gold standard" direct comparison in which patients selected according to the same detailed criteria are randomly assigned to receive DBS at one target or another is unlikely ever to be carried out with the sample size required. Some useful comparative data should be obtained in smaller studies in which two different targets can be stimulated in the same patients (with bilateral implantation of four electrodes per patient), since patients will be their own controls.

Mechanism of action of neurosurgical interventions

As to mechanisms of therapeutic action, the ventral anterior limb of the internal capsule/ventral striatum target has also been proposed to be part of longitudinal fiber pathways that are the targets of anterior capsulotomy and the more specific gamma ventral capsulotomy for OCD (Lopes et al. 2009). Interestingly, in terms of mechanism of action, mood and other depressive symptoms including anhedonia improved rapidly after ventral anterior limb of the internal capsule/ventral striatum stimulation in OCD patients. Moreover, mood symptoms worsened faster than obsessions and compulsions did when DBS was interrupted (Greenberg et al. 2010). Interestingly, stimulation in the same region has notably also produced rapid relief of anhedonia in patients who received DBS for major depression (Schlaepfer et al. 2008).

Patient selection

Appropriate patient selection is crucial for success for ablative procedure or DBS. At our sites, guidelines for assessing candidacy for clinical intervention specify that each patient must have (1) met DSM-IIIR criteria for OCD, (2) had severe OCD symptoms and functional impairment, and (3) failed a specific and rigorous regimen of medication and behavior therapy trials. In addition, the referring psychiatrist is required to agree to follow the patient after release from the hospital after the procedure. An assessment committee, which consists of psychiatrists, neurosurgeons, and neurologists, reviews each patient's records and determines whether preliminary approval for surgery is appropriate. Next, patients are directly interviewed and examined by a psychiatrist, a neurologist, and a neurosurgeon, and they complete additional tests and evaluations. They are then assessed using the Structured Clinical Interview for DSM-IV for diagnosis of axis I disorders and are also assessed with additional standardized instruments, including the Y-BOCS and the Beck Depression Inventory. Most surgical candidates have OCD that has been unresponsive to all available and appropriate psychotropic medication trials and behavior treatments. Each patient is required to have had adequate trials (at least 10 weeks at the maximally tolerated dose) of at least three of the SRIs (clomipramine, fluoxetine, sertraline, paroxetine, fluvoxamine, or citalopram) and augmentation of at least one of the previous drugs for one month with at least two of the following medications: lithium, clonazepam, buspirone, or a neuroleptic. All patients also must have had an adequate trial of behavior therapy consisting of at least 20 hours of exposure and response prevention therapy. Information regarding medication compliance history is obtained from the patient's referring psychiatrist and the patient's records, in addition to the history provided by the patient. The maximum dose tolerated is a subjective measure, in large part influenced by the patient's ability or willingness to tolerate adverse effects. The team attempts to ensure, through its communication with the patient and the referring physician, that previous treatment trials were not abandoned prematurely solely because of mild side effects. In a more general sense, patients who are characterized as poorly compliant (e.g., missing appointments, not taking their medications as prescribed, not genuine in their effort to participate in behavior therapy) are not deemed appropriate candidates for surgery. Patients who are accepted for neurosurgery provide informed consent for surgery and clinical follow-up.

Conclusions

Neurosurgical treatments remain an important option for appropriately selected patients with severe and otherwise intractable OCD. Although the effectiveness and safety of these procedures has improved, research in this area promises further advances. Neuroimaging techniques and use of laboratory behavioral measures might eventually aid in patient selection by predicting treatment response or (more speculatively) to individually tailor surgical interventions. The use of DBS offers the prospect of an adjustable and (usually) reversible method to relieve suffering and improve the quality of life in those with severe and treatment-refractory disorder. Neurosurgical treatments might even help to guide development of novel pharmacological therapies by advancing understanding of neurochemical systems within the relevant circuitry. Moreover, surgical treatments may shed light on dimensions of illness that cross categorical diagnoses, and on the mechanisms of therapeutic change that might also be relevant to several illnesses within the anxiety and affective disorder spectrum. Finally, there is the intriguing possibility that neurosurgery might in fact enhance the benefits of subsequent behavioral therapies that had proved ineffective before surgery.

How surgical interventions could accomplish that has become the subject of translational research bridging the behavioral and neurobiological levels of analysis. All of these lines of inquiry have potential implications for treatment development or evolution of existing therapies.

As is evident from the above, functional neuroimaging has played a key role in this intriguing disorder. Neuroimaging has established a role for frontal-basal ganglia-thalamic circuits and has been key in deepening our understanding of OCD. Moreover, the increasingly well-defined circuitry could serve not only to refine treatment (stereotactic ablation, DBS, newer and/or less-invasive stimulation methods) but also as a tool for characterizing intermediate phenotypes. Imaging, especially when applied in systematic study of neurosurgical outcomes across related diagnoses, could help to explore the relationship of OCD with other anxiety disorders, affective illnesses, behavioral addictions, and other related (OCD spectrum) conditions. Coming full circle, OCD circuitry models are being used to understand the effects of neurosurgical interventions for severely affected OCD patients who fail to respond to conventional behavioral and medication treatments. The models permit hypothesis testing that may help to refine existing neurosurgical approaches (lesion procedures or DBS) as well as other potential brain circuit-based interventions for OCD (such as transcranial magnetic stimulation, which remains little explored in the illness).

References

Abelson JL, Curtis GC, Sagher O, et al. (2005). Deep brain stimulation for refractory obsessive-compulsive disorder. *Biol Psychiatry* **57**: 510–516.

Alexander, GE, DeLong, MR, Strick, PL (1986). Parallel organization of functionally segregated circuits linking basal ganglia and cortex. *Ann Rev Neurosci* **9**: 357–381.

Alexander, GE, Crutcher, MD, DeLong, MR (1990). Basal ganglia-thalamocortical circuits: parallel substrates for motor, oculomotor, "prefrontal" and "limbic" functions. *Progr Brain Res* **85**: 119–146.

Anon. (1937). Surgery used on the soul-sick; relief of obsessions is reported. *New York Times*, p. 1.

Aouizerate, B, Cuny E, Martin-Guehl C, et al. (2004). Deep brain stimulation of the ventral caudate nucleus in the treatment of obsessive-compulsive disorder and major depression. Case report. *J Neurosurg* **101**: 682–686.

Ballantine HTJr., Bouckoms AJ, Thomas EK, Giriunas IE (1987). Treatment of psychiatric illness by stereotactic cingulotomy. *Biol Psychiatry* **22**: 807–819.

Bartha R, Stein MB, Williamson PC, *et al.* (1998). A short echo ^{1}H spectroscopy and volumetric MRI study of the corpus striatum in patients with obsessive-compulsive disorder and comparison subjects. *Am J Psychiatry* **155**: 1584–1591.

Baxter L, Schwartz J, Mazziotta J, *et al.* (1988). Cerebral glucose metabolic rates in nondepressed patients with obsessive compulsive disorder. *Am J Psychiatry* **145**: 1560–1563.

Baxter L, Jr., Schwartz J, Bergman KS, *et al.* (1992). Caudate glucose metabolic rate changes with both drug and behavior therapy for obsessive-compulsive disorder. *Arch Gen Psychiatry* **49**: 681–689.

Benkelfat C, Nordahl TE, Semple WE, *et al.* (1990). Local cerebral glucose metabolic rates in obsessive-compulsive disorder: patients treated with clomipramine. *Arch Gen Psychiatry* **47**: 840–848.

Binder DK, Iskandar BJ (2000). Modern neurosurgery for psychiatric disorders. *Neurosurgery* **47**: 9–21; discussion 21–23.

Bingley T, Leksell L, Meyerson BA, Rylander G (1977). Long term results of stereotactic capsulotomy in chronic obsessive-compulsive neurosis. In Sweet WH, Obrador Alcalde S, Martín-Rodríguez JG (eds.) *Proceedings of the Fourth World Congress of Psychiatric Surgery, September, Neurosurgical Treatment in Psychiatry, Pain, and Epilepsy Madrid*, 1975 (pp.287–299). Baltimore, MD: University Park Press.

Breiter HC, Rauch SL, Kwong KK, *et al.* (1996). Functional magnetic resonance imaging of symptom provocation in obsessive compulsive disorder. *Arch Gen Psychiatry* **53**: 595–606.

Bridges PK, Bartlett JR, Hale AS, *et al.* (1994). Psychosurgery: stereotactic subcaudate tractomy. An indispensable treatment. *Br J Psychiatry* **165**: 599–611; discussion 612–593.

Brody AL, Saxena S, Schwartz JM, *et al.* (1998). FDG-PET predictors of response to behavioral therapy and pharmacotherapy in obsessive-compulsive disorder. *Psychiatry Res* **84**: 1–6.

Cannistraro PA, Makris N, Howard JD, *et al.* (2007). A diffusion tensor imaging study of white matter in obsessive-compulsive disorder. *Depress Anxiety* **24**: 440–446.

Cho DY, Lee WY, Chen CC (2008). Limbic leukotomy for intractable major affective disorders: a 7-year follow-up study using nine comprehensive psychiatric test evaluations. *J Clin Neurosci* **15**: 138–142.

Cosgrove GR (2000). Surgery for psychiatric disorders. *CNS Spectr* **5**: 43–52.

Dougherty DD, Baer L, Cosgrove GR, *et al.* (2002). Prospective long-term follow-up of 44 patients who received cingulotomy for treatment-refractory obsessive-compulsive disorder. *Am J Psychiatry* **159**: 269–275.

Ebert D, Speck O, Konig A, *et al.* (1997). ^{1}H-magnetic resonance spectroscopy in obsessive-compulsive disorder: evidence for neuronal loss in the cingulate gyrus and the right striatum. *Psychiatry Res* **74**: 173–176.

El-Hai J (2005). *The Lobotomist: A Maverick Medical Genius and his Tragic Quest to Rid the World of Mental Illness*. Hoboken, NJ: Wiley.

Feldman RP, Alterman RL, Goodrich JT (2001). Contemporary psychosurgery and a look to the future. *J Neurosurg* **95**: 944–956.

Fins JJ (2003). From psychosurgery to neuromodulation and palliation: history's lessons for the ethical conduct and regulation of neuropsychiatric research. *Neurosurg Clin N Am* **14**: 303–319, ix–x.

Freeman W, Watts JW, Hunt T (1942). *Psychosurgery; Intelligence, Emotion and Social Behavior Following Prefrontal Lobotomy for Mental Disorders*. Springfield, IL: Charles C. Thomas.

Gilbert AR, Keshavan MS, Diwadkar V, *et al.* (2008). Gray matter differences between pediatric obsessive-compulsive disorder patients and high-risk siblings: a preliminary voxel-based morphometry study. *Neurosci Lett* **435**: 45–50.

Greenberg BD, Dougherty DD, Rauch SL. (2009). Neurosurgical treatments: lesion procedures and deep brain stimulation. In Sadock BJ, Sadock VA, Ruiz P (eds.) *Kaplan and Sadock's Comprehensive Textbook of Psychiatry, Ninth edition* (pp. 3314–3322). Philadelphia, PA: Lippincott, Williams & Wilkins.

Greenberg BD, Gabriels LA, Malone DA, Jr., *et al.* (2010). Deep brain stimulation of the ventral internal capsule/ventral striatum for obsessive-compulsive disorder: worldwide experience. *Mol Psychiatry* **15**: 64–79.

Hay P, Sachdev P, Cumming S, *et al.* (1993). Treatment of obsessive-compulsive disorder by psychosurgery. *Acta Psychiatr Scand* **87**: 197–207.

Herner T (1961). Treatment of mental disorders with frontal stereotactic thermo-lesions: a follow-up of 116 cases. *Acta Psychiatr Scand* **58**(Suppl 36): 1–140.

Hoehn-Saric R, Pearlson GD, Harris GJ, *et al.* (1991). Effects of fluoxetine on regional cerebral blood flow in obsessive compulsive patients. *Am J Psychiatry* **148**: 1243–1245.

Jenike MA, Breiter HC, Baer L, *et al.* (1996). Cerebral structural abnormalities in obsessive-compulsive disorder: a quantitative morphometric magnetic resonance imaging study. *Arch Gen Psychiatry* **53**: 625–632.

Kelly D, Richardson A, Mitchell-Heggs N, *et al.* (1973). Stereotactic limbic leucotomy: a preliminary report on forty patients. *Br J Psychiatry* **123**: 141–148.

Kim CH, Chang JW, Koo MS, *et al.* (2003). Anterior cingulotomy for refractory obsessive-compulsive disorder. *Acta Psychiatr Scand* **107**: 283–290.

Kim MC, Lee TK, Choi CR (2002). Review of long-term results of stereotactic psychosurgery. *Neurol Med Chir (Tokyo)* **42**: 365–371.

Knight G (1973). Further observations from an experience of 660 cases of stereotactic tractotomy. *Postgrad Med J* **49**: 845–854.

Kullberg G (1977). Differences in effects of capsulotomy and cingulotomy. In Sweet WH, Obrador WS, Martín-Rodríguez JG, eds. *Neurosurgical Treatment in Psychiatry, Pain, and Epilepsy* (pp. 301–208). Baltimore, MD: University Park Press.

Lopes AC, Greenberg BD, Noren G, *et al.* (2009): Treatment of resistant obsessive-compulsive disorder with ventral capsular/ventral striatal gamma capsulotomy: a pilot prospective study. *J Neuropsychiatry Clin Neurosci* **21**: 381–392.

Machlin SR, Harris GJ, Pearlson GD, *et al.* (1991). Elevated medial-frontal cerebral blood flow in obsessive compulsive patients: a SPECT study. *Am J Psychiatry* **148**: 1240–1242.

Mallet L, Polosan M, Jaafari N, *et al.* (2008). Subthalamic nucleus stimulation in severe obsessive-compulsive disorder. *N Engl J Med* **359**: 2121–2134.

McGuire PK, Bench CJ, Frith CD, *et al.* (1994). Functional anatomy of obsessive-compulsive phenomena. *Br J Psychiatry* **164**: 459–468.

Mindus P, Ericson K, Greitz T (1986). Regional cerebral glucose metabolism in anxiety disorders studied with positron emission tomography before and after psychosurgical intervention. A preliminary report. *Acta Radiol Suppl* **369**: 444–448.

Mindus P, Rasmussen SA, Lindquist C (1994). Neurosurgical treatment for refractory obsessive-compulsive disorder: implications for understanding frontal lobe function. *J Neuropsychiatry Clin Neurosci* **6**: 467–477.

Nordahl TE, Benkelfat C, Semple W, *et al.* (1989). Cerebral glucose metabolic rates in obsessive-compulsive disorder. *Neuropsychopharmacology* **2**: 23–28.

Nuttin B, Cosyns P, Demeulemeester H, Gybels J, Meyerson B (1999). Electrical stimulation in anterior limbs of internal capsules in patients with obsessive-compulsive disorder. *Lancet* **354**: 1526.

Okun MS, Bowers D, Springer U, *et al.* (2004). What's in a "smile?" Intra-operative observations of contralateral smiles induced by deep brain stimulation. *Neurocase* **10**: 271–279.

Pan HC, Sheehan J, Stroila M, Steiner M, Steiner L (2005). Late cyst formation following gamma knife surgery of arteriovenous malformations. *J Neurosurg* 2005 **102**(Suppl): 124–127.

Perani D, Colombo C, Bressi S, *et al.* (1995). FDG PET study in obsessive-compulsive disorder: a clinical metabolic correlation study after treatment. *Br J Psychiatry* **166**: 244–250.

Pool JL (1954). Psychosurgery in older people. *J Am Geriat Soc* **7**: 456–466.

Pressman JD (1998) *Last Resort: Psychosurgery and the Limits of Medicine.* Cambridge, UK: Cambridge University Press.

Price BH, Baral I, Cosgrove GR, *et al.* (2001). Improvement in severe self-mutilation following limbic leucotomy: a series of 5 consecutive cases. *J Clin Psychiatry* **62**: 925–932.

Rauch SL, Jenike MA, Alpert NM, *et al.* (1994). Regional cerebral blood flow measured during symptom provocation in obsessive-compulsive disorder using ^{15}O-labeled CO_2 and positron emission tomography. *Arch Gen Psychiatry* **51**: 62–70.

Rauch SL, Savage CR, Alpert NM, *et al.* (1997). Probing striatal function in obsessive-compulsive disorder: a PET study of implicit sequence learning. *J Neuropsychiatry Clin Neurosci* **9**: 568–573.

Rauch SL, Dougherty DD, Cosgrove GR, *et al.* (2001). Cerebral metabolic correlates as potential predictors of response to anterior cingulotomy for obsessive compulsive disorder. *Biol Psychiatry* **50**: 659–667.

Rauch SL, Shin LM, Dougherty DD, *et al.* (2002). Predictors of fluvoxamine response in contamination-related obsessive compulsive disorder: a PET symptom provocation study. *Neuropsychopharmacology* **27**: 782–791.

Robinson D, Wu H, Munne RA, *et al.* (1995) Reduced caudate nucleus volume in obsessive-compulsive disorder. *Arch Gen Psychiatry* **52**: 393–398.

Rubin RT, Villanueva-Myer J, Ananth J, *et al.* (1992). Regional xenon-133 cerebral blood flow and cerebral technetium-99m HMPAO uptake in unmedicated patients with obsessive-compulsive disorder and matched normal control subjects. *Arch Gen Psychiatry* **49**: 695–702.

Ruck C, Karlsson A, Steele JD, *et al.* (2008). Capsulotomy for obsessive-compulsive disorder: long-term follow-up of 25 patients. *Arch Gen Psychiatry* **65**: 914–921.

Saxena S, Brody AL, Maidment KM, *et al.* (1999). Localized orbitofrontal and subcortical metabolic changes and predictors of response to paroxetine treatment in obsessive-compulsive disorder. *Neuropsychopharmacology* **21**: 683–693.

Schlaepfer TE, Cohen MX, Frick C, *et al.* (2008). Deep brain stimulation to reward circuitry alleviates anhedonia in refractory major depression. *Neuropsychopharmacology* **33**: 368–377.

Schwartz JM, Stoessel PW, Baxter LR, Jr., Martin KM, Phelps ME (1996). Systematic changes in cerebral glucose metabolic rate after successful behavior modification treatment of obsessive-compulsive disorder. *Arch Gen Psychiatry* **53**: 109–113.

Shapira NA, Okun MS, Wint D, *et al.* (2006). Panic and fear induced by deep brain stimulation. *J Neurol Neurosurg Psychiatry* **77**: 410–412.

Swedo SE, Shapiro MB, Grady CL, *et al.* (1989). Cerebral glucose metabolism in childhood-onset obsessive-compulsive disorder. *Arch Gen Psychiatry* **46**: 518–523.

Swedo SE, Pietrini P, Leonard HL, *et al.* (1992). Cerebral glucose metabolism in childhood onset obsessive-compulsive disorder: revisualization during pharmacotherapy. *Arch Gen Psychiatry* **49**: 690–694.

Szeszko PR, Christian C, Macmaster F, *et al.* (2008). Gray matter structural alterations in psychotropic drug-naive pediatric obsessive-compulsive disorder: an optimized voxel-based morphometry study. *Am J Psychiatry* **165**: 1299–1307.

US National Commission (1977). *Psychosurgery: Report and Recommendations.* Bethesda, MD: National Commission for the Protection of Human Subjects of Biomedical and Behavioral Research.

Valenstein ES (1986). *Great and Desperate Cures: The Rise and Decline of Psychosurgery and Other Radical Treatments for Mental Illness.* New York: Basic Books.

Waziri R (1990). Psychosurgery for anxiety and obsessive-compulsive disorders. In Noyes R, Roth M, Burrows GD (eds.) *Handbook of Anxiety: The Treatment of Anxiety* (pp. 519–535). Amsterdam: Elsevier.

Chapter

3

Selective serotonin reuptake inhibitors in the treatment of obsessive-compulsive disorder

Signi A. Page and Robert Hudak

Introduction

While the clinical symptoms of obsessive-compulsive disorder (OCD) were described early in the twentieth century by Pierre Janet, decades passed before this disorder was recognized as a biological illness, resulting in a delay in medication being investigated for the treatment of OCD. As a result, the use of medications for OCD is a relatively recent phenomenon. Intravenous clomipramine, a serotonin reuptake inhibitor (SRI) that is a tricyclic antidepressant (TCA) was discussed as a possible treatment for OCD as early as 1970 (Rack and Chir 1970). While the study was inconclusive as to the role of clomipramine in the reduction of OCD symptoms, this pioneer study lead to further research into the benefits of medication treatment in OCD. The first placebo-controlled study that showed improvement in OCD symptoms without comorbid disorders was published in 1980 (Montgomery 1980) and additional studies the same year demonstrated that clomipramine improved OCD with comorbid depression (Marks et al. 1980; Thoren et al. 1980). This led to a marked increase in interest in investigations into possible OCD medical treatment throughout the following decade (Montgomery 1998), which ultimately culminated with the US Food and Drug Administration (FDA) approval of Anafranil, the brand name for the TCA clomipramine for the treatment of OCD as defined by the *Diagnostic and Statistical Manual of Mental Disorders,* 3rd edition revised (DSM-IIIR) in December of 1987. Further research has indicated the efficacy of additional medications, notably the selective serotonin reuptake inhibitors (SSRIs), in the treatment of OCD. Along with clomipramine, they are the first-line medications used in OCD therapy.

Initiating medications

The decision concerning when to start medications for OCD is a matter of clinical judgment and patient request. Because of its efficacy in OCD, behavioral therapy, specifically exposure with response prevention (ERP) should be offered as a first-line treatment for OCD. In particular, in patients without significant comorbid depression or anxiety, ERP may be the only treatment modality that is required, particularly if the symptoms are mild to moderate (American Psychiatric Association 2007). Medication should be considered if the symptoms are severe enough that the clinician and patient feel that they would be unable to perform the therapy or do the homework without pharmaceutical intervention. Therefore, most patients with moderate to severe OCD will be offered medication treatment in addition to ERP.

The presence of an active major depressive disorder poses problems with implementing ERP, necessitating a protocol involving only medication in the initial management of the OCD (Soomro 2003). However, patients still can respond to behavioral therapy if a comorbid depression is present (Foa et al. 1992); therefore, a patient's motivation to do therapy should be the primary driver in making the decision to prescribe ERP along with an SSRI in the presence of major depressive disorder. Medication is also indicated when the patient refuses to engage in behavioral therapy. In both circumstances, a medication trial may reduce the severity of the OCD symptoms enough that the person will eventually be able to successfully enter into a course of ERP. While combination treatment is not necessary for all patients (Cottraux et al. 2005), combining medications and therapy may lead to improved response rates in many OCD patients.

Clinical Obsessive-Compulsive Disorders in Adults and Children, ed. Robert Hudak and Darin D. Dougherty.
Published by Cambridge University Press. Copyright © Cambridge University Press 2011.

Some patients may respond well to medications as the sole course of therapy, usually based upon a history of successful treatment with medications only, although this is generally regarded as an exception.

In current clinical practice the first-line and mainstay medications used in OCD therapy include the SSRIs as well as the TCA clomipramine, an SRI that is not "selective" as it also acts on additional receptor sites. A large meta-analysis of 17 randomized controlled trials of SSRIs versus placebo showed that SSRIs showed advantages over placebo in weeks 6 through 13 for the treatment of OCD (Soomro et al. 2008). There have been studies to explore initiating additional medications along with the SSRI: a preliminary study using mirtazapine augmentation indicated that patients achieved clinical response earlier than with an SSRI alone; however, at the study endpoint both patient groups were equal (Pallanti et al. 2004). The current recommendation is that patients be placed on only one medication, an SSRI, at the start of treatment.

In conclusion, it should be noted while ERP is generally offered as a first-line treatment for all levels of severity in OCD patients, medications typically should be reserved as first-line treatment in patients whose symptoms are moderate to severe or who are diagnosed with comorbid major depressive disorder. An initial trial of a single SSRI is recommended for any patient beginning pharmaceutical intervention.

Medications

Clomipramine

Clomipramine has a long history of clinical use and is the most studied medication for OCD. The FDA approved its use for OCD in 1989, and it is one of four SRIs (the others being fluoxetine, fluvoxamine, and sertraline) also approved for use in children and adolescents. Clomipramine has been demonstrated to be superior to placebo in multiple controlled trials since the late 1980s (Katz et al. 1990; Clomipramine Collaborative Study Group 1991). Although its effectiveness has been demonstrated repeatedly, clinically it is seldom used first line because of concerns about tolerability.

Meta-analyses have attempted to answer the question of whether clomipramine performs better than the SSRIs against placebo. These studies have generally shown a larger effect size for clomipramine than for various SSRIs when each is compared with placebo

(Cox et al. 1993; Griest et al. 1995; Piccinelli et al. 1995; Stein et al. 1995; Abramowitz 1997; Ackerman and Greenland 2002; Eddy et al. 2004). However, these analyses were not based on head-to-head comparisons and were complicated by differences in patient samples among trials. Although superiority of clomipramine is generally found through these analyses, lower tolerability is often noted as a factor weighing against its first-line use. Head-to-head comparison trials with SSRIs (specifically fluoxetine, fluvoxamine, paroxetine, and sertraline) have had mixed results, with some trials demonstrating slight superiority of clomipramine and others slight superiority of the various SSRIs (Pigott et al. 1990; Jenike et al. 1990a; Freeman et al. 1994; Lopez-Ibor et al. 1996; Koran et al. 1996; Zohar and Judge, 1996; Mundo et al. 2000, 2001). Therefore, based on head-to-head trial data, clomipramine is generally considered equally effective to the SSRIs. Again, lower tolerability of clomipramine has been noted in these studies, although this was most notable in those studies using higher clomipramine doses relative to the doses of SSRIs used. Some studies show that the dropout rate for clomipramine is no different than that for SSRIs, indicating that its tolerability may be comparable to SSRIs in some patients (Greist et al. 1995a). Taken as a whole, the evidence from head-to-head trials of any SRIs, including both the SSRIs and clomipramine, has not demonstrated superiority of any one SRI over the others. Therefore, selection of a first-line medication is best made based on side effect profile, half-life, and potential interactions with other medications.

Side effects of clomipramine are caused by its anticholinergic, antihistaminergic, and antiadrenergic effects. Commonly noted effects are dry mouth, urinary retention, constipation, sedation, weight gain, and orthostatic hypotension. It is also associated with higher cardiac toxicity through prolongation of the QT interval and, therefore, should be used with caution in patients with known cardiac risk factors. Other side effects to consider include increased seizure risk with doses above 250 mg and the potential elevation of liver transanimases.

Clomipramine has never been tested in a controlled fixed-dose study to assess optimal doses; however, the cumulative results of studies to date suggest a dose of 250 mg to 300 mg results in an optimal effect.

Use of clomipramine as an augmentation agent in SSRI therapy is supported by evidence and expert opinion (March et al. 1997; Figueroa et al. 1998;

Pallanti *et al.* 1999) and, therefore, it is a commonly used augmentation agent for SSRIs. Similarly, there is also ample support in the literature for augmentation of clomipramine with SSRIs (March *et al.* 1997; Figueroa *et al.* 1998). The starting dose of clomipramine as an augmentation strategy is typically 25 mg/day and it may be increased as tolerated with doses as high as 150 mg having been demonstrated as successful for augmentation therapy (Pallanti *et al.* 1999). Care should be taken when adding clomipramine to SSRIs with significant P450 inhibition, particularly fluvoxamine, fluoxetine, and fluvoxamine.

Clomipramine is available in intravenous (IV) form although that formulation is not available in the USA. Administration IV enables higher plasma levels of clomipramine to be achieved as it avoids first-pass metabolism of the active compound to desmethylclomipramine. Use of IV clomipramine has been shown to be more effective than placebo in patients who previously did not respond to oral clomipramine (Fallon *et al.* 1998) and it appears to be more efficacious when the drug is pulse loaded as opposed to gradual dose increases (Koran *et al.* 1997). Because IV clomipramine use is not an option in the USA, the possibility exists of replicating its pharmacological profile, which has an increased clomipramine/desmethylclomipramine ratio, through avoidance of the first-pass effect. This is a strategy that has been noted clinically to work in treatment-resistant patients. The addition of fluvoxamine, a potent CYP1A2 inhibitor, will increase the clomipramine/desmethylclomipramine ratio. Szegedi *et al.* (1996) found the clomipramine/fluvoxamine combination was well tolerated, particularly when the total plasma clomipramine level was below 450 ng/ml defined as the combined clomipramine and desmethylclomipramine levels. The combination allowed an increase in clomipramine/desmethylclomipramine ratio in the subjects. It is recommended that clinicians using this protocol maintain total plasma clomipramine levels of 450 ng/ml or less, and that the goal clomipramine/desmethylclomipramine ratio should be 4:1 or greater, which is similar to the ratio obtained in the Szegedi study.

Selective serotonin reuptake inhibitors

Although there is a suggestion in the literature that the SSRIs may be slightly less effective than clomipramine, they are generally considered equally as effective, and

SSRIs remain the most frequently used first-line options because of their more tolerable side effect profiles. Doses used tend to be higher than those needed to treat depression, and fixed-dose studies clearly demonstrate superior efficacy with higher doses for fluoxetine, paroxetine, sertraline, and citalopram (Fineberg and Gale 2005), although a fixed-dose study has not been carried out for fluvoxamine. Correlations between plasma levels and response rates have not been demonstrated. Approximately 10–12 weeks on an appropriate dose is considered an adequate trial of efficacy for these medications when treating OCD, although some studies have demonstrated much earlier response times. Patients occasionally only begin to show response to the medication at the end of a 12 week trial. In those instances, extending the trial to 16 weeks or greater is warranted. Side effects are largely consistent among this group of medications and are discussed in further detail later in this chapter. Concerns related to specific medications are discussed below.

Fluvoxamine

Fluvoxamine is FDA approved for the treatment of OCD and has been demonstrated superior to placebo in multiple controlled trials (Goodman *et al.* 1989, 1996; Jenike *et al.* 1990b; Greist *et al.* 1995b; Hollander *et al.* 2003a), with average doses used typically between 250 and 300 mg. Earlier therapeutic response time, as early as two weeks after initiation of treatment, was noted in the trial using the highest starting dose of 100 mg (Hollander *et al.* 2003a). Most trials demonstrated a full clinical response by weeks 8–10.

In head-to-head comparator studies, fluvoxamine has been compared with clomipramine, citalopram, and paroxetine, although the majority of studies have used clomipramine as the comparator drug. The lack of placebo control groups complicates several of these studies, preventing calculation of the net drug effect. Studies comparing fluvoxamine and clomipramine have consistently demonstrated no difference in efficacy (Smeraldi *et al.* 1992; Freeman *et al.* 1994; Koran *et al.* 1996; Mundo *et al.* 2001). A small single-blind trial comparing fluvoxamine with paroxetine and citalopram showed no significant difference between outcomes in the three groups, suggesting similar effectiveness (Mundo *et al.* 1997).

Fluvoxamine has never been examined in a fixed-dose trial, but efficacy has been demonstrated throughout the dose range of 150 to 300 mg in various trials.

The controlled release formulation of fluvoxamine has demonstrated similar efficacy to the standard formulation, with onset of action of the controlled release form of the medication demonstrated as early as week two (Hollander *et al.* 2003a).

Its short half-life should be a consideration as it typically requires twice daily dosing with the standard formulation, potentially leading to difficulty with rapid withdrawal causing the SSRI discontinuation syndrome. Fluvoxamine also has a greater potential for drug–drug interactions compared with other SSRIs, which should be considered when deciding upon an individual patient's medication regimen.

Fluoxetine

Fluoxetine has an FDA approved indication for OCD. Superiority over placebo has been demonstrated in controlled trials (Montgomery *et al.* 1993; Tollefson *et al.* 1994), where doses between 40 and 60 mg have shown more benefit than a 20 mg dose. A study examining relapse rates during a 52 week follow-up period demonstrated that doses of 40 mg and below did not provide benefit over placebo in reducing relapse. A dose of 60 mg, however, did result in a significant reduction in relapse, suggesting that higher doses should be considered to prevent relapse over time (Romano *et al.* 2001). In clinical practice, there is anecdotal evidence of superior efficacy of doses as high as 80 mg over the 60 mg dose, although these higher doses have not been studied in clinical trials.

Two head-to-head comparator studies have demonstrated equivalent efficacy with clomipramine, although neither of these studies used a placebo control group to determine net drug effect (Pigott *et al.* 1990; Lopez-Ibor *et al.* 1996). Equivalence was also demonstrated with sertraline in a 24 week controlled trial, with some suggestion of earlier response in the sertraline group (Bergeron *et al.* 2002). None of these comparator studies noted a large difference in tolerance between the drugs studied.

Fluoxetine has the longest half-life of the SSRIs, two to four days. Additionally, the active metabolite, norfluoxetine, has a half-life of seven to nine days. The longer half-life results in fluoxetine having the least amount of discontinuation syndrome symptoms. In contrast, this long half-life may be responsible for any observed delay in response compared with other SSRIs as well as side effects such as agitation, which occur earlier in treatment with other SSRIs, cropping up later during fluoxetine treatment.

Fluoxetine is less serotonin specific than some other medications in the SSRI category, with the active metabolite having effects on norepinephrine reuptake as well as serotonin reuptake.

Paroxetine

Paroxetine has shown superiority to placebo in controlled trials (Zohar and Judge 1996; Kamijima *et al.* 2004; Hollander *et al.* 2003b) and is FDA approved for the treatment of OCD. One of these trials (Zohar and Judge 1996) also had an active comparator arm with clomipramine, and efficacy was comparable with the paroxetine arm. In these studies, doses above 60 mg were not tested. In general, doses between 40 and 60 mg were the most effective.

Paroxetine has the advantage of having been studied for long-term effectiveness over a six month period and has demonstrated a significantly reduced relapse rate compared with placebo during this six month extension phase (Hollander *et al.* 2003b).

Discontinuation syndrome is more likely with paroxetine because of its short half-life. Another factor to consider with use of this medication is the high risk of drug–drug interactions compared with many others in this class, because of its strong inhibition of CYP2D6.

Sertraline

Sertraline is also FDA approved for use in OCD. In placebo-controlled trials (Greist *et al.* 1995c; Kronig *et al.* 1999), doses as low as 50 mg had an effect discernable from placebo; however, more robust efficacy was seen with doses closer to 200 mg.

As mentioned above, sertraline was shown to be equipotent with clomipramine in a comparison trial, and responder and remission rates were comparable in a head-to-head trial with fluoxetine (Bergeron *et al.* 2002), although there was suggestion of earlier response times in the sertraline group. This may be because of the longer half-life of fluoxetine and not because of any advantages that sertraline has over other SSRIs. A regimen involving a rapid titration of medications has been studied using sertraline where a dose of 150 mg was reached by day five (Bogetto *et al.* 2002). Rapid titration resulted in a more rapid onset of response and was equally as well tolerated as a slower, more standard titration regimen.

Longer-term outcomes for up to two years of follow-up with flexible dosing (50–200 mg) demonstrated a continued decrease in scores on the Yale–Brown

Obsessive Compulsive Scale (Y-BOCS) after two years of continued treatment in one study (Rasmussen *et al.* 1997). However, in a later study, sertraline was not more successful than placebo in preventing relapse (Koran *et al.* 2002), possibly because more stringent criteria for defining relapse were used in this later trial.

Sertraline has also been tested in higher doses in 30 patients who did not respond to a 200 mg dose, and additional benefit was seen at doses between 250 and 400 mg in 40% of the patient sample (Ninan *et al.* 2006). Therefore, doses higher than 200 mg should be considered in OCD patients who have not responded to lower dosages.

Sertraline has a higher incidence of gastrointestinal side effects than other SSRIs, which may be a factor for some patients when choosing this medication. It should always be given with food. This not only reduces the possibility of the gastrointestinal side effects but also increases absorption of this medication.

Citalopram and escitalopram

Though not currently FDA approved for use in OCD, both citalopram and escitalopram are likely comparable to the other SSRIs and have been used successfully in clinical settings. Only one randomized controlled trial has been carried out comparing citalopram with placebo (Montgomery *et al.* 2001). This demonstrated significant efficacy at all dosages (20, 40, and 60 mg) with a trend for greater efficacy at the 60 mg dosage. Similar findings were replicated in another open-label study (Koponen *et al.* 1997).

Several open-label trials have demonstrated comparable efficacy between citalopram and other SSRIs. In a small trial, citalopram was similar to both paroxetine and fluvoxamine (Mundo *et al.* 1997). Another trial, which had arms for citalopram, paroxetine, fluvoxamine, and clomipramine, found no significant differences in responder rates between any of the study groups (Erzegovesi *et al.* 2001). Citalopram demonstrated some response in 14 of 18 patients who did not respond to adequate six month trials of other SSRIs (Marazziti *et al.* 2001); however, when more stringent response criteria were used in a subsequent study, this effect was not observed (Pallanti *et al.* 1999). Its IV use was shown in an open study to be well tolerated and to have rapid efficacy in a majority of treatment-resistant patients (Pallanti *et al.* 2002) and is worthy of further study. This modality is unavailable in the USA.

Escitalopram has had less opportunity to be studied in OCD, but it was demonstrated to be equally as effective as paroxetine in a controlled head-to-head trial (Dhillon *et al.* 2006). It was also shown to be superior to placebo in preventing relapse (Fineberg *et al.* 2007a).

Citalopram and escitalopram have less potential for drug–drug interactions than some of the other SSRIs, making it a good choice for patients with comorbidities requiring multiple medications.

Venlafaxine

Venlafaxine is a serotonin norepinephrine reuptake inhibitor (SNRI) that is not currently FDA approved for OCD and evidence is mixed on its efficacy in OCD. It has only been compared with placebo in OCD patients in one relatively small trial (Yaryure-Tobias and Neziroglu 1996). While there was no significant benefit over placebo, a trend towards better response in the venlafaxine group was noted. The trial was short in duration (eight weeks) and only used doses up to 225 mg, suggesting the possibility that larger doses and longer duration of treatment may prove to have greater benefit. However, in the absence of a placebo control arm, venlafaxine has recently demonstrated comparable efficacy to clomipramine (Albert *et al.* 2002) and paroxetine (Denys *et al.* 2003) in patients with OCD. A more robust placebo-controlled trial is needed to definitively clarify the potential role of venlafaxine as a treatment for OCD.

In one study, non-responders to venlafaxine or paroxetine were switched to the alternate medication, and the group switched to paroxetine did significantly better than the group switched to venlafaxine, although sample sizes were small and there was no placebo control group (Denys *et al.* 2004). Other studies have shown some evidence supporting efficacy of venlafaxine in patients who are non-responders to one or more SSRI trials (Hollander *et al.* 2003c). Doses up to 450 mg were used in this study; with a mean dose of 230 mg. Venlafaxine was also well tolerated in this trial, suggesting a potential use for this medication in patients who do not respond to trials of other SSRIs.

Because the data are mixed for venlafaxine at this time, including the possibility of decreased efficacy compared with SSRIs, this medication should not be considered a first-line medication for OCD. However, it can be considered an alternative medication if a patient does not respond to an adequate trial of

SSRIs or is intolerant of SSRIs. Factors to consider when using venlafaxine include its often severe discontinuation syndrome and a greater potential for toxicity in overdose. This toxicity occurs predominately when it is mixed with alcohol or other drugs and includes prolongation of the QT interval, bundle branch block, and QRS prolongation.

Choosing a specific medication

The medications that are currently approved by the FDA in the treatment of OCD include clomipramine, fluoxetine, sertraline, paroxetine, and fluvoxamine. The other two SSRIs, citalopram and escitalopram, do not have FDA approval but have demonstrated effectiveness in the treatment of OCD. The choice of specific SRI as a first-line drug for an individual patient is largely based on the side effect profile of the medications and of the specific comorbid conditions in the patient (Math and Reddy 2007). As in other psychiatric disorders, a family history of response to a specific medication may be a useful guide. In the absence of evidence for superiority of any individual SSRI in head-to-head trials, the switch from one medication to another in the case of nonresponse is made in the same manner. Because of the typical TCA side effect profile of clomipramine, it is not usually chosen as a first-line medication. As there is some evidence that it may be superior to the SSRIs, it can be used as a second-line medication if the patient has failed two or three appropriate trials of other SSRIs (Math and Reddy 2007); expert consensus guidelines suggest that two SSRIs should be tried before moving to clomipramine (March et al. 1997). Venlafaxine is not recommended as a first-line medication for OCD, but it may be useful to attempt a trial if the patient fails trials of SSRIs and clomipramine.

The side effects of sedation, orthostatic hypotension, anticholinergic effects, and potential lethality in overdose are the reasons that clomipramine is rarely chosen first for OCD treatment. Other side effects that may influence the choice of a particular drug include those for paroxetine, which has the highest chance of weight gain among the SSRIs as well as being the most anticholinergic (Maina et al. 2004). Sertraline is associated with a higher rate of gastrointestinal side effects, including diarrhea, and fluoxetine with higher amounts of agitation and insomnia (Math and Reddy 2007).

Drug–drug interactions may also be taken into consideration when choosing a specific medication. The action of the drug on the P450 system is the most important piece of information when evaluating drug interactions among this group. Fluvoxamine is a potent inhibitor of CYP1A2 and paroxetine and fluoxetine are potent inhibitors of CYP2D6. Sertraline, citalopram, and escitalopram are not as potent inhibitors of the P450 system and would be the preferred drugs in patients on multiple medications. The actions of the various SSRIs upon P450 isozymes are summarized in Table 3.1.

When prescribing medication for OCD, the physician should educate the patient as to the potential problem of consuming common and important inhibitors and substrates of the CYP isozymes. A substance that inhibits a specific isozyme can effect an increase in the enzyme's substrate. Erythromycin, amiodarone, and grapefruit inhibit CYP3A4; cimetidine is a strong inhibitor of both CYP2D6 and CYP1A2, and ciprofloxacin inhibits CYP1A2 (The Medical Letter, 2003). Important substrates of CYP isozymes include:

- 1A2: caffeine, theophylline, clozapine, clomipramine
- 2C19: proton pump inhibitors, diazepam

Table 3.1 Inhibition of specific cytochrome P450 activity

CYP isozyme	Citalopram	Fluoxetine	Fluvoxamine	Paroxetine	Sertraline
CYP1A2	+/−	+	+++	+	+/−
CYP2C19	?	++	+++		+
CYP2D6	+	+++	+	+++	+
CYP3A4	?	++	++	+/−	+/−

+/−, unlikely; ?, unknown; +, mild; ++, moderate; +++, substantial.
Sources: Skjelbo and Brosen (1992), Gram *et al.* (1993), Rasmussen *et al.* (1995), Harvey and Preskorn (1996), and the Evaluation of Genomic Applications in Practice and Prevention Working Group (2007).

- 2D6: many TCAs, beta-blockers, antiarrhythmic agents, atomoxetine, risperidone, codeine, hydrocodone
- 3A4: calcium channel blockers, erythromycin, alprazolam, midazolam, triazolam, hydroxymethylglutaryl-conezyme A (HMG-CoA) reductase inhibitors, HIV protease inhibitors, ziprasidone.

This list of P450 inhibitors and substrates is not meant to be a comprehensive list of medications and supplements but rather a general guide for clinicians to some of the more commonly seen medications in clinical practice. Psychiatrists are urged to consult the latest information available when making decisions concerning drug–drug interactions.

Dosage guidelines for medications

When starting a patient on SSRIs for OCD, the initial dose is typically no different than those used for other indications and generally follows the manufacturers' guidelines (Table 3.2). Common clinical practice involves starting at lower dosages when the patient has a comorbid panic or generalized anxiety disorder, as these patients may be more sensitive to or more

fearful of side effects such as agitation/akathesia. A lower initial dose is also warranted upon patient request because of fear of side effects or when reporting a prior history of sensitivity to medications. Elderly patients should also be started on lower dosages; maximum doses are the same as for this population as indicated for other adults. Most of the SSRIs are available in smaller dosages than the recommend starting dose, or come in liquid form allowing for individual titration. Medications that do not come in liquid forms can usually be compounded into smaller or individualized doses when necessary. Pharmacies that will compound medications can easily be found on the Internet through search engines.

After medications have been started, typical clinical practice is to titrate the SSRI to the highest tolerated dose, as patients with OCD generally require higher dosages of medications than those typically used in other disorders (Math and Reddy 2007). The SSRIs are usually titrated weekly or as tolerated. Table 3.2 has a list of the maximum dosages typically used in OCD treatment. Note that the highest recommended dosages may be higher than that approved by the FDA and by the manufacturer's insert; however, widespread clinical practice supports the use of higher dosing strategies. High doses used for periods greater than one year appear to be well tolerated in most cases and associated with symptomatic improvement (Pampaloni *et al.* 2009). Increased efficacy for higher dosages have been demonstrated for fluoxetine, paroxetine, sertraline, and citalopram (Fineberg and Gale 2005); although fixed-dose studies have not been performed for fluvoxamine or clomipramine (Denys 2006) experience indicates that the same higher dosing works with these medications as well.

Patients who do not respond to a lower dose of an SSRI will often respond to a higher dose of the same medication (Ninan *et al.* 2006). Since maximum benefit of the SSRI only occurs after 10–12 weeks on a medication (Fineberg and Gale 2005), most experts recommend that an adequate trial of an SSRI for OCD occurs only after the patient has tried the highest dose tolerated for a total of 12 weeks (March *et al.* 1997). Some patients may only just begin to show benefits at the end of a 12 week trial and in this scenario the medication should be continued for a minimum four additional weeks in order to realize the maximum effect. The question for clinicians when starting patients on medications, particularly medication naive patients, is whether to undertake a

Table 3.2 Dosage guidelines for serotonin reuptake inhibitors

Drug	Starting and incremental dose (mg/day)	Usual maximum dose (mg/day)	Occasionally prescribed maximum dose (mg/day)
Citalopram	20	80	120
Clomipramine	25	250	250[a]
Escitalopram	10	40	60
Fluoxetine	20	80	120
Fluvoxamine	50	300	450
Paroxetine	20	60	100
Sertraline	50	200	400

[a] Combined plasma levels of clomipramine plus desmethylclomipramine 12 hours after the dose should be kept below 500 ng/ml to minimize risk of seizures and cardiac conduction delay.
Source: Adapted from American Psychiatric Association (2007).

trial of the SSRI at a moderate dose initially or to titrate immediately to the highest dose tolerated. Such a decision largely rests on patient preference, severity of symptoms, and psychiatrist experience. Patients should be counseled that a full trial of a medication at a lower dose is still a minimum of 12 weeks. If they do not respond and require further titration to a higher dose, a medication trial for a single SSRI can take a significant portion of a year. In individuals with a prior history of good response at a lower dose, starting with a lower dose in subsequent trials may be suggested. Patients with a history of non-response to other SSRIs at a maximal dose should be considered a candidate for immediate titration to the highest dose of the current medication, as lower doses of different SSRIs are rarely successful in such patients. The use of the "rapid titration protocol," which is a cross-tapering protocol, can effect the change from the maximum dose of one SSRI to another in a timely manner.

Rapid titration protocol

Even when a patient fails an adequate trial of one SSRI, they still may respond to a different SSRI (Goodman *et al.* 1993; Ballenger 1999; Schruers *et al.* 2005). Switching medications is, therefore, an important strategy for the prescribing psychiatrist, even though this has not been investigated to any great degree. A small open-label study showed that some patients respond after a switch even when they have failed two prior trials (Hollander *et al.* 2002). A four year follow-up study showed that 30% of non-responders respond to a second trial, and only 15% of patients remained refractory after trials with five different SSRIs (Fontenelle *et al.* 2007). One of the difficulties psychiatrists encounter is the process of switching antidepressants once it has been decided that the patient either has not had an adequate response to the initial SSRI or has been unable to tolerate it. Most of the SSRIs require a slow tapering process when discontinuing in order to prevent SSRI discontinuation syndrome. Since an adequate trial of an SSRI for OCD usually involves a maximal dose, the tapering process can last weeks. After the tapering process is finished, a second SSRI will be initiated and titrated to a maximal dose. This titration process can also last weeks as well. Therefore, the process of switching SSRIs in OCD patients can last several weeks and sequential trials of medications can take many months (Ballenger 1999). This may lead to patient dissatisfaction as well as an increase in OCD symptoms during the

period of time that they are being maintained on minimal doses. For these reasons, an alternative method of switching SSRIs was developed to quickly and safely change SSRIs at elevated doses with a minimum of side effects. Clinical experience in a specialty OCD clinic has shown few side effects or problems with this protocol.

The use of this cross-tapering protocol enables the clinician to achieve the switch of SSRIs in only four days. It is noted that this method does not work with fluoxetine because of its extended half-life and is not recommended with clomipramine, but it does work with the other currently available SSRIs. Two medications classified as SNRIs (venlafaxine and duloxetine) are also included as this method works with them as well. Although they are unlikely to be used as first-line medications for OCD, this protocol can be used for medication switches in other illness such as depression.

The first step is for the psychiatrist to determine how many "units" of the SSRI the patient is currently taking (see Table 3.3). Note that one unit of the SSRI is in most cases simply the starting or minimal dose of the medication. A therapeutic trial for OCD with these SSRIs will typically involve four units of an SSRI, or four times the starting dose. After a failure of one SSRI, a trial of a second SSRI should also be performed at the maximal dose, which is again typically four units. The switch can be made by following the protocol in Table 3.4.

For example, if a patient has failed a therapeutic trial of sertraline at 400 mg (four units) and it has been decided to switch to citalopram, the protocol would occur as follows. On the first day, the patient would receive 300 mg sertraline and the remaining amount

Table 3.3 Conversion of the milligram equivalency of current medication into units

Drug	One unit (mg)
Sertraline	100
Paroxetine	20
Citalopram	20
Fluvoxamine	100
Escitalopram	10
Venlafaxine	100
Duloxetine	30

Table 3.4 Schedule for dosing of the switching medications for each day during rapid titration protocol

	Dose of 1st drug (units)	Dose of 2nd drug (units)
Day 1	3	1
Day 2	2	2
Day 3	1	3
Day 4 and beyond	0	4

would be replaced with a dose of 20 mg citalopram (one unit). On the second day, the patient would take 200 mg sertraline and 40 mg citalopram. For day number three, the patient takes 100 mg sertraline and 60 mg citalopram. On the fourth day and beyond, the patient will be taking 80 mg citalopram only.

Using this protocol to switch antidepressants enables a rapid switch of medications, saving time and helping to prevent relapse of the illness. Symptoms of SSRI discontinuation syndrome, as well as side effects from the rapid titration of the new SSRI, have been very unusual in clinical practice at the OCD specialty clinic over several years of the use of this technique.

Management of side effects

One of the primary concerns patients voice to their psychiatrists prior to starting medications concern potential side effects. Many of the adverse actions of these medications can be managed; however, the three complaints that are most likely to lead to patients requesting medication discontinuation are sexual side effects, weight gain, and apathy/amotivational difficulties. In addition to the common concerns of any individual facing antidepressant therapy, patients with OCD may have somatically focused obsessions that can increase their concern about medications. People who suffer from high levels of anxiety are often more attuned to somatic sensations and may be more worried about possible side effects. Because of the chronic nature of OCD, patients may be taking medications for extended periods of time; the psychiatrist, therefore, needs to be comfortable in discussing possible SSRI side effects with their patients and managing them when they occur. The higher doses of medications used for OCD also necessitate ongoing vigilance on the part of the psychiatrist. Interestingly,

it has been reported that side effects to SSRIs can be a positive predictor of drug response. Initial nervousness and sexual side effects are associated with an eventual positive response to medications. However, one should keep in mind that most patients do not report such side effects and their absence in no way precludes a positive response (Ackerman *et al.* 1999).

The following sections will outline commonly reported side effects of medication prescribed in the treatment of OCD and suggested management of these issues.

Gastrointestinal effects

Gastrointestinal side effects from SSRIs are common in adults and children, and are likely caused by serotonin receptors in the gastrointestinal tract. The symptoms most commonly seen are nausea, stomach pain, reflux symptoms, and diarrhea (Murphy *et al.* 2008). In most patients, the symptoms are transient and resolve in time. Usually, symptoms will resolve if the person is maintained at a constant dose of the medication for one to two weeks. These side effects can often be minimized by initiating the medications at lower dosages and recommending that patients take their medications with meals. One SSRI, sertraline, is actually better absorbed with meals so should always be taken with food regardless of gastrointestinal issues.

Agitation

Agitation or akathisia is a side effect that will occur early on in treatment, usually within the first two weeks of the initiation of treatment or an increase in dose. Contrary to what many clinicians believe, there is no evidence that this side effect is seen more often in patients with anxiety disorders, nor is there evidence that this is more common in SSRIs as opposed to TCAs (Sinclair *et al.* 2009). In adults, symptoms present in a similar manner to that seen in antipsychotic-induced akathisia, with motor restlessness and a physical sensation of anxiety. This can often be managed by lowering the dose temporarily until the agitation resolves, or switching to a different SSRI. In children and adolescents, agitation may manifest as behavioral activation, often described as a worsening of their clinical presentation: increases in impulsivity and talkativeness and/or hyperactivity (Murphy *et al.* 2008). Because of the possibility of an increase in suicidal behavior, in 2004 the FDA placed a black box warning on all antidepressants for children aged 18 and younger. In 2007 the FDA stated that this warning also applied to adults under the age of 25 years. No increase in the risk of suicide has been found in adults over the age of 25 (Gunnell *et al.* 2005). While it is not known if there is an increased risk of suicidal thoughts in patients with OCD not suffering from a comorbid mood disorder, careful monitoring for increases in suicidal thoughts or behaviors is important during the early phase of all antidepressant treatment or after an increase in dose (American Psychiatric Association 2007).

Excessive sweating

Excessive sweating or night sweats occur in 7–11% of people taking SSRIs (Garber and Gregory 1997). Many patients will report that the positive effects of the medication outweigh the negative effects of this excessive sweating. Therefore, conservative management is typically the only intervention required, such as suggesting that the patient has a change of night clothes readily available to them in the middle of the night for times when their clothes become soaked. Since tolerance does not typically develop to this side effect (Mavissakalian and Perel 2000), in the minority of instances where this side effect is severe enough to warrant more aggressive attention, a lowering of the dose or a switch to a different SSRI is indicated. Pharmacological treatment has been explored for antidepressant-induced sweating and case reports have looked at such medications as benztropine (Garber and Gregory 1997; Pierre and Guze 2000), cyproheptadine (Ashton and Weinstein 2002), and clonidine (Feder, 1995). However, at this point, the literature only involves random case reports and controlled studies are lacking. While treatment should focus on more conservative measures, benztropine would be an appropriate first choice if medication intervention is required (Marcy and Britton 2005).

Tachyphylaxis

After the acute phase of treatment for major depressive disorder is over and a patient has experienced a resolution of symptoms, it has been noted that some patients will experience reoccurrence of symptoms or a relapse. This phenomenon has been called "poop-out" or tachyphylaxis (Zimmerman and Thongy 2007). Studies have suggested that this is more likely to occur with a SSRI than in other classes of antidepressant (Postemak and Zimmerman 2005), although data are limited. If it is true that tachyphylaxis is more common with SSRI use, it is possible that this may occur in the

treatment of OCD as well, since SSRIs (in addition to clomipramine) are the medical treatment of choice. However, so far there has not been a study looking at the possibility of tachyphylaxis in OCD treatment; additionally, any such study would likely be complicated by the chronic nature of OCD. Because patients do report occasionally that their medications seem to "poop-out" over time, the clinician is advised to keep the possibility of tachyphylaxis in mind when evaluating patients who are experiencing an increase in OCD symptoms.

Movement disorders

It has been known that antidepressants are associated with extrapyramidal side effects, including myoclonus. Myoclonus (also known as positive myoclonus or myoclonic jerks) is defined as sudden, abrupt, brief, shock-like involuntary movements caused by muscular contractions and is a known side effect of both TCAs and SSRIs (Arya 1994; Vandel *et al.* 1997; Jiménez-Jiménez *et al.* 2004). While extrapyramidal effects are not common, they do occur and clinicians need to be aware of this possibility. Usually they can be managed by lowering the dose of the medication or by switching medications. Since this is likely not a class reaction, development of extrapyramidal side effects with one SSRI does not mean that a patient will develop similar problems with a different SSRI. Often, the movements will remit spontaneously (Vandel *et al.* 1997). Myoclonus usually occurs as a benign side effect, but it may also occur in the context of a serotonin syndrome.

Serotonin syndrome

Serotonin syndrome is a rare but serious medical condition caused by an excess of serotonin. It may occur from a wide variety of medications, and while classically it is associated with medication combinations, it can arise secondary to a single medication. It involves a constellation of symptoms including mental status changes, autonomic instability (such as tachycardia, hypertension, and hyperthermia), and neuromuscular abnormalities (such as myoclonus, hyperreflexia, hypertonicity, and rigidity) (Boyer and Shannon 2005). Treatment can involve supportive care or more intensive medical management depending on the severity of the syndrome.

Hyponatremia

Hyponatremia is manifested by muscle cramps, fatigue, confusion, and, in severe cases, seizures. Estimated rates vary, but 0.5% incidence per year can be expected. Higher rates are noted in populations with greater risks: advanced age, female gender, and concomitant use of diuretics (Moret *et al.* 2009; Reid and Barbui 2010). This will typically occur in the first few weeks of treatment or of a dosage change.

Discontinuation syndrome

The abrupt discontinuation of SSRI medication may result in a discontinuation syndrome, which can range from mild to severe in symptoms. Symptoms include dizziness, light-headedness, insomnia, fatigue, anxiety/agitation, nausea, headache, and sensory disturbance – often described as electrical sensations in the head or limbs (Zajecka *et al.* 1997). While uncomfortable and stressing, these symptoms are reversible and do not require aggressive medical management (Tamam and Ozpoyraz 2002). The symptoms are most likely to occur in medications with shorter half-lives, such as paroxetine, and are less likely with medications with long half-lives such as fluoxetine. The acute symptoms can be immediately managed by restarting the SSRI at the previous dose; the syndrome remits quickly with this intervention. A slow taper over a period of several weeks can mitigate the odds of reoccurrence. Some patients on high-risk medications have difficulty even with very slow tapers. In those instances, a successful strategy has been to switch to a lower-risk SSRI using the rapid titration protocol (see above). With this method, once the patient is stabilized on the new SSRI, the lower risk medication is subsequently tapered.

Gastrointestinal bleeding

Gastrointestinal bleeding has been reported as a side effect of SSRIs, likely because of an effect on platelet serotonin. The risk of bleeding appears to be increased with the concomitant use of non-steroidal anti-inflammatory drugs (Moret *et al.* 2009). Clinicians should be aware of this potential side effect particularly when a patient is on both classes of medication, and pharmacotherapy designed to reduce the risk of gastrointestinal bleeding should be considered in high-risk patients (Weinrieb *et al.* 2005).

Risk during pregnancy

Medication use in women is something the clinician treating OCD must always consider as OCD onset in women is usually in those of childbearing age. As a OCD is a chronic disorder, future planned and unexpected pregnancy could have a bearing on the choice of pharmacotherapy. A complete discussion of the risks of SSRI use in pregnancy is beyond the scope of this chapter, and it is recommended that the psychiatrist seek the latest information available when initiating informed consent with patients. The SSRIs do not seem to increase the risk of birth defects when exposure occurs during the first trimester, although after 20 weeks of gestation they may be associated with an increased risk of persistent pulmonary hypertension in the neonate (Reid and Barbui 2010). Some reports have noted that paroxetine is associated with an increase in congenital heart defects although the findings are inconclusive (Yonkers *et al.* 2009). Both SSRIs and TCAs prescribed in the third trimester may cause discontinuation effects – notably irritability – in the newborn, although this is usually mild and self-limiting (Reid and Barbui 2010).

Sexual side effects

There have been few studies examining the rate of sexual dysfunction as a result of SSRI use. Most of the studies involve patients with major depression, a complicating factor as depressed patients have perceived sexual dysfunction as a symptom of the illness. However, rates of 36–43% have been reported (Clayton *et al.* 2002) and psychiatrists must screen for these side effects because of their frequency. The most commonly reported sexual side effects are loss of libido, anorgasmia, and loss of physical arousal: erectile dysfunction in males and lack of lubrication in females (Murphy *et al.* 2008). Careful history taking is imperative; often complaints of erectile dysfunction in men are actually severe anorgasmia (Rosen *et al.* 1999). Treating those patients for erectile dysfunction will obviously have little effect. Unfortunately, there is a lack of controlled studies examining management options for sexual side effects. Typical recommendations include decreasing the dose of the medication to the lowest effective dose or waiting for symptoms to remit, which may occur within two months in approximately 10% of patients (American Psychiatric Association 2007). A drug holiday may work in many patients as long as the medication being prescribed is not fluoxetine (its long half-life precludes a successful drug holiday). The method used in an OCD specialty clinic involves having the patient skip their morning dose the day prior to planned sexual activity, as well as on the day itself. After the patient has engaged in intercourse, they may take that day's dose in the afternoon and then resume their normal schedule the following morning. This means that the patient will miss a total of only one dose of the medication. Patients should not use the drug holiday more than once a week. Clinical experience suggests that patients rarely experience discontinuation syndrome with this method (it is more likely with paroxetine or venlafaxine), and approximately one third report success.

A number of case reports but few controlled trials exist concerning medications to restore sexual function. Buproprion has been reported to improve sexual functioning at a dose of 300 mg/day (Clayton *et al.* 2004) but not at a dose of 150 mg/day (Debattista *et al.* 2005). Buspirone has been reported to work for SSRI-induced sexual side effects (Rosen *et al.* 1999) and clinical experience supports this as a safe therapy. Dosages used should be in the 20–60 mg range. Sildenafil has been shown to help to improve erectile dysfunction and anorgasmia (Nurnberg *et al.* 2003; Seidman *et al.* 2003). Other medications that have been tried include nefazadone, cyproheptadine, mirtazapine, yohimbine, ginko bilboa, and amphetamines (American Psychiatric Association 2007). These strategies can be explored in patients who are appropriate candidates and who give informed consent.

Apathy

Frontal lobe amotivational syndrome is characterized by apathy, affective blunting, and forgetfulness. It is most commonly seen with extended SSRI therapy and with the use of higher dosages (Murphy *et al.* 2008). Unlike other side effects, this does not improve with time. At times, the apathy or affective blunting can be so severe that the patient does not complain of any side effects: family members will instead report the difficulties to the clinician. Depression is included in the differential diagnosis: however, decreased mood and irritability are not present. Instead, the patient will report that they have a general lack of emotions and tend not to feel either happy or sad. Sedation is also a common complaint in these patients. Recommendations to treat this include lowering the dose or switching medications. An extensive literature search did not indicate research into drug treatment studies examining this problem, but experience in an OCD specialty clinic has found that modafinil can be a helpful medication in reversing this syndrome.

Weight gain

The SSRIs were initially thought to cause weight loss. However, it has been discovered that weight loss may occur only in the first six months of treatment; eventually weight gain is a more common phenomena with extended treatment (Ferguson 2001). Patients often report that weight gain happens even in the absence of a change in diet or exercise. All of the SSRIs can cause weight gain, although paroxetine is most likely to cause weight gain in both the short and long term (Pae and Patkar 2007).

Additional concerns

Other side effects that commonly occur with SSRI treatment include yawning, headache, dry mouth, dizziness, constipation, vivid dreams/nightmares, and tremors. These side effects can usually be addressed conservatively, by either waiting until the person develops tolerance, by lowering or switching medications, or with conservative management (e.g., acetaminophen for headaches or stool softeners for constipation). Of note, when patients develop yawning as an SSRI side effect, they often will report that they are suffering from sedation or fatigue, because of their misinterpretation of what excessive yawning indicates. A careful history is important in these instances to ensure that the proper issue is addressed.

Maintenance of treatment

As OCD is a chronic illness, many patients will require ongoing treatment. Once a patient obtains an adequate response to an SSRI, that medication should be continued for a minimum of one to two years. Behavioral therapy can be included in the maintenance plan, and patients show long-term improvements following ongoing behavioral therapy and medication management (Denys 2006). One study showed that behavioral therapy plus medications was equivalent to behavioral therapy plus placebo in a seven year follow-up (Rufer *et al.* 2005). Symptom relapse is lower at follow-up in patients who take SSRIs than in those taking placebo (Fineberg *et al.* 2007b). The dose of medications prescribed during maintenance should be the same dose used during the active phase of treatment (Romano *et al.* 2001), although many clinicians will need to lower doses in order to manage side effects such as sedation or sexual dysfunction. Regardless of whether patients continue behavioral therapy, many clinicians and patients will elect to continue medications on an ongoing basis past the minimum recommended one to two years because of clinical observations that reinstatement of medication upon relapse does not result in improvements to the same level as achieved prior to discontinuation (Figee and Denys 2009). In instances when patients opt for stopping their medications, it is recommended that the SSRI be tapered very slowly, over a period of four months or more, to minimize the risk of exacerbation.

Novel medications

Glutamatergic medications

The SSRIs, along with augmenting agents such as dopamine antagonists, have remained the cornerstone for medication treatment of OCD (Ch. 4 discusses augmenting agents). However, because of the chronic nature of OCD, as well as the high rate of treatment-resistant patients, novel medication strategies continue to be explored. One area that has received a significant amount of attention has been medications that inhibit glutamatergic neurotransmission. There is evidence of an excess of glutamatergic activity in OCD in the cortico-striato-thalamo-cortical circuitry (Pittenger et al. 2006). This has been noted in neuroimaging studies (Baxter 2001); cerebral spinal fluid analysis, which has showed higher glutamate activity in 18 OCD patients compared with 21 healthy controls (Chakrabarty et al. 2005); and genetic studies (Arnold et al. 2006; Dickel et al. 2006), which indicate an association between an altered gene for a glutamate transporter found in early-onset OCD in males but not females, although data here are mixed. There have been suggestions that the effect of SSRIs may be explained via a glutamatergic mechanism (Joel et al. 2005). As a result, trials have occurred involving medications that alter glutamate levels. While none of these medications is recommended for routine use at the time of publication, this remains an area of intense research and clinical interest.

The glutamate antagonist that has received the most attention has been riluzole, which is a benzothiazole used in the treatment of amyotrophic lateral sclerosis. Riluzole has been shown to be a well-tolerated medication with a good safety record in the treatment of this condition (Grant et al. 2007). The most common adverse event associated with riluzole is transient elevations in liver enzymes, seen in approximately 50% of patients taking the medication. In this population,

2% of these subjects will experience an increase in liver function tests greater than five times that of baseline tests. As a result, it is recommended that patients taking riluzole have liver function tests monitored monthly for the initial three months of use, every third month for the rest of the year, and periodically thereafter (Physicians Desk Reference 2006). In an open-label trial, six children with treatment-resistant OCD were given riluzole in addition to previously prescribed medication. Four of the participants had significant decline in OCD symptoms by the end of the 12 week trial and one of the remaining two subjects responded after an additional four week trial (Grant et al. 2007). The average dose of riluzole in the study was 101 mg. Thirteen adults received 100 mg riluzole a day in an additional open-label study. Seven patients had improvement in symptoms and five were classified as treatment responders (Coric et al. 2005). A case report has shown benefit in a patient with an eating disorder and pathological skin picking (Sasso et al. 2006). More trials are under way to examine this potentially useful medication further.

Memantine is a non-competitive N-methyl-D-aspartate (NMDA) receptor antagonist that is approved for the treatment of moderate to severe Alzheimer's disease. Memantine is thought to confer neuroprotection by limiting the negative effects of glutamatergic neurotoxicity (Aboujaoude et al. 2009). Six of fourteen patients with OCD responded to memantine addition to the prior medications in an open-label trial, although other reports have not observed this medication to help clinically (Pittenger et al. 2006).

N-Acetylcysteine is an amino acid commonly used for hepatoprotection in cases of acute acetaminophen overdose, and is thought to attenuate glutamatergic neurotransmission. A case report showed efficacy of this agent in a woman with treatment-refractory OCD (Lafleur et al. 2006) and efficacy was noted for trichotillomania in a double-blind placebo-controlled study (Grant et al. 2009).

D-Cycloserine is a glutamatergic partial NDMA receptor antagonist that is being studied as an adjunct to ERP. Kushner et al. (2007) have shown that administration of D-cycloserine two hours prior to ERP resulted in a more rapid decrease in distress associated with obsessions than occurring in a placebo group. Additional compounds are being explored to determine if they have glutamatergic and neuroprotective properties, such as beta-lactam antibiotics (Pittenger et al. 2006).

Clearly, evidence exists to support the benefits of glutamatergic medications in the treatment of OCD, and further study should clarify how these medications may eventually be adopted into the routine clinical treatment of OCD.

Other novel medications

Other novel pharmaceutical strategies have been explored for OCD. Monoamine oxidase inhibitors have been explored for OCD treatment. While they have not preformed well in trials compared with fluoxetine (Jenike *et al.* 1997), a small, non-placebo-controlled trial showed response to phenelzine compared with clomipramine (Vallejo *et al.* 1992). Some of this discrepancy may be explained by the suggestion that patients with symmetry obsessions may respond to monoamine oxidase inhibitors while patients with other types of obsession do not respond (Jenike *et al.* 1997). Treatment-resistant patients with symmetry obsessions who can tolerate the side effects of monoamine oxidase inhibitors, as well as the specialized diet required while taking them, may be candidates for a phenelzine trial.

Trials have also been conducted using drugs such as caffeine (Koran *et al.* 2009) and morphine (Koran *et al.* 2005). While these novel treatments cannot be recommended as routine options at this time, clearly the field of OCD pharmacology is an exciting and expanding one.

References

Aboujaoude E, Barry JJ, Gamel N (2009). Memantine augmentation in treatment-resistant obsessive-compulsive disorder: an open-label trial. *J Clin Psychopharmacol* **29**: 51–55.

Abramowitz JS (1997). Effectiveness of psychological and pharmacological treatments for obsessive-compulsive disorder: a quantitative review. *J Consult Clin Psychol* **65**: 44–52.

Ackerman DL, Greenland S (2002). Multivariate meta-analysis of controlled drug studies for obsessive-compulsive disorder. *J Clin Psychopharmacol* **22**: 309–317.

Ackerman DL, Greenland S, Bystritsky A (1999). Side effects as predictors of drug response in obsessive-compulsive disorder. *J Clin Psychopharmacol* **19**: 459–465.

Albert U, Aguglia E, Maina G, Bogetto F (2002). Venlafaxine versus clomipramine in the treatment of obsessive-compulsive disorder: a preliminary single-blind, 12-week, controlled study. *J Clin Psychiatry* **63**: 1004–1009.

American Psychiatric Association (1987). *Diagnostic and Statistical Manual of Mental Disorders*, 3rd edn. Washington, DC: American Psychiatric Press.

American Psychiatric Association (2007). *Practice Guidelines for the treatment of Patients with Obsessive Compulsive Disorder*. Washington, DC: American Psychiatric Press.

Arnold PD, Sicard T, Burroughs E, Richter MA, Kennedy JL (2006). Glutamate transporter gene *SLC1A1* associated with obsessive-compulsive disorder. *Arch Gen Psychiatry* **63**: 769–776.

Arya DK (1994). Extrapyramidal symptoms with selective serotonin reuptake inhibitors. *Br Med J* **165**: 728–733.

Ashton AK, Weinstein WL (2002). Cyproheptadine for drug-induced sweating. *Am J Psychiatry* **159**: 874–875.

Ballenger JC (1999). Current treatments of the anxiety disorders in adults. *Biol Psychiatry* **46**: 1579–1594.

Baxter LR (2001): Functional imaging of brain systems mediating obsessive-compulsive disorder. In Charney DS, Nestler EJ, Bunney BS (eds.) *Neurobiology of Mental Illness* (pp. 534–547). Oxford: Oxford University Press.

Bergeron R, Ravindran AV, Chaput Y, *et al.* (2002). Sertraline and fluoxetine treatment of obsessive-compulsive disorder: results of a double-blind, 6-month treatment study. *J Clin Psychopharmacol* **22**: 148–154.

Bogetto F, Albert U, Maina G (2002). Sertraline treatment of obsessive-compulsive disorder: efficacy and tolerability of a rapid titration regimen. *Eur Neuropsychopharmacol* **12**: 181–186.

Boyer EW, Shannon M (2005). The serotonin syndrome. *N Engl J Med* **352**: 1112–1120.

Chakrabarty K, Bhattacharyya S, Khanna S, Christopher R (2005). Glutamatergic dysfunction in OCD. *Neuropsychopharmacology* **30**: 1735–1740.

Clayton AH, Pradko JF, Croft HA, *et al.* (2002). Prevalence of sexual dysfunction among newer antidepressants. *J Clin Psychiatry* **63**: 357–366.

Clayton AH, Warnock JK, Kornstein SG, *et al.* (2004). A placebo-controlled trial of bupropion SR as an antidote for selective serotonin reuptake inhibitor-induced sexual dysfunction. *J Clin Psychiatry* **65**: 62–67.

Clomipramine Collaborative Study Group. (1991). Clomipramine in the treatment of patients with obsessive-compulsive disorder. *Arch Gen Psychiatry* **48**: 730–738.

Coric V, Taskiran S, Pittenger C, *et al.* (2005). Riluzole augmentation in treatment-resistant obsessive-compulsive disorder: an open-label trial. *Biol Psychiatry* 58: 424–428.

Cottraux J, Bouvard MA, Milliery M (2005). Combining pharmacotherapy with cognitive-behavioral interventions for obsessive-compulsive disorder. *Cogn Behav Ther* 34: 185–192.

Cox BJ, Swinson RP, Morrison B, Lee PS (1993). Clomipramine, fluoxetine, and behavior therapy in the treatment of obsessive-compulsive disorder: a meta-analysis. *J Behav Ther Exp Psychiatry* 24: 149–153.

Debattista C, Solvason B, Poirier J, Kendrick E, Loraas E (2005). A placebo-controlled, randomized, double-blind study of adjunctive bupropion sustained release in the treatment of SSRI-induced sexual dysfunction. *J Clin Psychiatry* 66: 844–848.

Denys D (2006). Pharmacotherapy of obsessive-compulsive disorder and obsessive-compulsive spectrum disorders. *Psychiatr Clin N Am* 29: 553–584, xi.

Denys D, van der Wee N, van Megen HJ, Westenberg HG (2003). A double-blind comparison of venlafaxine and paroxetine in obsessive-compulsive disorder. *J Clin Psychopharmacol* 23: 568–575.

Denys D, van Megen HJ, van der Wee N, Westenberg HG (2004). A double-blind switch study of paroxetine and venlafaxine in obsessive-compulsive disorder. *J Clin Psychiatry* 65: 37–43.

Dhillon S, Scott LJ, Plosker GL (2006). Escitalopram: a review of its use in the management of anxiety disorders. *CNS Drugs* 20: 763–790.

Dickel DE, Veenstra-VanderWeele J, Cox NJ, et al. (2006). Association testing of the positional and functional candidate gene *SLC1A1/EAAC1* in early-onset obsessive-compulsive disorder. *Arch Gen Psychiatry* 63: 778–785.

Eddy KT, Dutra L, Bradley R, Westen D (2004). A multidimensional meta-analysis of psychotherapy and pharmacotherapy for obsessive-compulsive disorder. *Clin Psychol Rev* 24: 1011–1030.

Erzegovesi S, Cavallini MC, Cavedini P, et al. (2001). Clinical predictors of drug response in obsessive-compulsive disorder. *J Clin Psychopharmacol* 21: 488–492.

Evaluation of Genomic Applications in Practice and Prevention Working Group (2007). Recommendations from the EGAPP Working Group: testing for cytochrome P450 polymorphisms in adults with nonpsychotic depression treated with selective serotonin reuptake inhibitors. *Genet Med* 9: 819–825.

Fallon BA, Liebowitz MR, Campeas R, et al. (1998). Intravenous clomipramine for obsessive-compulsive disorder refractory to oral clomipramine: a placebo-controlled study. *Arch Gen Psychiatry* 55: 918–924.

Feder R (1995). Clonidine treatment of excessive sweating. *J Clin Psychiatry* 56: 35.

Ferguson JM (2001). SSRI antidepressant medications: adverse effects and tolerability. *J Clin Psychiatry* 3: 22–27.

Figee M, Denys D (2009). New pharmacotherapeutic approaches to obsessive-compulsive disorder. *CNS Spectr* 14(Suppl 3): 13–23.

Figueroa Y, Rosenberg DR, Birmaher B, Keshavan MS (1998). Combination treatment with clomipramine and selective serotonin reuptake inhibitors for obsessive-compulsive disorder in children and adolescents. *J Child Adolesc Psychopharmacol* 8: 61–67.

Fineberg NA, Gale TM (2005). Evidence-based pharmacotherapy of obsessive-compulsive disorder. *Int J Neuropsychopharmacol* 8: 107–129.

Fineberg NA, Tonnoir B, Lemming O, Stein DJ (2007a). Escitalopram prevents relapse of obsessive-compulsive disorder. *Eur Neuropsychopharmacol* 17: 430–439.

Fineberg NA, Pampaloni I, Pallanti S, Ipser J, Stein DJ (2007b). Sustained response versus relapse: the pharmacotherapeutic goal for obsessive-compulsive disorder. *Int Clin Psychopharmacol* 22: 313–322.

Foa EB, Kozak MJ, Steketee GS, McCarthy PR (1992). Treatment of depressive and obsessive-compulsive symptoms in OCD by imipramine and behavior therapy. *Br J Clin Psychol* 31: 279–292.

Fontenelle LF, Nascimento AL, Mendlowicz MV, Shavitt RG, Versiani M (2007). An update on the pharmacological treatment of obsessive-compulsive disorder. *Expert Opin Pharmacother* 8: 563–583.

Freeman CP, Trimble MR, Deakin JF, Stokes TM, Ashford JJ (1994). Fluvoxamine versus clomipramine in the treatment of obsessive compulsive disorder: a multicenter, randomized, double-blind, parallel group comparison. *J Clin Psychiatry* 55: 301–305.

Garber A, Gregory RJ (1997). Benztropine in the treatment of venlafaxine induced sweating. *J Clin Psychiatry* 58: 176–177.

Goodman WK, Price LH, Rasmussen SA, et al. (1989). Efficacy of fluvoxamine in obsessive-compulsive disorder: a double-blind comparison with placebo. *Arch Gen Psychiatry* 46: 36–44.

Goodman WK, McDougle CJ, Barr LC, Aronson SC, Price LH (1993). Biological approaches to treatment-resistant obsessive compulsive disorder. *J Clin Psychiatry* 54(Suppl): 16–26.

Goodman WK, Kozak MJ, Liebowitz M, White KL (1996). Treatment of obsessive-compulsive disorder with fluvoxamine: a multicentre, double-blind, placebo-controlled trial. *Int Clin Psychopharmacol* 11: 21–29.

Gram LF, Hansen MG, Sindrup SH, *et al.* (1993). Citalopram: interaction studies with levomepromazine, imipramine, and lithium. *Ther Drug Monit* **15**: 18–24.

Grant JE, Odlaug BL, Kim SW (2009). *N*-Acetylcysteine, a glutamate modulator, in the treatment of trichotillomania: a double-blind, placebo-controlled study. *Arch Gen Psychiatry* **66**: 756–763.

Grant P, Lougee L, Hirschtritt M, Swedo S (2007). An open-label trial of riluzole, a glutamate antagonist, in children with treatment-resistant obsessive-compulsive disorder. *Child Adolesc Psychopharmacol* **17**: 761–767.

Greist JH, Jefferson JW, Kobak KA, Katzelnick DJ, Serlin RC (1995a). Efficacy and tolerability of serotonin transport inhibitors in obsessive-compulsive disorder. A meta-analysis. *Arch Gen Psychiatry.* **52**: 53–60.

Greist JH, Jenike MA, Robinson D, Rasmussen SA (1995b). Efficacy of fluvoxamine in obsessive-compulsive disorder: results of a multicentre, double blind, placebo controlled trial. *Eur J Clin Res* **7**: 195–204.

Greist J, Chouinard G, DuBoff E, *et al.* (1995c). Double-blind parallel comparison of three doses of sertraline and placebo in outpatients with obsessive-compulsive disorder. *Arch Gen Psychiatry* **52**: 289–295.

Gunnell D, Saperia J, Ashby D (2005). Selective serotonin reuptake inhibitors (SSRIs) and suicide in adults: meta-analysis of drug company data from placebo controlled, randomised controlled trials submitted to the MHRA's safety review. *BMJ* **330**: 385.

Harvey AT, Preskorn SH (1996). Cytochrome P450 enzymes: interpretation of their interactions with selective serotonin reuptake inhibitors. Part II. *J Clin Psychopharmacol* **16**: 345–355.

Hollander E, Bienstock CA, Koran LM, *et al.* (2002). Refractory obsessive-compulsive disorder: state-of-the-art treatment. *J Clin Psychiatry* **63**(Suppl 6): 20–29.

Hollander E, Koran LM, Goodman WK, *et al.* (2003a). A double-blind, placebo-controlled study of the efficacy and safety of controlled-release fluvoxamine in patients with obsessive-compulsive disorder. *J Clin Psychiatry* **64**: 640–647.

Hollander E, Allen A, Steiner M, *et al.* (2003b). Acute and long-term treatment and prevention of relapse of obsessive-compulsive disorder with paroxetine. *J Clin Psychiatry* **64**: 1113–1121.

Hollander E, Friedberg J, Wasserman S, *et al.* (2003c). Venlafaxine in treatment-resistant obsessive-compulsive disorder. *J Clin Psychiatry* **64**: 546–550.

Jenike MA, Baer L, Greist JH (1995a). Clomipramine versus fluoxetine in obsessive-compulsive disorder: a retrospective comparison of side effects and efficacy. *J Clin Psychopharmacol* **10**: 122–124.

Jenike MA, Hyman S, Baer L, *et al.* (1995b). A controlled trial of fluvoxamine in obsessive-compulsive disorder: implications for a serotonergic theory. *Am J Psychiatry* **147**: 1209–1215.

Jenike MA, Baer L, Minichiello WE, Rauch SL, Buttolph ML (1997). Placebo-controlled trial of fluoxetine and phenelzine for obsessive-compulsive disorder. *Am J Psychiatry* **154**: 1261–1264.

Jiménez-Jiménez FJ, Puertas I, de Toledo-Heras M (2004). Drug-induced myoclonus: frequency, mechanisms and management. *CNS Drugs* **18**: 93–104.

Joel D, Doljansky J, Roz N, Rehavi M (2005). Role of the orbital cortex and of the serotonergic system in a rat model of obsessive compulsive disorder. *Neuroscience* **130**: 25–36.

Kamijima K, Murasaki M, Asai M, *et al.* (2004). Paroxetine in the treatment of obsessive-compulsive disorder: randomized, double-blind, placebo-controlled study in Japanese patients. *Psychiatry Clin Neurosci* **58**: 427–433.

Katz RJ, DeVeaugh-Geiss J, Landau P (1990). Clomipramine in obsessive-compulsive disorder. *Biol Psychiatry* **28**: 401–414.

Koponen H, Lepola U, Leinonen E, *et al.* (1997). Citalopram in the treatment of obsessive-compulsive disorder: an open pilot study. *Acta Psychiatr Scand* **96**: 343–346.

Koran LM, McElroy SL, Davidson JR, *et al.* (1996). Fluvoxamine versus clomipramine for obsessive-compulsive disorder: a double-blind comparison. *J Clin Psychopharmacol* **16**: 121–129.

Koran LM, Sallee FR, Pallanti S (1997). Rapid benefit of intravenous pulse loading of clomipramine in obsessive-compulsive disorder. *Am J Psychiatry* **154**: 396–401.

Koran LM, Hackett E, Rubin A, *et al.* (2002). Efficacy of sertraline in the long-term treatment of obsessive-compulsive disorder. *Am J Psychiatry* **159**: 88–95.

Koran LM, Aboujaoude E, Bullock KD, *et al.* (2005). Double-blind treatment with oral morphine in treatment-resistant obsessive-compulsive disorder. *J Clin Psychiatry* **66**: 353–359.

Koran LM, Aboujaoude E, Gamel NN (2009). Double-blind study of dextroamphetamine versus caffeine augmentation for treatment-resistant obsessive-compulsive disorder. *J Clin Psychiatry* **70**: 1530–1535.

Kronig MH, Apter J, Asnis G, *et al.* (1999). Placebo-controlled, multicenter study of sertraline treatment for obsessive-compulsive disorder. *J Clin Psychopharmacol* **19**: 172–176.

Kushner MG, Won KS, Donahue C, *et al.* (2007). D-Cycloserine augmented exposure therapy for obsessive compulsive disorder. *Biol Psychiatry* **62**: 835–838.

Lafleur DL, Pittenger C, Kelmendi B, *et al.* (2006). *N*-Acetylcysteine augmentation in serotonin reuptake inhibitor refractory obsessive-compulsive disorder. *Psychopharmacology (Berl)* **184**: 254–256.

Lopez-Ibor JJ Jr., Saiz J, Cottraux J, *et al.* (1996). Double-blind comparison of fluoxetine versus clomipramine in the treatment of obsessive compulsive disorder. *Eur Neuropsychopharmacol* **6**: 111–118.

Maina G, Albert U, Salvi V, Bogetto F (2004). Weight gain during long-term treatment of obsessive-compulsive disorder: a prospective comparison between serotonin reuptake inhibitors. *J Clin Psychiatry* **65**: 1365–1371.

Marazziti D, Dell'Osso L, Gemignani A, *et al.* (2001). Citalopram in refractory obsessive-compulsive disorder: an open study. *Int Clin Psychopharmacol* **16**: 215–219.

March JS, Frances A, Carpenter D, Kahn DA (1997). The Expert Consensus Guideline Series: treatment of obsessive-compulsive disorder. *J Clin Psychiatry* **58**(Suppl 4): 3–72.

Marcy TR, Britton ML (2005). Antidepressant-induced sweating. *Ann Pharmacother* **39**: 748–752.

Marks IM, Stern RS, Mawson D, Cobb J, McDonald R (1980). Clomipramine and exposure for obsessive compulsive rituals. *Br J Psychiatry* **136**: 1–25.

Math SB, Reddy CJ (2007). Issues in the pharmacological treatment of obsessive-compulsive disorder. *J Clin Pract* **61**: 1188–1197.

Mavissakalian MR, Perel JM (2000). The side effects burden of extended imipramine treatment of panic disorder. *J Clin Psychopharmacol* **20**: 547–555.

Montgomery SA (1980). Clomipramine in obsessional neurosis: a placebo controlled trial. *Pharmaceut Med* **1**: 189–192.

Montgomery SA (1998). Psychopharmacology of obsessive-compulsive disorder. *CNS Spectr* **3**(Suppl 1): 33–37.

Montgomery SA, McIntyre A, Osterheider M, for the Lilly European OCD Study Group (1993). A double-blind, placebo-controlled study of fluoxetine in patients with DSM-III-R obsessive-compulsive disorder. *Eur Neuropsychopharmacol* **3**: 143–152.

Montgomery SA, Kasper S, Stein DJ, Bang HK, Lemming OM (2001). Citalopram 20 mg, 40 mg and 60 mg are all effective and well tolerated compared with placebo in obsessive-compulsive disorder. *Int Clin Psychopharmacol* **16**: 75–86.

Moret C, Isaac M, Briley M (2009). Problems associated with long term treatment of selective serotonin reuptake inhibitors. *J Psychopharmacol* **23**: 967–974.

Mundo E, Bianchi L, Bellodi L (1997). Efficacy of fluvoxamine, paroxetine, and citalopram in the treatment of obsessive-compulsive disorder: a single-blind study. *J Clin Psychopharmacol* **17**: 267–271.

Mundo E, Maina G, Uslenghi C (2000). Multicentre, double-blind, comparison of fluvoxamine and clomipramine in the treatment of obsessive-compulsive disorder. *Int Clin Psychopharmacol* **15**: 69–76.

Mundo E, Rouillon F, Figuera ML, Stigler M (2001). Fluvoxamine in obsessive-compulsive disorder: similar efficacy but superior tolerability in comparison with clomipramine. *Hum Psychopharmacol* **16**: 461–446.

Murphy TK, Segarra A, Storch EA, Goodman WK (2008). SSRI adverse events: how to monitor and manage. *Int Rev Psychiatry* **20**: 203–208.

Ninan PT, Koran LM, Kiev A, *et al.* (2006). High-dose sertraline strategy for nonresponders to acute treatment for obsessive-compulsive disorder: a multicenter double-blind trial. *J Clin Psychiatry* **67**: 15–22.

Nurnberg HG, Hensley PL, Gelenberg AJ, *et al.* (2003). Treatment of antidepressant-associated sexual dysfunction with sildenafil: a randomized controlled trial. *JAMA* **289**: 56–64.

Pae CU, Patkar AA (2007). Paroxetine: current status in psychiatry. *Expert Rev Neurother* **7**: 107–120.

Pallanti S, Quercioli L, Paiva RS, Koran LM (1999). Citalopram for treatment-resistant obsessive-compulsive disorder. *Eur Psychiatry* **14**: 101–106.

Pallanti S, Quercioli L, Koran LM (2002). Citalopram intravenous infusion in resistant obsessive-compulsive disorder: an open trial. *J Clin Psychiatry* **63**: 796–801.

Pallanti S, Quercioli L, Bruscoli M (2004). Response acceleration with mirtazapine augmentation of citalopram in obsessive-compulsive disorder patients without comorbid depression: a pilot study. *J Clin Psychiatry* **65**: 1394–1399.

Pampaloni I, Sivakumaran T, Hawley C, *et al.* (2009). High-dose selective serotonin reuptake inhibitors in OCD: a systematic retrospective case notes survey. *J Psychopharmacol* 2009 (epub ahead of print; doi:10.1177/0269881109104850).

Physicians Desk Reference (2006). Montvale NJ: PDR Network, Thomson http://www.pdr.net/login/Login.aspx (accessed 26 July 2010).

Piccinelli M, Pini S, Bellantouono C, *et al.* (1995). Efficacy of drug treatment in obsessive-compulsive disorder: a meta-analytic review. *Br J Psychiatry* **166**: 424–443.

Pierre JM, Guze BH (2000). Benztropine for venlafaxine-induced night sweats. *J Clin Psychopharmacol* **20**: 269.

Pigott TA, Pato MT, Bernstein SE, *et al.* (1990). Controlled comparisons of clomipramine and fluoxetine in the treatment of obsessive-compulsive disorder: behavioral and biological results. *Arch Gen Psychiatry* 47: 926–932.

Pittenger C, Krystal JH, Coric V (2006). Glutamate-modulating drugs as novel pharmacotherapeutic agents in the treatment of obsessive-compulsive disorder. *Neurotherapeutivs* 3: 69–81.

Postemak M, Zimmerman M (2005). Dual reuptake inhibitors incur lower rates of tachyphylaxis than selective serotonin reuptake inhibitors. *J Clin Psychiatry* 66: 705–707.

Rack M, Chir D (1970). Experience with intravenous clomipramine. In Salzman L (ed.) *Obsessional States and their Treatment with Anafranil* (pp. 10–13). Macclesfield, UK: Geigy.

Rasmussen BB, Maenpaa J, Pelkonen O, *et al.* (1995). Selective serotonin reuptake inhibitors and theophylline metabolism in human liver microsomes: potent inhibition by fluvoxamine. *Br J Clin Pharmacol* 39: 151–159.

Rasmussen S, Hackett E, DuBoff E, *et al.* (1997). A 2-year study of sertraline in the treatment of obsessive-compulsive disorder. *Int Clin Psychopharmacol* 12: 309–316.

Reid S, Barbui C (2010). Long term treatment of depression with selective serotonin reuptake inhibitors and newer antidepressants. *BMJ* 340: c1468.

Romano S, Goodman W, Tamura R, Gonzales J (2001). Long-term treatment of obsessive-compulsive disorder after an acute response: a comparison of fluoxetine versus placebo. *J Clin Psychopharmacol* 21: 46–52.

Rosen RC, Lane RM, Menza M (1999). Effects of SSRIs on sexual function: a critical review. *J Clin Psychopharmacol* 19: 67–85.

Rufer M, Hand I, Alsleben H, *et al.* (2005). Long-term course and outcome of obsessive-compulsive patients after cognitive-behavioral therapy in combination with either fluvoxamine or placebo: a 7-year follow-up of a randomized double-blind trial. *Eur Arch Psychiatry Clin Neurosci* 255: 121–128.

Sasso DA, Kalanithi PS, Trueblood KV, *et al.* (2006). Beneficial effects of the glutamate-modulating agent riluzole on disordered eating and pathological skin-picking behaviors. *J Clin Psychopharmacol* 26: 685–687.

Schruers K, Koning K, Luermans J, Haack MJ, Griez E (2005). Obsessive-compulsive disorder: a critical review of therapeutic perspectives. *Acta Psychiatr Scand* 111: 261–271.

Seidman SN, Pesce VC, Roose SP (2003). High-dose sildenafil citrate for selective serotonin reuptake inhibitor-associated ejaculatory delay: open clinical trial. *J Clin Psychiatry* 64: 721–725.

Sinclair LI, Christmas DM, Hood SD, *et al.* (2009). Antidepressant-induced jitteriness/anxiety syndrome: systematic review. *Br J Psychiatry* 194: 483–490.

Skjelbo E, Brosen K (1992). Inhibitors of imipramine metabolism by human liver microsomes. *Br J Clin Pharmacol* 34: 256–261.

Smeraldi E, Erzegovesi S, Bianchi I, *et al.* (1992). Fluvoxamine vs clomopramine treatment in obsessive-compulsive disorder: a preliminary study. *New Trends Exp Clin Psychiatry* 8: 63–65.

Soomro GM (2003). Obsessive compulsive disorder. *Clin Evidence* 10: 1172–1187.

Soomro GM, Altman DG, Rajagopal S, Oakley Browne M (2008). Selective serotonin re-uptake inhibitors (SSRIs) versus placebo for obsessive compulsive disorder (OCD). *Cochrane Database of Systematic Reviews* (1): CD001765.

Stein DJ, Spadaccni E, Hollander E (1995). Meta-analysisof pharmacotherapy trials for obsessive-compulsive disorder. *Int Clin Psychopharmacol* 10: 11–18.

Szegedi A, Wetzel H, Leal M, Härtter S, Hiemke C (1996). Combination treatment with clomipramine and fluvoxamine: drug monitoring, safety, and tolerability data. *J Clin Psychiatry* 57: 257–264.

Tamam L, Ozpoyraz N (2002). Selective serotonin reuptake inhibitor discontinuation syndrome: a review. *Adv Ther* 19: 17–26.

The Medical Letter (2003). 45(Issue W1158B), June 9 http://www.medicalletter.org/restricted/articles/w1158b.pdf (access available to subscribers only).

Thoren P, Asberg M, Cronholm B, Jornestedt L, Traskman L (1980). Clomipramine treatment in obsessive-compulsive disorder, a controlled trial. *Arch Gen Psychiatry* 37: 1281–1285.

Tollefson GD, Rampey AH Jr., Potvin JH, *et al.* (1994). A multicenter investigation of fixed-dose fluoxetine in the treatment of obsessive-compulsive disorder. *Arch Gen Psychiatry* 51: 559–567.

Vallejo J, Olivares J, Marcos T, Bulbena A, Menchon JM (1992). Clomipramine versus phenelzine in obsessive-compulsive disorder: a controlled clinical trial. *Br J Psychiatry* 161: 665–670.

Vandel P, Bonin B, Leveque E, Sechter D and Bizouard P (1997). Tricyclic antidepressant-induced extrapyramidal side effects. *Eur Neuropsychopharmacol* 7: 207–212.

Weinrieb RM, Auriacombe M, Lynch KG, Lewis JD (2005). Selective serotonin re-uptake inhibitors and the risk of bleeding. *Expert Opin Drug Saf* 4: 337–344.

Yaryura-Tobias JA, Neziroglu FA (1996). Venlafaxine in obsessive-compulsive disorder. *Arch Gen Psychiatry* 53: 653–654.

Yonkers KA, Wisner KL, Stewart DE, *et al.* (2009). The management of depression during pregnancy: a report from the American Psychiatric Association and the American College of Obstetricians and Gynecologists. *Obstet Gynecol* **114**: 703–713.

Zajecka J, Tracy KA, Mitchell S (1997). Discontinuation symptoms after treatment with serotonin reuptake inhibitors: a literature review. *J Clin Psychiatry* **58**: 291–297.

Zimmerman M, Thongy T (2007). How often do SSRIs and other new-generation antidepressants lose their effect during continuation treatment? Evidence suggesting the rate of true tachyphylaxis during continuation treatment is low. *J Clin Psychiatry* **68**: 1271–1276.

Zohar J, Judge R (1996). OCD Paroxetine Study Investigators: Paroxetine versus clomipramine in the treatment of obsessive-compulsive disorder. *Br J Psychiatry* **169**: 468–474.

Chapter

4

Augmentation of serotonin reuptake inhibitors in the treatment of obsessive-compulsive disorder

Andrew Goddard and Yong-Wook Shin

Introduction

Obsessive-compulsive disorder (OCD) is the fourth commonest mental disorder after depression, alcohol and substance misuse, and social phobia, with a mean lifetime prevalence of up to 3% in the general population (Karno *et al.* 1988). The OCD symptoms are time consuming and cause severe functional impairment, debilitating both to the patients and their family (Calvocoressi *et al.* 1995). The natural course of untreated OCD patients only leads to one fifth of the full remission rate (Skoog and Skoog 1999) and most untreated patients show a high rate of unemployment, less productivity, lower marriage rate, and many negative effects on their family members (Rasmussen and Eisen 1992; Leon *et al.* 1995; Koran *et al.* 1996). The current treatments of choice for OCD are behavioral therapy and serotonin reuptake inhibitors (SRI). Clomipramine, a potent SRI and the later selective SRIs (SSRIs) will all be referred to here as SRIs in a broader sense. While SRIs such as fluoxetine, paroxetine, sertraline have been used for the treatment of OCD (Kelly and Myers 1990), approximately half of adult and pediatric OCD patients still do not respond to SRI therapy (Insel and Murphy 1981; Goodman and Price 1992; March *et al.* 1998; Liebowitz *et al.* 2002; March 2004). This has prompted searches for more effective pharmacological strategies for patients who fail to respond, or to respond adequately, to SRI treatment.

This chapter will look at several options for augmentation therapy for those patients with "treatment-resistant" OCD. Since there is no consensus or standardized criteria for treatment response in OCD, early studies referred to in the chapter have defined "treatment-resistance" using mixed terms such as refractory, failure, or non-responsive. However, despite the various terms, most studies have used similar criteria for treatment resistance: having less than 25%, sometimes 35%, reduction in the total score on the Yale–Brown Obsessive Compulsive Scale (Y-BOCS) or not having "much" or "very much improved" on the Clinical Global Impression Improvement (CGI-I) scale after having sufficient SRI treatment during 12 weeks or more. This chapter loosely follows the same criteria when using the term treatment resistant in introducing individual studies.

Augmentation with antipsychotics in adult OCD

The use of antipsychotics in OCD patients was reported as early as in 1950s (Trethowan and Scott 1955), based on the fact that some patients had lack of insight and not infrequently obsessions that were so unreasonable as to resemble overvalued idea or delusional ideas (Matsunaga *et al.* 2002). The high comorbidity with tic disorder, in which antipsychotics were effective, also encouraged the use of antipsychotics for OCD patients. However, antipsychotics alone did not improve OCD symptoms and sometimes even worsened the symptoms (Andrade 1998). Ironically, it was only after SRIs became the treatment of choice for OCD that antipsychotics were again considered as having beneficial effects in OCD, via augmentation of SRI therapy.

Typical antipsychotics

The news that antipsychotics could be a good augmentation agent for the patients who do not respond to SRI

Clinical Obsessive-Compulsive Disorders in Adults and Children, ed. Robert Hudak and Darin D. Dougherty.
Published by Cambridge University Press. Copyright © Cambridge University Press 2011.

treatment was first reported by McDougle *et al.* in 1990. They reported an uncontrolled open-label study in which 9 of 17 OCD patients who had been unresponsive on more than seven weeks of fluvoxamine treatment with or without lithium showed response to the antipsychotics added to the fluvoxamine with or without lithium. The lack of response to SRI treatment was defined by the authors as (1) less than 35% reduction on the Y-BOCS total score, (2) no better than "minimally improved" on of the CGI-I score, and (3) reached consensus among the treating doctors and the authors about the unimproved state of the patients. In the same year, the same group reported a case series showing that pimozide augmentation improved the patients who had not responded to fluvoxamine (Delgado *et al.* 1990). The case series showed that only combined therapy with pimozide and fluvoxamine could initiate and maintain improvement, while pimozide or fluvoxamine alone had failed to improve the patient.

A further report from this group in 1994 described the results of double-blind placebo-controlled study in which haloperidol was given to the patients who had not responded to at least eight weeks of previous fluvoxamine treatment (McDougle *et al.* 1994). The mean dosage of 6 mg haloperidol or placebo was given to the 34 treatment-resistant patients for four weeks. In the results, 11 of 17 patients who were treated with haloperidol responded, showing 35% or greater improvement or less than 16 points in a final score as measured by Y-BOCS. None of the 17 patients given placebo responded. However, approximately 30% of patients treated with haloperidol required propranolol for the management of akathisia despite the prophylactic use of benztropine. It should be noted that, in this study, haloperidol augmentation was only effective for the patients with comorbidity of chronic tic disorders but not in those without tics.

Another study also showed the efficacy of haloperidol to augment SRI for treatment-resistant OCD (Li *et al.* 2005). This double-blind placebo-controlled crossover study compared the efficacy of augmentation with risperidone (an atypical antipsychotic, see below) and haloperidol. Over nine weeks, the patients were given two weeks of 1 mg/day risperidone, 2 mg/day haloperidol, or placebo in a crossover design. Between the phases, a 1-week placebo washout period intervened. The two weeks of haloperidol treatment showed significant reduction in Y-BOCS total score compared with placebo, with mean total score below 15. Two

weeks of risperidone treatment did not have this effect. Interestingly, haloperidol showed an efficacy despite the short two weeks of treatment. However, it was disappointing that of the 12 patients, five patients terminated the haloperidol phase before finishing the haloperidol treatment because of dystonia or severe lethargy.

Risperidone

There are three double-blind placebo-controlled studies that show risperidone could be a good augmentation agent for treatment-resistant OCD. The first controlled study of risperidone augmentation for the treatment-resistant OCD (McDougle *et al.* 2000) included patients who had not responded to 12 weeks of SRI treatment including at least eight weeks of the maximum tolerated doses of SRI. The criteria of non-responsiveness to the SRI were the same as used in the haloperidol study described above (McDougle *et al.* 1990): less than 35% reduction on the Y-BOCS total score, no better than "minimally improved" of CGI-I score, and having consensus among the treating doctor and the authors. The average dose of risperidone was 2.2 mg during the six weeks of treatment. Among the 18 risperidone-treated patients, nine responded by showing reduction of Y-BOCS total score from a mean of 27.5 to one of 13.3 points. None of the 15 patients responded in the placebo group. The symptom improvement began at week 3 and slowly improved thereafter. In this study, there was no report of significant adverse event. Unlike the haloperidol study, there was no association between comorbid tic disorder and treatment response in the study of risperidone.

Hollander *et al.* (2003) reported the results of risperidone augmentation in patients who had not responded to at least 12 weeks of two or more SRI trials. Of the ten patients treated with risperidone, four showed a CGI-I of "very much improved" or "much improved" and more than 25% reduction on Y-BOCS total score after eight weeks of treatment. None of the placebo-treated patients responded. The average dosage of risperidone was 2.25 mg/day. The authors also reported that the four responders maintained improvement until the end of the additional three months of follow-up, on a mean dosage of 2.6 mg/day, without any extrapyramidal symptoms or weight gain. The difference between the risperidone and placebo groups did not reach significance, probably as a result of the small sample size of the study. However, risperidone augmentation still showed a trend ($p = 0.065$) in reducing

Y-BOCS total score and a significance in reducing Y-BOCS obsession score.

Erzegovesi et al. (2005) used a very low dose of risperidone, 0.5 mg/day, for augmentation. In this double-blind placebo-controlled study, patients had been treated during 12 weeks of open label with up to 300 mg fluvoxamine daily before augmentation. Both partial responders and non-responders to fluvoxamine participated in the augmentation phase, being given a fixed dose of 0.5 mg risperidone. After six weeks of combined therapy, only fluvoxamine-resistant patients showed significant improvement to risperidone augmentation. Interestingly, those who had some response to fluvoxamine became worse with risperidone augmentation. Among the 10 fluvoxamine-resistant patients, five responded to risperidone, while only two responded to placebo. A few patients reported mild sedation and increase of appetite, but none of the patients discontinued medication. The remarkable finding of the study was the differential response to risperidone. It suggests the possibility that there might be a different pharmacodynamic effect between subgroups of patients with OCD, which will be further discussed below.

Several other studies, including case studies, retrospective, and open-label studies, have also reported efficacy of low-dose risperidone augmentation, mostly no more than 3 mg/day (McDougle et al. 1995a; Ravizza et al. 1996; Saxena et al. 1996; Stein et al. 1997; Kawahara et al. 2000).

Olanzapine

There are two double-blind placebo-controlled studies in which olanzapine was used as augmentation for treatment-resistant OCD. The two studies showed contrary results. Bystritsky et al. (2004) reported on a study where the participants had not responded to at least 12 weeks of two or more SRI trials and at least one trial of behavioral therapy. They received flexible doses of olanzapine, starting from 2.5 mg/day and titrated up to a mean dose of 11.2 mg/day at week six or the last week of treatment. The olanzapine-treated patient had a mean decrease of 4.2 points and placebo-treated patient had an increase of 0.54 points in Y-BOCS total score, which was a significant difference between the groups. In the olanzapine-treated group, 6 out of 13 patients responded, showing more than 25% improvement in Y-BOCS. They had average score of 13.3 points after six weeks of treatment. None of the 13 patients in the placebo group responded. Two patients dropped out from the olanzapine group: one because

of weight gain and the other for "lack of effect" and sedation.

The other double-blind placebo-controlled study comprised patients who were partial or non-responders to eight weeks of fluoxetine treatment (Shapira et al. 2004). The partial response was defined as showing 25% or greater reduction in Y-BOCS score but having symptoms of at least moderate level in CGI severity and residual symptoms greater than 16 points on Y-BOCS total score. Patients were given olanzapine augmentation for six weeks with the maximal dose fixed at 10 mg/day. In the olanzapine group, 5 out of 22 patients responded, showing 35% or greater improvement in Y-BOCS score, whereas 4 out of 22 patients in the placebo group, responded. There was no significant difference between groups. This negative result of olanzapine augmentation differs from many other studies reporting positive results. Maina et al. (2008) reported a comparison of the efficacy of risperidone and olanzapine in augmentation for treatment-resistant OCD. Both groups showed significant improvement after eight weeks of augmentation treatment. Other open-label studies reporting the effectiveness of olanzapine in augmenting SRI for treatment-resistant OCD include those by Weiss et al. (1999), Bogetto et al. (2000), D'Amico et al. (2003), and Marazziti et al. (2005).

In two ways the study by Shapira et al. (2004) differs from other studies of antipsychotic augmentation. One was that the maximal daily dose of fluoxetine was fixed to 40 mg, which was quite low compared with other studies: below the minimal daily dose (60 mg) in one study (Hollander et al. 2003). Many other studies used a maximal daily dose of at least 80 mg fluoxetine. The other was that the study had eight weeks of fluoxetine treatment before olanzapine augmentation. Most other controlled studies had at least 12 weeks of treatment with the SRI before augmentation. These differences have led to the inclusion of many undertreated patients in both the olanzapine and the placebo group, which could have weakened the power to detect group difference. This explanation is supported by the fact that both groups showed significant improvement over the six weeks of augmentation period. Therefore this study requires cautious interpretation. Despite these issues, this study was the largest controlled study using olanzapine augmentation. Further large controlled studies are needed to examine this negative result of olanzapine augmentation in treatment-resistant OCD patients.

Quetiapine

In a single-blind placebo-controlled study, OCD patients who had not responded to 12 weeks of SRI significantly improved with quetiapine augmentation (Atmaca *et al.* 2002). In this study, 10 out of 14 patients responded after receiving quetiapine for eight weeks. The response was defined as showing more than 30% of reduction in Y-BOCS total score. None responded among the 13 placebo-treated patients.

Three double-blind placebo-controlled studies of quetiapine augmentation have showed contradictory results. The study by Denys *et al.* (2004) comprised patients who had not responded to at least eight weeks of maximum tolerated level of two or more SRI trials, showing less than 25% reduction in Y-BOCS total score. They were given quetiapine or placebo for eight weeks. Quetiapine was started at 50 mg/day and increased up to 300 mg/day with a fixed dosing schedule. The quetiapine-treated patients showed greater improvement on the Y-BOCS score than the placebo group, from the fourth week onward. The mean reduction on Y-BOCS total score for quetiapine-treated patients was 9.0 points after eight weeks of treatment, which was significantly greater than the mean 1.8 points of the placebo group. A response was seen in 8 of the 20 quetiapine-treated patients and 2 of the 20 placebo-treated patients. There was no dropout for adverse events but somnolence was observed in most of the quetiapine-treated patients and frequently it was rated as moderate or severe. Dry mouth, weight gain, and dizziness were also reported in more than 30% of quetiapine-treated patients. These results are similar to those of previous open-label studies reporting an efficacy of quetiapine augmentation in treatment-resistant OCD (Denys *et al.* 2002; Mohr *et al.* 2002).

However, the other two double-blind placebo-controlled studies (Carey *et al.* 2005; Fineberg *et al.* 2005) and another open-label study (Sevincok and Topuz 2003) reported different results. A more recent study by Kordon *et al.* (2008) also failed to show a significant effect.

Carey *et al.* (2005) did not detect a significant effect of quetiapine augmentation in patients who had not previously responded to 12 weeks of open-label study with a SRI, including at least six weeks on the maximum tolerated dose of the SRI. Non-responsiveness was defined as less than 25% reduction on the Y-BOCS total score or no better than "minimally improved" of CGI-I score. During the augmentation period, the patients received placebo or a flexible dose of quetiapine. Quetiapine started from 25 mg/day for one week and was titrated up to an average dose of 168.75 mg/day at week six of treatment. The quetiapine-treated patients showed 7.10 points reduction and the placebo-treated patients showed 7.17 point on the Y-BOCS total score at week six; 8 out of 20 quetiapine-treated patients and 10 out of 21 placebo-treated patients responded. Generally, quetiapine was well tolerated without serious adverse events, but two patients dropped out in the olanzapine-treated group because of severe sedation.

Fineberg *et al.* (2005) reported the results of a 16 week randomized double-blind placebo-controlled study of quetiapine augmentation with patients who had not responded to at least 12 weeks of SRI treatment at the maximum tolerated dose. Non-responsiveness was defined as less than 25% improvement on Y-BOCS total score. Quetiapine was started at 25 mg/day and gradually titrated up to 400 mg/day, with a mean dose of 215 mg/day at endpoint. After 16 weeks of combined therapy, mean reduction on Y-BOCS total score was 3.4 points in the quetiapine group and 1.4 points in the placebo group, with no significant different between the groups. A response was seen in 3 of the 11 quetiapine-treated patients and 1 of the 10 placebo-treated patients. One patient dropped out because of dry mouth and fatigue after quetiapine treatment.

Amisulpiride

One open-label study has reported efficacy of amisulpiride for augmentation of SRI (Metin *et al.* 2003). In this study, amisulpride was given to patients who showed no response to at least 12 weeks of two or more SRIs. Amisulpiride was started at 200 mg/day and titrated up to 600 mg/day, with a mean dose of 325 mg/day. In the enrolled 20 patients, there was significant reduction in Y-BOCS total score after 12 weeks of augmentation, from baseline score of average 26.7 to 12.5 points at the end of treatment. If the 25% reduction in Y-BOCS score is used for criteria of response, 19 out of 20 patients responded to amisulpiride augmentation. None discontinued the study. Weight gain, mild sedation, and asthenia were the adverse events that more than 30% of patients reported.

Aripiprazole

There has not yet been a systematic study for aripiprazole although there is one uncontrolled study and case reports for treatment-resistant OCD. However, the results of these studies are included here as they are consistent. There are four case reports. The first (Friedman *et al.* 2007) concerned an OCD patient who had not showed response to at least eight weeks of clomipramine treatment. After adding aripiprazole at a fixed dose of 15 mg/day, the patient showed continual symptom improvement until the endpoint of 16 weeks of augmentation. The Y-BOCS total score was changed from 32 at baseline to 6 points at the week 16. The other three case reports also describe an effect with aripiprazole augmentation in patients who had failed to respond not only to SRIs but also to the combined therapy of SRI and a second-generation antipsychotic drug. One patient, who had not responded adequately to various SRI and antipsychotics including risperidone and olanzapine, showed remarkable improvement in OCD symptoms after aripiprazole augmentation (da Rocha and Correa 2007). Another who had failed for more than 20 years on various SRIs or combined treatment of SRI and antipsychotics, achieved remission with aripiprazole augmentation (Sarkar *et al.* 2008). In the last case, aripiprazole monotherapy was used for a patient with OCD and Tourette's syndrome who had been refractory to various antipsychotics and SRI in both diagnoses for more than 20 years. Using aripiprazole alone showed dramatic improvement in OCD symptoms (Winter *et al.* 2008). The results of these cases are consistent with the one open-label study showing aripiprazole monotherapy was effective in treatment of OCD (Connor *et al.* 2005).

Miscellaneous agents

Clozapine and ziprasidone have been reported as lacking efficacy in augmentation for treatment-resistant OCD (McDougle *et al.* 1995b; Savas *et al.* 2008). Many other agents, such as lithium, tryptophan, buspirone, or trazodone, have also showed no efficacy for OCD patients in double-blind studies (Mattes 1986; McDougle *et al.* 1991; Pigott *et al.* 1992a, 1992b). Some new agents are now being studied to assess their potential for augmenting SRIs. One agent that has shown most promising results is an antiglutamatergic agent, riluzole. Pittenger *et al.* (2008) have reported riluzole augmentation for 13 treatment-resistant OCD patients. By 12 weeks of treatment, 6 of 13 patients showed 35% or greater reduction in Y-BOCS total score. Riluzole was well tolerated and no patient discontinued medication.

This promising result was almost identical with that of their previous study (Coric *et al.* 2005). Other than riluzole, D-cycloserine, a partial agonist at the N-methyl-D-aspartate (NMDA) glutamatergic receptor, and ondansetron, a 5-HT$_3$ antagonist, were reported to be effective in the treatment of OCD (Hewlett *et al.* 2003; Wilhelm *et al.* 2008). In their double-blind controlled study, Wilhelm *et al.* (2008) reported that augmentation with D-cycloserine enhanced the efficacy of behavioral therapy for OCD patients; however, this result contradicts that of another double-blind placebo-controlled study that reported no efficacy of D-cycloserine on enhancing the effect of behavioral therapy (Coric *et al.* 2005; Storch *et al.* 2007). Other glutamate modulating drugs such as memantine (Pasquini and Biondi 2006) and dronabinol (Schindler *et al.* 2008) have also been reported to have some efficacy on treatment-resistant OCD. Ondansetron monotherapy was reported to be effective for some medication-free OCD patients (Hewlett *et al.* 2003).

Augmentation with antipsychotics for children and adolescents with OCD

There are few studies for augmentation of antipsychotics in children and adolescents, maybe because of the worry of the safety of medications. Only three studies, including a case report, were found investigating antipsychotic augmentation in children and adolescents. In an open uncontrolled trial using no quantitative measure, risperidone was used to augment SRI for four pediatric patients (Fitzgerald *et al.* 1999). In this study, none of the children had responded to SRI but they improved after risperidone augmentation. An open-label uncontrolled study has been carried out with adolescent patients, mean age 16.6 years, who had shown no or minimal improvement previously with two SRIs and cognitive-behavioral therapy (CBT). The patients were given risperidone, starting with 0.5 mg/day and titrated up to a maximum of 2.0 mg/day for 12 weeks in addition to the SRI and CBT (Thomsen 2004). Non-response was defined as a reduction of less than 25% on the Child-Y-BOCS (CY-BOCS) or a total score of above 20 points at the endpoint There was a response to augmentation in 4 of the 17 patients, but although this was significant, the degree of reduction as measured by CY-BOCS was not large: from an average 24.2 points to 19.9 points. Eight patients had weight gain of more than 10% of their body weight and in one patient there was 33.3% weight gain. Four had sedation.

A case report described a 13-year-old child with OCD who improved with an initial treatment with low-dose aripiprazole but the response stagnated after tapering out the aripiprazole (Storch et al. 2008). He further improved with re-administration of aripiprazole, up to 5 mg/day, when the residual symptoms almost subsided. No significant adverse effects were reported during the five month follow-up period.

Other than the antipsychotics, riluzole and buspirone have been tried to augment SRI in child and adolescent OCD. In an open-label study, riluzole was given to six child and adolescent OCD patients, aged 8–16 years, who were resistant to at least one previous SRI. Four of the six patients responded by showing 30% or greater reduction in CY-BOCS total score after 12 weeks of augmentation. No adverse event was reported (Grant et al. 2007). Buspirone was tried for six adolescents with treatment-resistant OCD; three showed clinical improvement with buspirone augmentation of an SRI (Thomsen and Mikkelsen 1999).

Pharmacological mechanism of augmentation

The antipsychotic drugs used in augmentation have included typical antipsychotics, second-generation agents, and newer antipsychotics such as aripiprazole; in addition glutamate-modulating agents have shown anti-OCD effects in some patients with treatment-resistant OCD. These drugs have different pharmacodynamic actions, affecting the serotonin, dopamine, and glutamatergic neurotransmitter systems. By considering the possible mechanism by which augmentation occurs, it may be possible to suggest a pathophysiology for OCD.

The target molecule of the SRI is the serotonin transporter (SERT), which takes up the serotonin molecule and releases it into the intrasynaptic space. As there is no degrading enzyme in this space for serotonin (contrary to dopamine or norephinephrine, which are degraded by catechol-O-methyltransferase), SERT is very important to control the concentration of serotonin in the synaptic cleft. By blocking the action of SERT, an SRI increases the concentration of serotonin in the extracellular space of the synapse. Since the 5-HT_{1A}-autoreceptor, which inhibits serotonin release in response to increased extracellular concentration of serotonin, becomes desensitized, the long-term use of

an SRI eventually increases serotonin release (Szabo and Blier 2001).

Increased serotonin release cannot be interpreted as having a direct treating affect in OCD because lowering serotonin concentration by a tryptophan-depleted diet did not cause symptom aggravation (Berney et al. 2006; Külz et al. 2007). It is more likely that there is a change in the postsynaptic 5-HT receptor with long-term use of SRI, which allows the therapeutic effect in OCD (Goddard et al. 2008).

As seen in Fig. 4.1, there are a number of different subtypes of postsynaptic serotonin receptor.

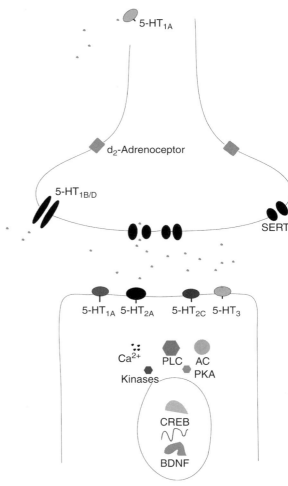

Fig. 4.1 Serotonin modulation in the synapse. Serotonin (5-HT) released into the synapse acts at the various 5-HT receptors on the postsynaptic membrane to modulate the activation cascade in the postsynaptic neuron. Serotonin is removed from the synaptic space by the serotonin transporter SERT. PLC, phospholipase C; PKA, protein kinase A; AC, acetylcholine; CREB, cAMP response element-binding protein; BDNF, brain-derived neurotrophic factor.

Importantly, agonistic action is not therapeutic at every receptor type. The activation of $5\text{-}HT_{2A}$ receptors opposes the therapeutic effects achieved by the activation of other 5-HT receptors (Marek et al. 2003). It is known that risperidone and olanzapine have potent $5\text{-}HT_2$ receptor antagonism. Therefore, mechanism of augmentation of these drugs could be through this antagonism (McDougle et al. 2000; Marek et al. 2003; Goddard et al. 2008). However, since clozapine monotherapy has no efficacy in augmenting SRI and clozapine has a strong affinity for $5\text{-}HT_2$ receptors, thus blocking $5\text{-}HT_{2A}$ and/or $5\text{-}HT_{2C}$ receptors, sole $5\text{-}HT_2$ antagonism may not be beneficial to OCD. If $5\text{-}HT_2$ receptor antagonism at the same time as agonistic action at other types of 5-HT receptor is associated with antiobsessional effect, aripiprazole, which has $5\text{-}HT_1$ agonist and probably $5\text{-}HT_2$ antagonist action (Swainston et al. 2004), might be an promising agent for OCD patients.

The efficacy of haloperidol and pimozide in treatment-resistant OCD (McDougle et al. 1994) cannot be explained by $5\text{-}HT_2$ receptor antagonism since they do not have this action. Increased dopaminergic activity has been reported to be involved in the pathophysiology of OCD: OCD patients have higher dopamine transporter densities and lower dopamine:D_2 receptor binding ratios compared with controls (Kim et al. 2003), which suggests increased dopaminergic activity in OCD (Skapinakis et al. 2007). Haloperidol and pimozide, both D_2 receptor antagonists, may act as augmenting agents through this antagonism. Since monotherapy with these drugs has shown no efficacy to reduce OC symptoms, D_2 receptor antagonism could be beneficial only in combination with serotonin reuptake inhibition. However, it should be noted that a dopaminergic mechanism involved in the pathophysiology in OCD might not be unidirectional, since dopamine antagonists could improve or aggravate OCD symptoms (Khullar et al. 2001; Alevizos et al. 2002; Stamouli and Lykouras 2006).

The potential efficacy of antiglutamatergic agents such as riluzole or memantine suggests that hyperactivity of the glutamate system could have a role in the pathogenesis of OCD. There is some evidence for glutamate abnormality in OCD. For example, elevated glutamate in cerebrospinal fluid was found in unmedicated OCD patients (Chakrabarty et al. 2005) and the OC symptom-like grooming behavior could be simulated by the knock-out mouse lacking a cytoskeletal protein found in the cortico-striatal glutamatergic neurons (Welch et al. 2007).

Issues in practicing augmentation

Published studies have provided a number of useful methods to optimize the benefits of augmentation in clinical practice. In the study of Shapira et al. (2004), which failed to show the efficacy of olanzapine in augmenting SRI, 25.6% of the patients who had not responded to eight weeks of maximum 40 mg fluoxetine did responded to continuing SRI monotherapy. That is contrasting to the less than 5% response rate in the study using maximum dose of SRI for 12 weeks (Bloch et al. 2006). This is indirect evidence that more than 12 weeks of maximum-tolerated dose of SRI is required before starting augmentation.

There was a dose-dependent response rate for risperidone in augmenting SRI. Saxena et al. (1996) reported an average dose of 2.75 mg/day risperidone showed a 23.8% of response rate, which was higher than the 12.5% seen when a dose of 1.25 mg/day was used. Nevertheless, most of the studies, including the previous one, showing the efficacy of risperidone for OCD patients used an average dose below 3 mg/day. Titration usually started with 0.5 mg/day and slowly increased to the target dose (Saxena et al. 1996; Stein et al. 1997). For olanzapine, the maximal dose was not more than 10 mg/day. Some authors have argued that upward titration of risperidone could be more beneficial if the antiobsessional effect is mediated via dopamine D_2 receptor antagonism (Ramasubbu 2002). However, pharmacodynamic studies of the therapeutic mechanism do not support this hypothesis. The low dose of atypical antipsychotics leads to $5\text{-}HT_{2A}$ receptor antagonism in the medial frontal cortex, which seems to be therapeutic. However, higher doses of atypical antipsychotics result in $5\text{-}HT_{2A}$ receptor antagonism in the orbitofrontal cortex, which seems to be countertherapeutic (Tundo et al. 2007; Goddard et al. 2008). With regard to titration in augmentation, it is noteworthy that there was a case report of immediate aggravation of OCD symptoms after rapid titration of risperidone augmentation (Andrade 1998). There have also been a number of reports that rapid titration of risperidone caused increased incidence of adverse events (Brody 1996; Brown 1997).

Most studies of augmentation reported the time to response to be from days to within a month (McDougle et al. 1995a; Saxena et al. 1996; Stein et al. 1997). Because the number of treatment responders did not increase after four weeks of augmentation with antipsychotic drugs, it is unlikely that patients who fail to respond by the end of one month of antipsychotic augmentation will improve with continuation (Bloch *et al.* 2006). However, it has also been shown that, in patients who showed a response, the longer the augmentation trial continued the better was the outcome. Therefore, some have insisted on the need for observing for at least eight weeks before deciding whether the augmenting agent is effective or not (Skapinakis *et al.* 2007).

Obsessive-compulsive disorder is frequently combined with tic disorder, depression, substance abuse, or other psychiatric disorders. In the study by McDougle *et al.* (1990) showing the efficacy of typical antipsychotics on treatment-resistant OCDs, the response rate was significantly higher in patients with comorbid tic disorder or schizotypal personality disorder than in those without these comorbidities. However, that association of efficacy and comorbidity with tic disorder was not observed for treatment with second-generation antipsychotics. In fact, in the study of Saxena *et al.* (1996), the patients with tic disorder rarely responded to risperidone and had the highest rate of adverse events, which is in striking contrast to the study of haloperidol, which reported the most favorable response to haloperidol in the patients with tic disorder (McDougle *et al.* 1990). Risperidone or quetiapine (McDougle *et al.* 2000; Denys *et al.* 2004) augmentation seems to lower symptoms of depression or anxiety as measured by the Hamilton Depression Rating Scale or Anxiety Rating Scale,, respectively, while haloperidol augmentation had no effect on mood or anxiety (McDougle *et al.* 1994). However, there was no difference in the change in depression or anxiety between groups, as measured by these two scales, in the olanzapine augmentation study (Bystritsky *et al.* 2004).

There is one report that patients with the hoarding symptom responded better with addition of antipsychotics (Pallanti and Quercioli 2006); therefore, it is possible that treatment-refractory patients with hoarding symptom may respond better to antipsychotics.

Most of the studies on augmentation do not report significant adverse events using the augmentation agents, apart from sedation, weight gain, and akathisia.

To predict the response to antipsychotic augmentation is very important in a clinical setting. Denys *et al.* (2004) have insisted that a higher Y-BOCS obsessional subscale score could predict favorable response to antipsychotic augmentation. They showed that responders to quetiapine augmentation had higher Y-BOCS obsessional subscale scores than non-responders. A more favorable result for obsessional symptoms compared with compulsion was also observed in the risperidone augmentation study by Li *et al.* (2005) and in a very early study with chlorpromazine monotherapy (Trethowan and Scott 1955). A small open-label study has shown more pronounced improvement in compulsion symptoms when an SRI was augmented with aripiprazole (Connor *et al.* 2005).

Conclusions

Haloperidol and risperidone showed robust clinical efficacy compared with placebo in augmentation therapy of treatment-refractory OCD whereas other agents such as olanzapine and quetiapine have shown inconsistent results (Bloch *et al.* 2006; Skapinakis *et al.* 2007). At present, it can be said that antipsychotics are the only proven augmenting agents for treatment-refractory OCD. Typical antipsychotics, however, have limited use for OCD patients because of the high likelihood of serious side effects such as tardive dyskinesia in long-term use. Therefore, risperidone and olanzapine are preferred agents for the management of treatment-resistant OCD. The rather inconsistent results, and adverse effect such as severe weight gain found with olanzapine, make risperidone more favorable as the first-line agent for the augmentation of treatment-resistant OCD. Aripiprazole seems promising but a large-scale double-blind controlled study is mandatory to confirm its efficacy. However, it is also true that more than half of all patients who were enrolled in augmentation studies failed to respond to the augmentation strategies. In such patients, an augmentation strategy with aripiprazole or an antiglutamatergic agent would be a reasonable alternative.

References

Alevizos B, Lykouras L, Iannis Z, *et al.* (2002). Risperidone-induced obsessive-compulsive symptoms: a series of six cases. *J Clin Psychopharmacol* **22**: 461–467.

Andrade C (1998). Risperidone may worsen fluoxetine-treated OCD. *J Clin Psychiatry* **59**: 255–256.

Atmaca M, Kuloglu M, Tezcan E, *et al.* (2002). Quetiapine augmentation in patients with treatment resistant obsessive-compulsive disorder: a single-blind, placebo-controlled study. *Int Clin Psychopharmacol* **17**: 115–119.

Berney A, D. Sookman, Leyton SN, *et al.* (2006). Lack of effects on core obsessive-compulsive symptoms of tryptophan depletion during symptom provocation in remitted obsessive-compulsive disorder patients. *Biol Psychiatry* **59**: 853–857.

Bloch MH, Landeros-Weisenberger A, Kelmendi BK, *et al.* (2006). A systematic review: antipsychotic augmentation with treatment refractory obsessive-compulsive disorder. *Mol Psychiatry* **11**: 622–632.

Bogetto F, Bellino S, Vaschetto P, Ziero S (2000). Olanzapine augmentation of fluvoxamine-refractory obsessive-compulsive disorder (OCD): a 12-week open trial. *Psychiatry Res* **96**: 91–98.

Brody AL (1996). Acute dystonia induced by rapid increase in risperidone dosage. *J Clin Psychopharmacol* **16**: 461–462.

Brown ES (1997). Extrapyramidal side effects with low-dose risperidone. *Can J Psychiatry* **42**: 325–326.

Bystritsky A Ackerman DL, Rosen RM, *et al.* (2004). Augmentation of serotonin reuptake inhibitors in refractory obsessive-compulsive disorder using adjunctive olanzapine: a placebo-controlled trial. *J Clin Psychiatry* **65**: 565–568.

Calvocoressi L, Lewis B, Harris M, *et al.* (1995). Family accommodation in obsessive-compulsive disorder. *Am J Psychiatry* **152**: 441–443.

Carey PD, Vythilingum B, Seedat S, *et al.* (2005). Quetiapine augmentation of SRIs in treatment refractory obsessive-compulsive disorder: a double-blind, randomised, placebo-controlled study [ISRCTN83050762]. *BMC Psychiatry* **5**: 44.

Chakrabarty K, Bhattacharyya S, Christopher R, Khanna S (2005). Glutamatergic dysfunction in OCD. *Neuropsychopharmacology* **30**: 1735–1740.

Connor KM, Payne VM, Gadde KM, Zhang W, Davidson JR (2005). The use of aripiprazole in obsessive-compulsive disorder: preliminary observations in 8 patients. *J Clin Psychiatry* **66**: 49–51.

Coric V, Taskiran S, Pittenger C, *et al.* (2005). Riluzole augmentation in treatment-resistant obsessive-compulsive disorder: an open-label trial. *Biol Psychiatry* **58**: 424–428.

D'Amico G, Cedro C, Muscatello MR, *et al.* (2003). Olanzapine augmentation of paroxetine-refractory obsessive-compulsive disorder. *Prog Neuropsychopharmacol Biol Psychiatry* **27**: 619–623.

da Rocha FF, Correa H, (2007). Successful augmentation with aripiprazole in clomipramine-refractory obsessive-compulsive disorder. *Prog Neuropsychopharmacol Biol Psychiatry* **31**: 1550–1551.

Delgado PL, Goodman WK, Price LH, Heninger GR, Charney DS (1990). Fluvoxamine/pimozide treatment of concurrent Tourette's and obsessive-compulsive disorder. *Br J Psychiatry* **157**: 762–765.

Denys D, van Megen H, Westenberg H (2002). Quetiapine addition to serotonin reuptake inhibitor treatment in patients with treatment-refractory obsessive-compulsive disorder: an open-label study. *J Clin Psychiatry* **63**: 700–703.

Denys D, de Geus F, van Megen HJ, Westenberg HG (2004). A double-blind, randomized, placebo-controlled trial of quetiapine addition in patients with obsessive-compulsive disorder refractory to serotonin reuptake inhibitors. *J Clin Psychiatry* **65**: 1040–1048.

Erzegovesi S, Guglielmo E, Siliprandi F, Bellodi L (2005). Low-dose risperidone augmentation of fluvoxamine treatment in obsessive-compulsive disorder: a double-blind, placebo-controlled study. *Eur Neuropsychopharmacol* **15**: 69–74.

Fineberg NA, Sivakumaran T, Roberts A, Gale T (2005). Adding quetiapine to SRI in treatment-resistant obsessive-compulsive disorder: a randomized controlled treatment study. *Int Clin Psychopharmacol* **20**: 223–226.

Fitzgerald KD, Stewart CM, Tawile V, Rosenberg DR (1999). Risperidone augmentation of serotonin reuptake inhibitor treatment of pediatric obsessive compulsive disorder. *J Child Adolesc Psychopharmacol* **9**: 115–123.

Friedman S, Abdallah TA, Oumaya M, Rouillon F, Guelfi JD (2007). Aripiprazole augmentation of clomipramine-refractory obsessive-compulsive disorder. *J Clin Psychiatry* **68**: 972–973.

Goddard AW, Shekhar A, Whiteman AF, McDougle CJ (2008). Serotoninergic mechanisms in the treatment of obsessive-compulsive disorder. *Drug Discov Today* **13**: 325–332.

Goodman WK, Price LH (1992). Assessment of severity and change in obsessive compulsive disorder. *Psychiatr Clin N Am* **15**: 861–869.

Grant P, Lougee L, Hirschtritt M, Swedo SE (2007). An open-label trial of riluzole, a glutamate antagonist, in children with treatment-resistant obsessive-compulsive disorder. *J Child Adolesc Psychopharmacol* **17**: 761–767.

Hewlett WA, Schmid SP, Salomon RM (2003). Pilot trial of ondansetron in the treatment of 8 patients with obsessive-compulsive disorder. *J Clin Psychiatry* **64**: 1025–1030.

Hollander E, Baldini Rossi N, Sood E, Pallanti S (2003). Risperidone augmentation in treatment-resistant obsessive-compulsive disorder: a double-blind, placebo-controlled study. *Int J Neuropsychopharmacol* **6**: 397–401.

Insel TR, Murphy DL (1981). The psychopharmacological treatment of obsessive-compulsive disorder: a review. *J Clin Psychopharmacol* **1**: 304–311.

Karno M, Golding JM, Sorenson SB, Burnam MA (1988). The epidemiology of obsessive-compulsive disorder in five US communities. *Arch Gen Psychiatry* **45**: 1094–1099.

Kawahara T, Ueda Y, Mitsuyama Y (2000). A case report of refractory obsessive-compulsive disorder improved by risperidone augmentation of clomipramine treatment. *Psychiatry Clin Neurosci* **54**: 599–601.

Kelly MW, Myers CW (1990). Clomipramine: a tricyclic antidepressant effective in obsessive compulsive disorder. *DICP* **24**: 739–744.

Khullar A, Chue P, Tibbo P (2001). Quetiapine and obsessive-compulsive symptoms (OCS): case report and review of atypical antipsychotic-induced OCS. *J Psychiatry Neurosci* **26**: 55–59.

Kim CH, Koo MS, Cheon KA, *et al.* (2003). Dopamine transporter density of basal ganglia assessed with [^{123}I] IPT SPECT in obsessive-compulsive disorder. *Eur J Nucl Med Mol Imaging* **30**: 1637–1643.

Koran LM, Thienemann ML, Davenport R, *et al.* (1996). Quality of life for patients with obsessive-compulsive disorder. *Am J Psychiatry* **153**: 783–788.

Kordon A, Wahl K, Koch N, *et al.* (2008). Quetiapine addition to serotonin reuptake inhibitors in patients with severe obsessive-compulsive disorder: a double-blind, randomized, placebo-controlled study. *J Clin Psychopharmacol* **28**: 550–554.

Külz AK, Meinzer, S, Kopasz M, Voderholzer U (2007). Effects of tryptophan depletion on cognitive functioning, obsessive-compulsive symptoms and mood in obsessive-compulsive disorder: preliminary results. *Neuropsychobiology* **56**: 127–131.

Leon AC, Portera L, Weissman MM (1995). The social costs of anxiety disorders. *Br J Psychiatry* **166**(Suppl 27): 19–22.

Li X, May RS, Tolbert LC, *et al.* (2005). Risperidone and haloperidol augmentation of serotonin reuptake inhibitors in refractory obsessive-compulsive disorder: a crossover study. *J Clin Psychiatry* **66**: 736–743.

Liebowitz MR, Turner SM, Piacentini J, *et al.* (2002). Fluoxetine in children and adolescents with OCD: a placebo-controlled trial. *J Am Acad Child Adolesc Psychiatry* **41**: 1431–1438.

Maina G, Pessina E, Albert U, Bogetto F (2008). Eight-week, single-blind, randomized trial comparing risperidone versus olanzapine augmentation of serotonin reuptake inhibitors in treatment-resistant obsessive-compulsive disorder. *Eur Neuropsychopharmacol* **18**: 364–372.

Marazziti D, Pfanner C, Dell'Osso B, *et al.* (2005). Augmentation strategy with olanzapine in resistant obsessive compulsive disorder: an Italian long-term open-label study. *J Psychopharmacol* **19**: 392–394.

March JS (2004). Cognitive-behavioral therapy, sertraline, and their combination for children and adolescents with obsessive-compulsive disorder: the Pediatric OCD Treatment Study (POTS) randomized controlled trial. *JAMA* **292**: 1969–1976.

March JS, Biederman J, Wolkow R, *et al.* (1998). Sertraline in children and adolescents with obsessive-compulsive disorder: a multicenter randomized controlled trial. *JAMA* **280**: 1752–1756.

Marek GJ, Carpenter LL, McDougle CJ, Price LH (2003). Synergistic action of 5-HT$_{2A}$ antagonists and selective serotonin reuptake inhibitors in neuropsychiatric disorders. *Neuropsychopharmacology* **28**: 402–412.

Matsunaga H, Kiriike N, Matsui T, Oya K, Iwasaki Y (2002). Obsessive-compulsive disorder with poor insight. *Compr Psychiatry* **43**: 150–157.

Mattes JA (1986). A pilot study of combined trazodone and tryptophan in obsessive-compulsive disorder. *Int Clin Psychopharmacol* **1**: 170–173.

McDougle CJ, Goodman WK, Price LH, *et al.* (1990). Neuroleptic addition in fluvoxamine-refractory obsessive-compulsive disorder. *Am J Psychiatry* **147**: 652–654.

McDougle CJ, Price LH, Goodman WK, Charney DS, Heninger GR (1991). A controlled trial of lithium augmentation in fluvoxamine-refractory obsessive-compulsive disorder: lack of efficacy. *J Clin Psychopharmacol* **11**: 175–184.

McDougle CJ, Goodman WK, Leckman JF, *et al.* (1994). Haloperidol addition in fluvoxamine-refractory obsessive-compulsive disorder. A double-blind, placebo-controlled study in patients with and without tics. *Arch Gen Psychiatry* **51**: 302–308.

McDougle CJ, Fleischmann RL, Epperson CN, *et al.* (1995a). Risperidone addition in fluvoxamine-refractory obsessive-compulsive disorder: three cases. *J Clin Psychiatry* **56**: 526–528. [Comment in *J Clin Psychiatry* 1996 **57**: 594–595.]

McDougle CJ, Barr LC, Goodman WK, *et al.* (1995b). Lack of efficacy of clozapine monotherapy in refractory obsessive-compulsive disorder. *Am J Psychiatry* **152**: 1812–1814.

McDougle CJ, Epperson CN, Pelton GH, Wasylink S, Price LH (2000). A double-blind, placebo-controlled study of risperidone addition in serotonin reuptake inhibitor-refractory obsessive-compulsive disorder. *Arch Gen Psychiatry* **57**: 794–801.

Metin O, Yazici K, Tot S, Yazici AE (2003). Amisulpiride augmentation in treatment resistant obsessive-compulsive disorder: an open trial. *Hum Psychopharmacol* **18**: 463–467.

Mohr N, Vythilingum B, Emsley RA, Stein DJ (2002). Quetiapine augmentation of serotonin reuptake inhibitors in obsessive-compulsive disorder. *Int Clin Psychopharmacol* **17**: 37–40.

Pallanti S, Quercioli L (2006). Treatment-refractory obsessive-compulsive disorder: methodological issues, operational definitions and therapeutic lines. *Prog Neuropsychopharmacol Biol Psychiatry* **30**: 400–412.

Pasquini M, Biondi M (2006). Memantine augmentation for refractory obsessive-compulsive disorder. *Prog Neuropsychopharmacol Biol Psychiatry* **30**: 1173–1175.

Pigott TA, L'Heureux F, Hill JL, et al. (1992a). A double-blind study of adjuvant buspirone hydrochloride in clomipramine-treated patients with obsessive-compulsive disorder. *J Clin Psychopharmacol* **12**: 11–18.

Pigott TA, L'Heureux F, Rubenstein CS, et al. (1992b). A double-blind, placebo controlled study of trazodone in patients with obsessive-compulsive disorder. *J Clin Psychopharmacol* **12**: 156–162.

Pittenger C, Kelmendi B, Wasylink S, Bloch MH, Coric V (2008). Riluzole augmentation in treatment-refractory obsessive-compulsive disorder: a series of 13 cases, with long-term follow-up. *J Clin Psychopharmacol* **28**: 363–367.

Ramasubbu R (2002). Antiobsessional effect of risperidone add-on treatment in serotonin reuptake inhibitor-refractory obsessive-compulsive disorder may be dose-dependent. *Arch Gen Psychiatry* **59**: 472; author reply 472–473.

Rasmussen SA, Eisen JL (1992). The epidemiology and clinical features of obsessive compulsive disorder. *Psychiatr Clin N Am* **15**: 743–758.

Ravizza L, Barzega G, Bellino S, Bogetto F, Maina G (1996). Therapeutic effect and safety of adjunctive risperidone in refractory obsessive-compulsive disorder (OCD). *Psychopharmacol Bull* **32**: 677–682.

Sarkar R, Klein J, Kruger S (2008). Aripiprazole augmentation in treatment-refractory obsessive-compulsive disorder. *Psychopharmacology (Berl)* **197**: 687–688.

Savas HA, Yumru M, Ozen ME (2008). Quetiapine and ziprasidone as adjuncts in treatment-resistant obsessive-compulsive disorder: a retrospective comparative study. *Clin Drug Investig* **28**: 439–442.

Saxena S, Wang D, Bystritsky A, Baxter LR Jr. (1996). Risperidone augmentation of SRI treatment for refractory obsessive-compulsive disorder. *J Clin Psychiatry* **57**: 303–306.

Schindler F, Anghelescu I, Regen F, Jockers-Scherubl M (2008). Improvement in refractory obsessive compulsive disorder with dronabinol. *Am J Psychiatry* **165**: 536–537.

Sevincok L, Topuz A (2003). Lack of efficacy of low doses of quetiapine addition in refractory obsessive-compulsive disorder. *J Clin Psychopharmacol* **23**: 448–450.

Shapira NA, Ward HE, Mandoki M, et al. (2004). A double-blind, placebo-controlled trial of olanzapine addition in fluoxetine-refractory obsessive-compulsive disorder. *Biol Psychiatry* **55**: 553–555.

Skapinakis P, Papatheodorou T, Mavreas V, et al. (2007). Antipsychotic augmentation of serotonergic antidepressants in treatment-resistant obsessive-compulsive disorder: a meta-analysis of the randomized controlled trials. *Eur Neuropsychopharmacol* **17**: 79–93.

Skoog G, Skoog I (1999). A 40-year follow-up of patients with obsessive-compulsive disorder. *Arch Gen Psychiatry* **56**: 121–127.

Stamouli S, Lykouras L (2006). Quetiapine-induced obsessive-compulsive symptoms: a series of five cases. *J Clin Psychopharmacol* **26**: 396–400.

Stein DJ, Bouwer C, Hawkridge S, Emsley RA (1997). Risperidone augmentation of serotonin reuptake inhibitors in obsessive-compulsive and related disorders. *J Clin Psychiatry* **58**: 119–122.

Storch EA, Merlo LJ, Bengtson M, et al. (2007). D-Cycloserine does not enhance exposure-response prevention therapy in obsessive-compulsive disorder. *Int Clin Psychopharmacol* **22**: 230–237.

Storch EA, Lehmkuhl H, Geffken GR, Touchton A, Murphy TK (2008). Aripiprazole augmentation of incomplete treatment response in an adolescent male with obsessive-compulsive disorder. *Depress Anxiety* **25**: 172–174.

Swainston Harrison T, Perry CM (2004). Aripiprazole: a review of its use in schizophrenia and schizoaffective disorder. *Drugs* **64**: 1715–1736.

Szabo ST, Blier P (2001). Effect of the selective noradrenergic reuptake inhibitor reboxetine on the firing activity of noradrenaline and serotonin neurons. *Eur J Neurosci* **13**: 2077–2087.

Thomsen PH (2004). Risperidone augmentation in the treatment of severe adolescent OCD in SSRI-refractory cases: a case-series. *Ann Clin Psychiatry* **16**: 201–207.

Thomsen PH, Mikkelsen HU (1999). The addition of buspirone to SSRI in the treatment of adolescent obsessive-compulsive disorder. A study of six cases. *Eur Child Adolesc Psychiatry* **8**: 143–148.

Trethowan WH, Scott PA (1955). Chlorpromazine in obsessive-compulsive and allied disorders. *Lancet* **268**: 781–785.

Tundo A, Salvati L, Busto G, Di Spigno D, Falcini R (2007). Addition of cognitive-behavioral therapy for nonresponders to medication for obsessive-compulsive disorder: a naturalistic study. *J Clin Psychiatry* **68**: 1552–1556.

Weiss EL, Potenza MN, McDougle C, Epperson CN (1999). Olanzapine addition in obsessive-compulsive disorder refractory to selective serotonin reuptake inhibitors: an open-label case series. *J Clin Psychiatry* **60**: 524–527.

Welch JM, Lu J, Rodriguiz RM, *et al.* (2007). Cortico-striatal synaptic defects and OCD-like behaviours in Sapap3-mutant mice. *Nature* **448**: 894–900.

Wilhelm S, Buhlmann U, Tolin DF, *et al.* (2008). Augmentation of behavior therapy with D-cycloserine for obsessive-compulsive disorder. *Am J Psychiatry* **165**: 335–341; quiz 409.

Winter C, Heinz A, Kupsch A, Ströhle A (2008). Aripiprazole in a case presenting with Tourette syndrome and obsessive-compulsive disorder. *J Clin Psychopharmacol* **28**: 452–454.

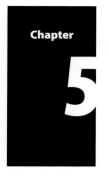

Chapter

5

Obsessive-compulsive disorder and comorbid mood disorders

Jonathan S. Abramowitz

Introduction

Obsessive compulsive disorder (OCD) is a psychological disorder that primarily involves *obsessions* – recurrent unwanted or senseless thoughts, images, or impulses that evoke anxiety (e.g., a persistent doubt that one is contaminated because he had a wet dream) – and *compulsive rituals* – overt behaviors (e.g., taking a 45-minute shower) or mental acts (e.g., ritualistic praying) that are performed to reduce obsessional distress (American Psychiatric Association, 2000). Compulsive rituals, although linked (at least in the sufferer's mind) to the obsessions they are designed to neutralize (e.g., washing to reduce fears of contamination, checking to alleviate doubts about causing a fire), are clearly excessive in relation to the obsessional concern (e.g., hand washing for 15 minutes after using the bathroom), or performed according to strict self-imposed rules and regulations (e.g., counting to 10 while checking). Patients also engage in avoidance behavior that is aimed at reducing distress and lessening the need for compulsive behaviors. Consistent research indicates that obsessions and rituals typically conform to the following themes: contamination/decontamination; responsibility for harm, sex, religion, and violence; and the need for order or symmetry (e.g., McKay *et al.* 2004; Abramowitz *et al.* 2010a). Although hoarding – the irresistible urge to collect, and failure to discard, possessions of little practical value – has been considered a symptom of OCD, emerging research suggests that hoarding is most likely an overlapping (in some instances), but distinct phenomenon (e.g., Abramowitz *et al.* 2008).

Data from large epidemiologic studies show that the lifetime prevalence of OCD is between 2 and 3% in adults (Fireman *et al.* 2001). The obsessional distress, avoidance, and rituals typically cause significant personal suffering and functional impairment. Areas of life such as school, work, social, leisure, and family role functioning may be moderately to severely impaired. Unfortunately, individuals with OCD often do not receive appropriate treatment until long after the onset of the disorder (perhaps between 5 and 10 years). Therefore, when the relatively high prevalence and associated functional impairment are considered along with the time lag between symptom onset and when treatment is finally obtained, it can be seen that this condition is a significant public health concern.

Individuals with OCD are also at an increased risk for developing comorbid axis I and axis II psychopathology, with anxiety and mood disorders among the most commonly co-occurring problems. This chapter focuses on the comorbidity of OCD and mood disorders: unipolar and bipolar. After reviewing the rates of comorbidity between OCD and mood disorders, the impact of comorbidity on the clinical presentation of OCD is described. Next, the effect of mood disorder comorbidity on the psychological treatment of OCD using cognitive-behavioral treatment (CBT) is covered. Lastly, the chapter focuses on recommendations for how routine CBT can be adapted in instances where a person with OCD presents with a comorbid mood disorder. A case example is included to illustrate the treatment of a depressed individual with OCD.

Comorbidity and clinical characteristics

Unipolar depression

Major depressive disorder (MDD) is a condition characterized by one or more major depressive episodes without a history of manic, mixed, or hypomanic episodes (American Psychiatric Association 2000). A

Clinical Obsessive-Compulsive Disorders in Adults and Children, ed. Robert Hudak and Darin D. Dougherty.
Published by Cambridge University Press. Copyright © Cambridge University Press 2011.

Table 1 Rates of major depressive disorder in samples of adults with obsessive-compulsive disorder

Study	DSM	No.	Comorbidity (%)
Antony et al. (1998)	IV	87	24
Yaryura-Tobias et al. (1996)	IIIR	391	29
Crino and Andrews (1996)*	IIIR	108	50
Ricciardi and McNally (1995)	IIIR	125	21
Andrews et al. 2002	IV	641	17
Nestadt et al. (2001)	IV	80	54
Sanderson et al. (1990)	IIIR	12	33

DSM, *Diagnostic and Statistical Manual of Mental Disorders.*

major depressive episode is a period of at least two weeks in which the individual consistently experiences depressed mood or a loss of interest or pleasure in daily activities; which represents a change from the person's normal mood. Further, the change in mood negatively impacts social, occupational, educational, or other important areas of functioning. The criteria for a major depressive episode also include the presence of at least five of the following symptoms: significant weight loss, insomnia, psychomotor agitation or retardation, fatigue, feelings of worthlessness or excessive or inappropriate guilt, diminished ability to concentrate, and recurrent suicidal ideation.

Given the personal distress and functional impairment associated with OCD, it is not surprising that individuals suffering with this condition are likely to show signs and symptoms of depressive disorders. Table 5.1 shows the rates of MDD among adult OCD samples in recent studies. Across seven countries, the lifetime prevalence of MDD among OCD patients ranges from 12.4 to 60.3%. In the eastern USA, researchers found a lifetime comorbidity rate of 54.1%, and a concurrent comorbidity rate of 36% (e.g., Nestadt et al. 2001). Studies on the temporal nature of this comorbidity pattern indicate that in most (but not all) instances, OCD symptoms predate the depressive symptoms (Bellodi et al. 1992; Demal et al. 1993). This suggests that the mood disturbance often occurs as a response to the distress and functional impairment associated with obsessions and compulsions.

The presence of depression appears to impact the presentation of OCD symptoms. Depressed OCD patients, for example, have an earlier age of OCD onset and more severe obsessions and compulsions than their non-depressed counterparts (e.g., Hong et al. 2004; Tükel et al. 2006; Abramowitz et al. 2007). Depressive symptoms seem to be more strongly associated with the severity of obsessions than with compulsive rituals (Ricciardi and McNally 1995), and may be specifically associated with the occurrence of sexual and religious obsessions (Hong et al. 2004; Hasler et al. 2005). This is consistent with finding that sexual and religious obsessions are experienced as more distressing than are other OCD symptoms (Abramowitz et al. 2003a; McKay et al. 2004).

Depressed OCD patients also show more severe general anxiety symptoms and higher rates of other comorbid conditions (e.g., anxiety disorders) than do OCD patients without depression (Ricciardi and McNally, 1995; Tükel et al. 2002; Hong et al. 2004; Tükel et al. 2006; Abramowitz et al. 2007). A study examining the cognitive–behavioral correlates of comorbid OCD and depression found that, relative to non-depressed OCD patients, those with depression more strongly overestimated the significance of their intrusive obsessional thoughts (Abramowitz et al. 2007). For example, the presence of an unwanted obsessional image of harm befalling a loved one might be interpreted as indicating that the person is bad or dangerous. This finding has implications for the treatment of OCD using cognitive-behavioral methods (discussed later in this chapter), as one aim of this treatment approach is to help the individual to correct mistaken interpretations of his or her obsessional intrusive thoughts.

Postpartum occurrence of OCD and depression

Both OCD and depression tend to occur at higher than expected rates among pregnant and (especially) postpartum women (Abramowitz *et al.* 2003b, 2010b), and the obsessional thoughts in postpartum OCD often concern harm befalling the fragile infant (e.g., images of dropping the baby down the stairs; Abramowitz *et al.* 2003c). Research and clinical observations both point to a relationship between these two conditions; for example, the observation that many perinatal women who experience OCD symptoms find the obsessive thoughts particularly distressing, leading them to report experiencing many of the symptoms of MDD.

Empirical investigations also support the idea of a relationship between postpartum OCD symptoms – particularly unwanted thoughts and fears of harming the infant – and postpartum depression. For example, Jennings *et al.* (1999) compared the prevalence of unwanted harm-related obsessional thoughts in a group of 100 women with postpartum depression, versus 46 women who had recently given birth but had no psychiatric diagnoses. Of the 41% of depressed mothers who reported harm-related thoughts, 20% experienced them as just "passing" thoughts. The thoughts were "repetitious" in 12% of these individuals, and they elicited "precautions" (e.g., avoiding being alone with the infant) in 4%. Among the postpartum women without depression, only 6.5% reported unwanted harm-related thoughts, and all of these were described as "passing" thoughts.

Although a relationship between postpartum depression and OCD symptoms – particularly upsetting intrusive (obsessional) thoughts regarding intentionally or accidentally harming the newborn – might exist, it is not known whether depressive symptoms are a cause or an effect of the obsessional thoughts. Given that depression involves unwanted and/or self-destructive thoughts, it is possible that obsessional problems (e.g., unwanted thoughts of harm) are symptoms of postpartum depression. Alternatively, it is plausible that the presence of such unwanted obsessional thoughts indicates the presence of OCD, yet this is distressing to the point that it also gives rise to depressive symptoms. Finally, it is possible that both OCD and depression occur coincidentally, each the result of a third variable (or variables; e.g., biological factors). Further study is warranted to clarify this relationship, which may have a bearing on clinical management of these disorders in the postpartum.

Bipolar mood disorder

Bipolar disorder is a chronic and lifelong mood disorder in which the individual experiences extreme shifts in mood, energy, and functioning, which may be subtle or dramatic and which typically vary over the course of the person's life (American Psychiatric Association 2000). It is characterized by recurring episodes of mania and depression that can last from days to months; these often begin in adolescence or early adulthood, and occasionally in children. The symptoms of a manic episode may include either an elated, happy mood or an irritable, angry, unpleasant mood; increased physical and mental activity and energy; racing thoughts and flight of ideas; increased talking and more rapid speech than normal; ambitious, often grandiose plans; inappropriate risk taking; impulsive activity such as spending sprees, sexual indiscretion, and alcohol abuse; and decreased sleep without experiencing fatigue.

In contrast to MDD, there has been much less research on the overlap between OCD and bipolar disorder. The rate of lifetime comorbid bipolar disorder in clinical samples of OCD patients appears to range from 3.8% to 21.5%, with a higher prevalence of bipolar disorder type II (which involves depression and hypomania rather than full-blown mania; 7.8–17.7%; Lensi *et al.* 1996). Compared with individuals with OCD and no bipolar disorder, obsessional patients with bipolar disorder tend to have a more gradual onset of their OCD symptoms and a more episodic course (Perugi *et al.* 1997) that is associated with greater functional impairment (Tükel *et al.* 2006). One study found less severe obsessions and compulsions among those with comorbid bipolar disorder than among non-comorbid patients (Zutshi *et al.* 2007). Whereas one study found that OCD patients with comorbid bipolar disorder had a higher than expected rate of sexual and religious obsessions and a lower rate of checking rituals compared with non-comorbid OCD patients (Perugi *et al.* 1997), other researchers have reported reduced rates of religious obsessions (Zutshi *et al.* 2007) and increased rates of symmetry obsessions and repeating, counting, and ordering/arranging rituals among such patients (Hasler *et al.* 2005; Tükel *et al.* 2006; Maina *et al.* 2007).

As is the case with OCD–MDD comorbidity, the combination of OCD and bipolar disorder is associated with the presence of additional mood and anxiety disorders, particularly social anxiety and generalized anxiety disorder (Perugi *et al.* 1997; Tükel *et al.* 2006; Zutshi *et al.* 2007), substance use disorders, and higher rates of cluster A and B personality disorders, with narcissistic and antisocial personality disorders more frequent among the comorbid patients (Maina *et al.* 2007). Despite some inconsistencies in the reported rates of symptom themes, the existing research literature suggests that OCD patients with bipolar disorder differ in a number of ways from OCD patients without this comorbidity. This raises the possibility that there is some degree of shared pathophysiology between OCD and bipolar disorder. But in the absence of any evidence to support this notion, strong conclusions cannot be drawn.

Psychological treatment

Behavioral and cognitive therapies for OCD

The importance of recognizing that people with OCD often suffer from comorbid mood disorders is highlighted by the fact that comorbidity impacts treatment response, particularly to exposure and response prevention therapy (ERP) – a form of CBT and the most effective treatment that exists for OCD (e.g., Foa *et al.* 2005). The ERP approach entails repeated and prolonged confrontation with obsessional stimuli (exposure therapy) and help with refraining from compulsive rituals (response prevention). For example, a patient with contamination fears and compulsive hand washing is coached to confront feared "contaminants" that actually pose low levels of risk (e.g., touching a shoe, using a public restroom) while simultaneously refraining from cleaning or washing (e.g., limited contact with water during the treatment period). As alluded to above, ERP is a highly effective therapy for OCD, producing an average of 60–70% reduction in obsessions and compulsions (Franklin *et al.* 2000). A drawback of this approach, however, is that patients must deliberately provoke obsessional anxiety and resist urges to ritualize. Because ERP requires compliance with these demanding procedures, approximately 25% of patients either refuse this form of therapy or terminate prematurely. Moreover, ERP is highly focused on alleviating obsessional anxiety and the need for compulsive rituals, and

it does not directly address comorbid problems such as depression and mania.

Cognitive conceptualizations of OCD have led to the inclusion of cognitive therapy (CT) strategies along with ERP in treatment manuals for OCD (e.g., Salkovskis and Warwick 1985; Steketee 1999). In CT, a number of verbal and skill-development techniques are used to educate individuals about the nature of OCD, and to help them to correct mistaken interpretations of obsessional thoughts and related stimuli. For example, someone who experiences recurrent sexual obsessions (e.g., thoughts of raping a colleague) would be helped to recognize that unwanted or upsetting thoughts are normal occurrences that happen in virtually 100% of the population. Thus, rather than thinking that the presence of such an obsession means that the event will happen, or that the person is vile or a pervert, the patient is taught to see his or her obsessions as senseless but normal and meaningless intrusive thoughts. In doing so, patients are helped to correct a number of key cognitive distortions present in OCD (e.g., the need for certainty, an inflated sense of responsibility). In addition to verbally challenging these dysfunctional ways of thinking, patients test out the validity of these (and corrected) beliefs using behavioral experiments that are similar to exposure exercises. The efficacy of CT is suggested by a number of outcome studies, yet CT does not appear to be quite as effective as ERP for OCD.

Effects of comorbidity on psychological treatment

Some studies have reported a relationship between depression and outcome of psychological treatment for OCD: the more severe the depressive symptoms, the less improvement following treatment with ERP (Foa *et al.* 1983). One explanation for this relationship is that severely depressed patients overreact when presented with feared stimuli during exposure exercises. The typical response to exposure is initially an increase in subjective distress, followed by a gradual natural decline in anxiety (i.e., habituation). If depressed individuals are highly reactive, however, they might not experience the natural reduction in anxiety. Other studies, however, have reported no relationship between comorbid depression and outcome (Basoglu *et al.* 1988). One likely explanation for these inconsistent results is that only *severe* depression hinders outcome of ERP. Indeed, many of the existing predictor studies were secondary analyses of larger controlled treatment trials in which patients with severe depression had been excluded (to maximize experimental control). Thus the range of depression severity on the continuous measures used in predictor analyses was restricted, perhaps obfuscating a relationship between severe depression and poor treatment outcome.

A more definitive, prospective study (Abramowitz et al. 2000) investigated the relationship between pretreatment levels of depression and outcome of ERP within a large clinic-based sample of OCD patients ($n = 87$) with a wide range of depression severity. When patients with OCD were grouped on the basis of their baseline Beck Depression Inventory (BDI) scores, the most severely depressed patients (e.g., BDI ≥ 30) evidenced significantly lower rates of improvement with ERP than those with moderate, mild, or no depression (BDI < 30). This finding leads to the conclusion that OCD patients with comorbid MDD would show less improvement than those with no clinical diagnosis of depression. Accordingly, in two studies examining the effects of concurrent diagnoses on outcome of ERP (Steketee et al. 2001; Abramowitz and Foa 2000), the presence of MDD was related to poorer outcome on symptom variables and social functioning at post-treatment and at follow-up.

There are no existing studies on the effects of bipolar comorbidity on response to exposure-based treatment for OCD. One reason for this is that studies evaluating psychological treatments for OCD have usually excluded patients with bipolar disorders since the manic symptoms have a tendency to interfere with normal perception, cognition, and judgment, and perhaps impede patients' ability to follow treatment instructions on their own or attend to the cognitive changes that ERP aims to facilitate. Clinically, it is recommended that patients with bipolar disorder first receive treatment to bring their manic symptoms under control before attempting ERP for OCD. When this approach is used, individuals can often make good progress in reducing their OCD symptoms when they begin ERP. The author, for example, has had success using ERP with several bipolar OCD patients whose manic symptoms were well controlled on medication. The treatment of these individuals was essentially the same as for OCD patients without any comorbid conditions.

Because there is strong evidence that unipolar depression hinders the outcome of ERP, the remainder of this chapter will focus on treating individuals with OCD and comorbid MDD.

Treating depressed OCD patients

Psychological treatment manuals developed for OCD (for either ERP or CT) have not routinely addressed the common comorbid depressive symptoms that are now known to present challenges. The prevalence of depression in OCD and the evidence that severe depression impedes response to ERP, however, suggest the need to develop and apply specific strategies for OCD patients with comorbid MDD. Such an advance would reduce the sheer amount of therapy and increase the cost effectiveness for these patients, who are often referred for treatment of their depression *before* beginning a course of treatment.

Possible treatment approaches for depressed OCD patients

Medication

Antidepressant medications, such as the serotonin reuptake inhibitors (SRIs), are the most widely used treatments for both depression and OCD. Intuitively, the use of these agents should improve outcome for depressed OCD patients. Three studies have addressed whether antidepressants offer an advantage over ERP for this population. First, in a post hoc analysis, Marks et al. (1980) found that clomipramine helped severe depression and OCD symptoms more than did placebo. However, the comparison included only five patients taking clomipramine and five placebo, and the statistical analysis was conducted at the four-week point, which may not have been enough time for clomipramine to take effect in all patients. In the second study, Foa et al. (1992) examined whether using imipramine prior to ERP would facilitate improvement in OCD symptoms. In their prospective study, mildly and severely depressed OCD patients received either pill placebo or imipramine for six weeks prior to ERP. Results indicated that although imipramine improved symptoms of depression, it did not potentiate the effects of ERP on OCD symptoms. The third study was that by Abramowitz et al. (2000) described above, which included a comparison between severely depressed OCD patients who either were or were not using SRI medications during ERP. No differences between groups were reported, although the small size of the severely depressed group in that study (11) limits the generalizability of this finding. Consequently, to date there is no compelling evidence that medication potentiates the effects of ERP with severely depressed OCD patients.

A possible explanation for the above conclusion is that because SRI medications are the most widely used therapy for OCD, patients with OCD have often already tried these medications before presenting for psychotherapy. The many depressed OCD patients in treatment studies might have been "treatment resistant," thus putting a ceiling on the effects of medications for OCD. Nevertheless, since the average improvement with SRI medication is somewhat modest (approximately 20–40%; Abramowitz *et al.* 2009), there is a need to consider non-medication strategies for augmenting psychological treatment for depressed OCD patients.

Cognitive therapy

Perhaps CT techniques that are used for postpartum depression could be added to ERP for depressed OCD patients. Indeed, CT yields high responder rates, few adverse effects, and good durability of gains in depressed patients (e.g., Elkin *et al.* 1989). The use of CT for depression involves identifying and challenging overly negative beliefs about oneself, the world, and the future that lead to overly negative and biased interpretations of events, giving rise to feelings of extreme hopelessness, helplessness, and personal failure. Numerous studies report significant and lasting improvement in dysphoric mood and other MDD symptoms following CT. Typically, 50–70% of MDD patients who complete CT no longer meet criteria for MDD at post-treatment, and only 20–30% show significant relapse at follow-up (Craighead *et al.* 1992).

Another reason CT is a good choice to use in the treatment of depressed OCD patients is efficiency: that is, the skills and techniques used to reduce depression (e.g., identifying and challenging beliefs) are largely the same as those used in CT protocols developed for reducing OCD symptoms – although the content is different. For example, cognitive restructuring can be used to modify dysfunctional cognitions relevant to OCD (e.g., "thinking is as bad as doing"), as well as those relevant to depression (e.g., "I am a failure as a human being"). Thus, patients would learn to make use of the same skill to reduce both MDD and OCD symptoms.

Perhaps engaging in CT to reduce depressive symptoms prior to beginning ERP alleviates some depressive symptoms and helps the patient to increase motivation and compliance with difficult exposure therapy assignments, thereby enhancing reductions in OCD symptoms. However, the effects of adding CT to traditional ERP programs for OCD have yet to be systematically evaluated in a sample of OCD patients with comorbid MDD. An ongoing study at our center, however, aims to examine the effectiveness of using CT for depression and OCD to augment traditional ERP in the management of this more treatment-resistant subpopulation of OCD patients. The case description below illustrates the use of CT in combination with ERP for the treatment of depressed OCD patients.

Case example

Case description

Elaine was a 26-year-old woman from the southeastern USA who came to our outpatient clinic seeking treatment for "depression and obsessive thoughts." She stated that her obsessive thoughts about her new baby were "ruining her life." Elaine and her husband of three years, Joe, had recently given birth to their first child, a son named Ryan. But Elaine was avoiding interacting with Ryan, especially if Joe wasn't around to "supervise." This was because Elaine was having thoughts that she might sexually molest the baby when no one was looking. She was unable to bathe Ryan, change his diaper, or breastfeed him. Assessment using the Yale–Brown Obsessive Compulsive Scale (Y-BOCS) and Symptom Checklist indicated prominent sexual obsessions, mental rituals (e.g., praying), and rituals involving asking for reassurances from her mother and husband that she would "never do such a thing." Specific obsessional thoughts included images of the baby's penis and impulses to touch his genitals. Elaine was very religious and spent hours praying that she wouldn't act on her unwanted thoughts. She also repeatedly asked others questions such as "Do you think I will molest the baby?" and "What does it mean that I think about doing such evil things?" Elaine's pretreatment score on the Y-BOCS severity scale was 27, indicating fairly severe OCD symptoms.

A diagnostic interview confirmed both a diagnosis of OCD and of major depression. Elaine had experienced some minor OCD symptoms as a teenager, but her anxiety got noticeably worse during her pregnancy; and her symptoms spiked after Ryan was born. For the last few months, Elaine reported feeling down, having decreased energy, decreased interest in activities or hobbies, and feelings of worthlessness, hopelessness, and passive suicidal thinking. Her Beck Depression Inventory (BDI) score was 29 and her Hamilton Depression Rating Scale (HDRS) score was 20, suggesting clinical depression of moderate severity.

Elaine had never received treatment for OCD or depression except to speak with the pastor at her church. After several sessions with the pastor, she saw the advertisement for our clinic and decided to contact us. After an assessment and discussion of treatment options, Elaine was quite ambivalent about beginning therapy, primarily because she feared engaging in exposure exercises. Her therapist explained how treatment would indeed be a challenge but would progress at a level Elaine was comfortable with and that she would never be forced into doing exposure practices. Instead, it would be the therapist's job to help Elaine to see how trying ERP would help her to achieve relief from her symptoms even if it meant "investing anxiety up front in a calmer future." After some discussion with her family, Elaine opted to enter our program.

Course of treatment

Treatment involved 16 90-minute twice-weekly sessions over the course of eight weeks. During the first two treatment sessions, the therapist continued to collect information about Elaine's depressive symptoms and she was introduced to the cognitive model of emotional disorders wherein negative emotions are considered to be evoked by dysfunctional interpretations of situations. It became clear that Elaine's depression was secondary to her OCD symptoms; she described feeling guilty, worthless, and like a "bad mother" as a result of her unwanted sexual obsessions. She believed that, deep down, she was becoming a sexual predator and that it was only a matter of time before she eventually gave in and ended up sexually assaulting her own child. Elaine attributed her problems to demonic possession and often berated herself for not being a good enough servant of God. Cognitive therapy for depression was begun and the therapist taught Elaine to recognize cognitive errors including "overgeneralizing," "catastrophizing," and "discounting the positive." Elaine was helped to generate more realistic appraisals of herself and her future. For example, "I am a terrible mother" was modified to "I want what's best for my baby, but am having problems with

OCD that make me have recurring thoughts about strange things."

Elaine was instructed in how to use daily thought diaries to practice identifying and modifying dysfunctional thoughts on her own. She also worked with her therapist to develop a routine of activities that she enjoyed (behavioral activation), such as watching certain humorous television shows and renting movies she liked. It became clear that Elaine felt that how others perceived her as a parent was very important. Numerous cognitive therapy worksheets were dedicated to thoughts regarding the importance of what others thought of her and her ability to be a good parent. Thus, Elaine was helped to reduce the emphasis she placed on what she *thought* others might be thinking of her.

Sessions three and four involved learning to apply the cognitive model (and CT) to OCD symptoms. In particular, Elaine was taught that just about everyone experiences intrusive thoughts of one sort or another, but that such thoughts do not mean anything significant or threatening about the thinker. Instead, Elaine was helped to see how she was misappraising the presence and meaning of her sexual thoughts. A model of OCD in which normal obsessional thoughts get misinterpreted as overly significant, leading to anxiety, was outlined. Anxiety then leads to urges to avoid Ryan, engage in compulsive prayer, and ask for excessive reassurance from her family. These avoidance behaviors and rituals, which reduce anxiety in the short term, paradoxically reinforce obsessional anxiety in the long run because they lead to greater preoccupation with the unwanted thoughts, and the sense that the thoughts are "out of control." Elaine understood the conceptual model, and it came as a relief to learn that others also experience strange intrusive thoughts from time to time. She understood that once she realized that her sexual thoughts about Ryan were not dangerous, her urges to engage in avoidance, excessive prayer, and reassurance-seeking would be diminished, and that her anxiety preoccupation with the unwanted thoughts would similarly decline.

In the fourth session, an exposure hierarchy was developed collaboratively. After a thorough discussion of the rationale for therapeutic exposure and response prevention, Elaine agreed to confront over the remaining 11 sessions a number of situations that she had been avoiding, while also attempting to gradually drop her compulsive behaviors.

Elaine continued to practice cognitive restructuring for depressive symptoms during (and between) the first several sessions. During the fifth visit she reported that her mood was improved, that she felt a good deal of confidence in her therapist, and that she was hopeful of improving with continued therapy. Exposure began with confronting objects such as diapers and pictures of babies from magazines. Elaine was instructed to allow unwanted sexual thoughts to enter her mind and just "hang out" there. She was also told to allow herself to worry about molesting Ryan; she needed to confront, rather than avoid, these thoughts and ideas. Although Elaine had some difficulty refraining from compulsive praying rituals at first, by the seventh treatment session, she had cut her prayer to acceptable levels, such as before bedtime, and was not asking Joe for reassurance about her unwanted thoughts. Joe had attended an early exposure session and had been instructed by the therapist in how to offer supportive reinforcement for successful exposure practice, rather than giving reassurance that "everything would be OK." At the eighth session a mid-treatment evaluation revealed a Y-BOCS score of 20, BDI score of 13, and a HDRS score of 10.

Sessions 9 through 16 included reviewing exposure and cognitive therapy homework assignments as well as conducting in-session exposure practice with gradually more difficult situations. With some reluctance, Elaine was able to confront most items on her exposure hierarchy including changing Ryan, playing with him while he was naked, giving him a bath, and putting lotion on his penis. She also was able to allow her unwanted intrusive thoughts to enter her mind without needing to resist or suppress them. Although urges to say prayers about these thoughts sometimes occurred, Elaine understood the importance of resisting these urges and practicing exposure to her fear cues. She reported being able to spend more and more time with Ryan, and being alone with him. She also began to feel more worthwhile as a parent, and her feelings of being a bad mother had disappeared. An important aspect of Elaine's reduction in depression was the genuine recognition and reinforcement she received from her family, who had observed her hard work and improvement over the course of therapy.

At the end of treatment, Elaine's Y-BOCS score was 11, indicating a near 60% reduction in OCD symptoms. Her BDI score was 7 and her Hamilton score was 4, both within normal range. She felt much more in control of her obsessional and depressive symptoms. Elaine also felt able to continue her trajectory of improvement after the end of therapy. Three months following the end of treatment, Elaine's Y-BOCS score was 12. She arranged to see her therapist for four additional sessions to practice exposure to a few situations that continued to give her trouble, including bathing and changing Ryan. She was only infrequently asking for assurances and was no longer praying about her intrusive thoughts.

Clinical issues

The case of Elaine indicates that CBT using CT methods to augment traditional ERP procedures holds potential for treating OCD patients with comorbid major depression. At least for this particular individual, the 16-session, twice-weekly comprehensive treatment regimen appeared to improve the tolerability of anxiety-evoking exposure assignments so that she was able to engage in (and benefit from) them. Given Elaine's disposition to ERP during her initial assessment, it is likely that she would have had difficulty with compliance (if not discontinued therapy altogether) if ERP had been begun immediately. Instead, by introducing CT first, Elaine had the opportunity to (1) establish rapport with her therapist, (2) see that the therapist understood her OCD symptoms, (3) come to better understand her own obsessional thoughts in a less threatening way, and (4) develop cognitive coping strategies to reduce her depressive symptoms and prepare for ERP exercises. It is interesting to speculate whether these factors contributed to Elaine's engagement in the more difficult aspects of the therapy. Indeed, some have advocated that CT strategies should be used routinely to help patients to confront feared situations during exposure (Abramowitz 2006).

Elaine's depression was quite straightforward and clearly secondary to her OCD. That is, she was primarily depressed about having OCD. Very likely, reduction in her OCD symptoms toward the middle and later stages of treatment resulted in further improvements in her depression. In some instances, however, patients' depressive symptoms represent primary complaints in their own right, over and above the distress associated with having OCD. For example, one patient we evaluated had experienced depression for several years before the onset of her OCD. An important question concerns whether patients whose depressive symptoms are related to the distress or functional impairment associated with OCD would fare better in CBT for OCD than would patients for whom OCD and depression represent truly unrelated diagnoses.

Although this single case provides reason for cautious optimism, much work is required before more firm conclusions regarding the effectiveness of this treatment can be made. Additionally, important questions need to be answered in order to determine the clinical and cost effectiveness of this treatment approach. For example, it will be necessary to determine whether or not this comprehensive treatment package is more effective than ERP, CT, or SRI medication alone, or that it is superior to the combination of psychotherapy and medication in this population.

Conclusions

Obsessive-compulsive disorder is a heterogeneous disorder not only in terms of its symptom presentation but also in that patients often present with additional diagnoses. Mood disorders are among the most common comorbidities. The presence of either unipolar depression or bipolar disorder affects the presentation of OCD in terms of its overall severity, types of obsession and ritual manifested, and the degree of functional disability. Most importantly, mood disorders predict poorer outcome of psychological treatment for OCD. Whereas patients with OCD and bipolar disorder should not be treated with cognitive or behavioral methods unless their manic symptoms are well controlled, those with comorbid MDD can respond to ERP, although their response is likely to be attenuated as a function of the severity of their depression. The introduction of CT techniques, which are effective in the treatment of unipolar depression, is one strategy that might improve depressed OCD patients' response to ERP. Given that SRI medications are effective in the treatment of OCD, pharmacotherapy might also be suggested in such cases. Importantly, when depression is so severe that patients have extreme psychomotor retardation or suicidal ideation, alternative treatment approaches (e.g., hospitalization) should be considered.

References

Abramowitz JS (2006). *Understanding and Treating Obsessive-Compulsive Disorder: A Cognitive-Behavioral Approach*. Mahway NJ: Lawrence Erlbaum.

Abramowitz JS, Foa EB (2000). Does comorbid major depressive disorder influence outcome of exposure and response prevention for OCD? *Behav Ther* **31**: 795–800.

Abramowitz JS, Franklin ME, Street G, Kozak M, Foa EB (2000). Effects of comorbid depression on response to treatment for obsessive-compulsive disorder. *Behav Ther* **31**: 517–528.

Abramowitz J, Franklin M, Schwartz S, Furr J (2003a). Symptom presentation and outcome of cognitive-behavior therapy for obsessive-compulsive disorder. *J Consult Clin Psychol* **71**: 1049–1057.

Abramowitz JS, Schwartz SA, Moore KM, Luenzmann KR (2003b). Obsessive-compulsive symptoms in pregnancy and the puerperium: A review of the literature. *J Anxiety Disord* **17**: 461–478.

Abramowitz JS, Schwartz SA, Moore KM (2003c). Obsessional thoughts in postpartum females and their partners: Content, severity and relationship with depression. *J Clin Psychol in Medical Settings* **10**: 157–164.

Abramowitz JS, Storch EA, Keely M, Cordell E (2007). Obsessive-compulsive disorder with comorbid major depression: What is the role of cognitive factors? *Behav Res Ther* **45**: 2257–2267.

Abramowitz JS, Wheaton MG, Storch EA (2008). The status of hoarding as a symptom of obsessive-compulsive disorder. *Behav Res Ther* **46**: 1026–1033.

Abramowitz JS, Taylor S, McKay D (2009). Obsessive-compulsive disorder. *Lancet* **374**: 491–499.

Abramowitz JS, Deacon B, Olatunji BO, *et al.* (2010a). Assessment of obsessive-compulsive symptoms: development and evaluation of the Dimensional Obsessive-Compulsive Scale. *Psychol Assess* **22**: 180–198.

Abramowitz JS, Meltzer-Brody S, Leserman J, *et al.* (2010b). Obsessional thoughts and compulsive behaviors in sample of women with postpartum mood symptoms. *Arch Women Mental Health* doi: 10.1007/s00737-010-0172-4.

American Psychiatric Association (1994). *Diagnostic and Statistical Manual of Mental Disorders*, 4th edn. Washington, DC: American Psychiatric Press.

Andrews G, Slade T, Issakidis C (2002). Deconstructing current comorbidity: data from the Australian National Survey of Mental Health and Well-being. *Br J Psychiatry* **181**: 306–314.

Antony MM, Downie F, Swinson RP (1998). Diagnostic issues and epidemiology and obsessive-compulsive disorder. In Swinson RP, Antony M, Rachman S, Richter M (eds.) *Obsessive-Compulsive Disorder: Theory, Research, and Treatment* (pp. 3–32). New York: Guilford Press.

Basoglu M, Lax. T, Kasvikis Y, Marks I (1988). Predictors of improvement in obsessive-compulsive disorder. *J Anxiety Disord* **2**: 299–317.

Bellodi L, Scioto G, Diaferia G, Ronchi P, Smiraldi E (1992). Psychiatric disorders in families of patients with obsessive-compulsive disorder. *Psychiatry Res* **42**: 111–120.

Craighead W, Evans D, Robins C (1992). Unipolar depression. In Turner SM, Calhoun KS, Adams H, (eds.) *Handbook of Clinical Behavior Therapy*, 2nd edn (pp. 99–116). New York: Wiley.

Crino R, Andrews G (1996). Obsessive-compulsive disorder and axis I comorbidity. *J Anxiety Disord* **19**: 37–46.

Demal U, Lenz G, Mayrhofer A, Zapotoczky, H-G, Zitterl W (1993). Obsessive-compulsive disorder and depression. A retrospective study on course and interaction. *Psychopathology* **26**: 145–150.

Elkin I, Shea M, Watkins, IS, *et al.* (1989). National Institute of Mental Health Treatment of Depression Collaborative Research program: General effectiveness of treatments. *Arch Gen Psychiatry* **46**: 971–982.

Fireman B, Koran L, Leventhal J, Jacobson A (2001). The prevalence of clinically recognized obsessive-compulsive disorder in a large health maintenance organization. *Am J Psychiatry* **158**: 1904–1910.

Foa EB, Grayson JB, Steketee GS, *et al.* (1983). Success and failure in the behavioral treatment of obsessive-compulsives. *J Consult Clin Psychol* **51**: 287–297.

Foa EB, Kozak MJ, Steketee G, McCarthy PR (1992). Treatment of depressive and obsessive-compulsive symptoms in OCD by imipramine and behavior therapy. *Br J Clin Psychol* **31**: 279–292.

Foa, EB, Liebowitz MR, Kozak MJ, *et al.* (2005). Randomized, placebo-controlled trial of exposure and ritual prevention, clomipramine, and their combination in the treatment of obsessive-compulsive disorder. *Am J Psychiatry* **162**: 151–161.

Franklin ME, Abramowitz JS, Kozak MJ, Levine J, Foa EB (2000). Effectiveness of exposure and ritual prevention for obsessive-compulsive disorder: a comparison of randomized and clinic patients. *J Consult Clin Psychol* **68**: 594–602.

Hasler G, LaSalle-Ricci V, Ronquillo J (2005). Obsessive-compulsive symptom dimensions show specific relationships to psychiatric comorbiditiy. *Psychiatry Res* **135**: 121–132.

Hong J, Samuels J, Bienvenu OJ, *et al.* (2004). Clinical correlates of recurrent major depression in obsessive-compulsive disorder. *Depress Anxiety* **20**: 86–91.

Jennings KD, Ross S, Pepper S, Elmore M (1999). Thoughts of harming infants in depressed and nondepressed mothers. *J Affect Disord* **54**: 21–28.

Lensi P, Cassano G, Correddu G (1996). Obsessive-compulsive disorder: familial-developmental history, symptomatology, comorbidity and course with special reference ti gender-related pathogenetic differences. *Br J Psychiatry* **169**: 101–107.

Maina G, Albert H, Pessina E, Bogetto F (2007). Bipolar obsessive-compulsive disorder and personality disorders. *Bipolar Disord* **9**: 722–729.

Marks IM, Stern R, Mawson D, Cobb J, McDonald R (1980). Clomipramine and exposure for obsessive-compulsive rituals I. *Br J Psychiatry* **136**: 1–25.

McKay D, Abramowitz JS, Calamari JE, *et al.* (2004). A critical evaluation of obsessive-compulsive disorder subtypes: Symptoms versus mechanisms. *Clin Psychol Rev* **24**: 283–313.

Nestadt G, Samuels J, Riddle M, *et al.* (2001). The relationship between obsessive-compulsive disorder and anxiety and affective disorders: Results from the Johns Hopkins OCD Family Study. *Psychol Med* **31**: 481–487.

Perugi G, Akiskal H, Pfanner C, *et al.* (1997). The clinical impact of bipolar disorder and unipolar affective comorbidity on obsessive-compulsive disorder. *J Affect Disord* **46**: 15–23.

Ricciardi JN, McNally RJ (1995). Depressed mood is related to obsessions but not compulsions in obsessive-compulsive disorder. *J Anxiety Disord* **9**: 249–256.

Salkovskis PM, Warwick HM (1985). Cognitive therapy of obsessive-compulsive disorder: treating treatment failures. *Behav Psychother* **13**: 243–255.

Sanderson W, DiNardo P, Rapee R, Barlow D (1990). Syndrome comorbidity in patients diagnosed with a DSM-III-R anxiety disorder. *J Abnorm Psychol* **99**: 308–312.

Steketee GS (1999). Therapist Protocol for Overcoming Obsessive-Compulsive Disorder: *A Behavioral and Cognitive Protocol for the Treatment of OCD*. Oakland, CA: New Harbinger.

Steketee GS, Chambless DL, Tran G (2001). Effects of axis I and II comorbidity on behavior therapy outcome for obsessive-compulsive disorder and agoraphobia. *Compr Psychiatry* **42**: 76–86.

Tükel R, Polat A, Ozdemir O, Sksut D, Turksoy N (2002). Comorbid conditions in obsessive-compulsive disorder. *Compr Psychiatry* **43**: 204–209.

Tükel R, Meteris H, Koyuncu A, Tecer A, Yazici O (2006). The clinical impact of mood disorder comorbidity on obsessive-compulsive disorder. *Eur Arch Psychiatry Clin Neurosci* **256**: 240–245.

Yaryura-Tobias J, Todaro J, Gunes M, *et al.* (1996). Comorbidity versus continuum of axis I disorders in OCD. In *Proceedings of the Annual Meeting of the Association for Advancement of Behavior Therapy*, November, New York.

Zutshi A, Kamath P, Reddy Y (2007). Bipolar and nonbipolar obsessive-compulsive disorder: a clinical exploration. *Compr Psychiatry* **48**: 245–251.

Chapter

6

Obsessive-compulsive symptoms in schizophrenia: clinical characterization and treatment

Michael Poyurovsky

Schizophrenia and obsessive-compulsive disorder (OCD) are distinct nosological entities with discrete underlying mechanisms, clinical presentations, and treatments. Nevertheless, they share some demographic and clinical characteristics and pathophysiological mechanisms (Table 6.1). The lifetime prevalence is about 1% for schizophrenia and 2–3% for OCD. Both are lifelong conditions associated with periods of exacerbations and remissions; affect men and women equally, and have a similar age-at-onset distribution with a trend towards earlier age of onset for OCD. Increasingly sophisticated translational, neurophysiological, and neuroimaging research have deepened our understanding of the neurobiology of both disorders and show a substantial overlap between schizophrenia and OCD in structural and functional brain abnormalities: the prefrontal and anterior cingulate cortex, striatum and thalamus are consistently implicated in both disorders. There is also common ground for the pharmacotherapy of schizophrenia and OCD, based on the involvement of dopamine, serotonin, and glutamate neurotransmitter systems in the pathophysiology of both disorders. Hence, it is not surprising that OCD and schizophrenia coexist in a proportion of patients that extends beyond random co-occurrence between the two disorders.

This chapter evaluates recent findings pertaining to the phenomenological characterization and diagnostic boundaries of distinct but partially overlapping subgroups on the putative schizophrenia–OCD axis. Tentative therapeutic approaches and challenges of pharmacotherapy in these difficult-to-treat patient populations are presented. Finally, future directions of investigation in schizophrenia–OCD comorbidity relevant to clinical practice are discussed.

Clinical characteristics

Epidemiology

Obsessive-compulsive symptoms (OCS)/OCD were identified in patients with schizophrenia well before the introduction of the *Diagnostic and Statistical Manual of Mental Disorders* (DSM). Founders of clinical psychiatry (Westphal, Mayer-Gross, and Bleuler) considered OCS a possible feature of the prodromal phase of schizophrenia, with chronic obsessions as an actual manifestation of the disorder. Hoch and Polatin (1949) highlighting the clinical significance of OCS in schizophrenia along with other neurotic symptoms (e.g., phobias, depersonalization, pan-anxiety), deemed them within a "pseudo-neurotic" subtype of schizophrenia. Allowing diagnosis of schizophrenia in the presence of "pseudo-neurotic" features, sometimes without characteristic schizophrenia symptoms, led to a substantial broadening of diagnostic boundaries of schizophrenia, limiting both reliability and validity of diagnosis. In contrast, according to a hierarchical rule, formalized in psychiatric nosology in DSM-III, OCD was not diagnosed in the presence of schizophrenia since it was "due to" a disorder higher on the hierarchy. These exclusion criteria temporarily delayed research on the comorbidity between schizophrenia and OCD. The publication of DSM-IV accepted the possibility of co-occurrence of schizophrenia and OCD and stating that "if another Axis I disorder is present, the content of the obsessions or the compulsions should not be restricted to it." By permitting multiple axis I diagnoses, DSM-IV draws attention to the presence of additional and potentially treatable "non-schizophrenic" syndromes (i.e., depression, OCD, panic disorder) in

Table 6.1 Comparative characteristics of schizophrenia and obsessive-compulsive disorder

	Schizophrenia	OCD
Prevalence (%)	1	2–3
Male/female ratio	1/1	1/1
Age of onset	2nd–3rd decade	1st–2nd decade
Course	Chronic with remissions	Wax and wane
Involved brain regions	Cortex: prefrontal, temporal, anterior cingulate, thalamus, hippocampus, striatum	Cortex: prefrontal, anterior cingulate, thalamus, striatum
Neurotransmitter systems	Dopamine/serotonin/glutamate	Serotonin/dopamine/glutamate
Treatment	Antipsychotic agents (add-on serotonin reuptake inhibitors)	Serotonin reuptake inhibitors (add-on antipsychotic agents)

patients with a primary diagnosis of schizophrenia (Bermanzohn *et al.* 2000).

Initially, OCS were thought to occur in a minority (1.1–3.5%) of patients with schizophrenia and were considered a positive prognostic indicator, protecting against "personality disintegration" and "malignant schizophrenic course" (Stengel 1945; Rosen 1956). Fenton and McGlashan (1986), and later Berman and colleagues (1995), challenged this view. Applying operationally defined behavioral criteria (Fenton and McGlashan 1986), both groups found a significantly higher rate of OCS in schizophrenia (12.8–25%) and a poorer prognosis for schizo-obsessive patients. These investigations prompted further research to evaluate the prevalence of obsessive-compulsive phenomena in schizophrenia.

Using the Structured Clinical Interview for DSM-IV (SCID) and rigorous DSM-IV criteria for both schizophrenia and OCD, the majority of contemporary studies reveal a considerably higher rate of OCD in schizophrenia patients than initially suggested. Epidemiological surveys and studies based on clinical samples estimate that roughly 20% of schizophrenia patients also exhibit OCD (Table 6.2). The wide estimate range is accounted for by variations in the definition of obsessive–compulsive features (disorder versus symptoms), diagnostic criteria applied (categorical versus dimensional), the patient population studied (inpatients, outpatients, or community residents), research methodologies (chart review or direct interview; lay or clinician assessments) and the phase of the schizophrenic illness (first admission versus chronic stage). Despite these methodological

differences, reports from research groups worldwide provide compelling evidence suggesting that the rate of occurrence of OCD in schizophrenia is considerably higher than in the general population (2.3%) (Ruscio *et al.* 2010). Notably, Niehaus *et al.* (2005) evaluating the prevalence of OCD in Xhosa-speaking schizophrenia patients in South Africa found that only 3 (0.5%) of 509 patients met criteria for OCD. These findings contrasted starkly with most OCD comorbidity data in schizophrenia patients of Caucasian ethnicity. Both schizophrenia and OCD are disorders with significant commonality across different cultures and ethnic groups. Nevertheless, a variation in the phenomenology of schizophrenia across ethnic groups, and a lower prevalence of OCD in some ethnic communities have also been reported (Weissman *et al.* 1994; Emsley *et al.* 2002). If replicated, the provoking findings of Niehaus *et al.* (2005) might support the hypothesis that cultural and/or genetic factors play a role in protecting against comorbid OCD in schizophrenia in certain ethnic groups. Finally, when the diagnostic threshold is relaxed from DSM-IV OCD to OCS, an even higher proportion of schizophrenia patients exhibits clinically significant obsessions and/or compulsions. A high prevalence of subthreshold OCD symptoms has recently been revealed in the National Comorbidity Survey Replication (28.2%; Ruscio *et al.* 2010), suggesting that the health burden of obsessive–compulsive phenomena is significantly greater than the DSM-IV OCD prevalence implies.

A critical question is whether the high prevalence of OCD in schizophrenia is a result of chronic illness, hospitalization or the OCD-inducing potential of

Table 6.2 Rate of occurrence of obsessive-compulsive disorder/symptoms in schizophrenia

Authors	Country	Study sample size and type	Study design, diagnostic criteria for schizophrenia and OCD	Prevalence of OCD/OCS in schizophrenia
Epidemiological sample				
Karno et al. (1988)	USA	18 500; community residents	Survey interview; DSM-III	OCD 12.2%
Bland et al. (1987)	USA	20; community residents	DSM-III for OCS	OCS 59.2%
Regier et al. (1990)	USA	20 861; community residents	Survey interview	OCD 23.7%
First-episode or recent-onset schizophrenia				
Strakowski et al. (1993)	USA	10; inpatients	SCID, DSM-IIIR	OCD 20%
Poyurovsky et al. (1999)	Israel	50; inpatients	SCID; DSM-IV	OCD 14%
Craig et al. (2002)	USA	225; inpatients	SCID; DSM-IIIR	OCD 3.8%; OCS 16.2%
de Haan et al. (2005)	Holland	113; inpatients	SCID-P; DSM-IV	OCD 29.2%; OCS 15%
Sim et al. (2006)	Singapore	142; inpatients	SCID; DSM-IV	OCD 6.3%
Chronic schizophrenia				
Fenton and McGlashan (1986)	USA	163; inpatients	Operational criteria for OCS	OCS 12.9%
Berman et al. (1995)	USA	108; outpatients	Operational criteria for OCS	OCS 26.5%
Eisen et al. (1997)	USA	77; outpatients	SCID; DSM-IV	OCD 7.8%
Porto et al. (1997)	USA	50; outpatients	SCID-P; DSM-IV	OCD 26%; OCS 20%
Cassano et al. (1998)	Italy	31; inpatients	SCID, DSM-IIIR	OCD 29%
Dominquez et al. (1999)	Mexico	52; outpatients	Chart review, self-rated MOCI for OCS	OCS 32.7%
Meghani et al. (1998)	USA	192; outpatients	SCID and self-report measures	OCD 31.7%
Cosoff et al. (1998)	Australia	60; inpatients	SCID; DSM-IIIR	OCD 13%
Higuchi et al. (1999)	Japan	45; inpatients/ outpatients	SCID; DSM-IIIR	OCD 20%
Kruger et al. (2000)	Germany	76; inpatients	SCID; DSM-IIIR	OCD 15.8%
Tibbo et al. (2000)	Canada	52; outpatients	SCID; DSM-IV	OCD 25%
Lysaker et al. (2000)	USA	46; outpatients	Chart review	OCD 45%
Bermanzohn et al. (2000)	USA	37; outpatients	SCID; DSM-IV	OCD 29.7%
Poyurovsky et al. (2000)	Israel	68; inpatients	SCID; DSM-IV	OCD 23.5%
Fabisch et al. (2001)	Austria	150; inpatients	Operational criteria for OCS	OCS 10%
Bayle et al. (2001)	France	40; inpatients/ outpatients	Clinical diagnosis	OCD 35%
Goodwin et al. (2003)	USA	184; inpatients	DIGS; DSM-IIIR	OCD 5.4%

Table 6.2 (cont.)

Authors	Country	Study sample size and type	Study design, diagnostic criteria for schizophrenia and OCD	Prevalence of OCD/OCS in schizophrenia
Ohta et al. (2003)	Japan	71; inpatients/outpatients	SCID, DSM-IV	OCD 18.3
Pallanti et al. (2004)	Italy	80; outpatients	SCID; DSM-IV	OCD 22.5%
Kayahan et al. (2005)	Turkey	100; outpatients	SCID; DSM-IV	OCD 30%; OCS 64%
Byerly et al. (2005)	USA	100; outpatients	SCID; DSM-IV	OCD 23%; OCS 30%
Ongür and Goff (2005)	USA	118; outpatients	SCID; DSM-IV	OCD 8.8%
Adolescent schizophrenia				
Nechmad et al. (2003)	Israel	50; inpatients	SCID; DSM-IV	OCD 26%
Ross et al. (2006)	USA	83; outpatients	Kiddie-SADS-PL; DSM-IV	OCD 20%
Elderly schizophrenia				
Poyurovsky et al. (2005)	Israel	50; inpatients	SCID; DSM-IV	OCD 16%

SCID, Structured Clinical Interview for DSM-Patient Edition; OCD/OCS, obsessive-compulsive disorder/symptoms; MOCI, Maudsley Obsessive-Compulsive Inventory; DIGS, Diagnostic Interview for Genetic Studies; Kiddie-SADS-PL, Schedule for Affective Disorders and Schizophrenia for school-age children-present and lifetime version.

second-generation antipsychotics (SGAs). First-episode research methodology addresses this issue by estimation of obsessive–compulsive phenomena in drug-naive schizophrenia patients experiencing their first psychotic episode. As shown in Table 6.2, a comparable rate of OCD was noted in first-episode, predominantly drug-naive patients, indicating that OCD apparently is not consequent to primary schizophrenia-related factors.

Overall, reports since the mid 1990s are remarkably consistent in demonstrating that the odds for OCD in schizophrenia patients are considerably higher than would be expected in random epidemiological comorbidity, suggesting a pathophysiological linkage between the two disorders.

Phenomenology of OCD in schizophrenia

Research into schizophrenia–OCD comorbidity has been hampered by questionable reliability and validity of the identification of OCS in schizophrenia. This uncertainty is accounted for by the existing overlap between obsessions and delusions and/or formal thought disorders, as well as compulsions and schizophrenic mannerisms and stereotypic behavior.

According to DSM-IV criteria, OCD is characterized by recurrent, persistent, and intrusive thoughts; images or impulses (obsessions); and repetitive actions (compulsions) or mental rituals that are aimed at preventing or reducing anxiety and distress that arise from obsessions. Obsessive thoughts are "a product of the patients' own mind" and are recognized to be unreasonable and excessive, as opposed to "thought insertion," which is symptomatic of schizophrenia. Sometimes, obsessions can be distinguished from delusions by the person's insight into the nature of the impairment (ego-dystonic obsession versus ego-syntonic delusion), affect (obsession-associated anxiety versus delusion-associated paranoid affect) or associated actions (repetitive rituals versus delusional persecutory behavior). Accordingly, distinction of obsessions from the schizophrenia symptom of "thought insertion" is based on the evaluation of thought possession (own versus alien), agency thinking (own versus alien) and ego-boundary (intact versus permeated) (Mullins and Spence 2003). In clinical reality, however, the existing overlap between delusional and obsessive phenomena poses a significant diagnostic challenge. Patients with "pure" OCD may exhibit varying degrees of insight ranging from total lack of insight to full insight (Eisen and Rasmussen

1993). Poor insight has been found in a substantial proportion (10–36%) of OCD patients (Catapano *et al.* 2001; Matsunaga *et al.* 2002). Moreover, delusional transformation of obsessions has been described (Insel and Akiskal 1986). Alternatively, the concept of delusion as a complete loss of insight was challenged by the demonstration of dimensions of delusions, and the term "recovering delusion" was used to highlight the possibility of the patients' partial awareness of the falsity of the delusional idea (Appelbaum *et al.* 1999). The concept of "obsessive delusions" was put forward to refer to a complex symptom phenomenon, obsessional in form and delusional in content (Bermanzohn *et al.* 1997). Hallucinations may also become the "intrusive focus" of a patients' attention and have been referred to as "compulsive hallucinations" (Bermanzohn *et al.* 1997).

Although the identification of OCS in schizophrenia, and the distinction of obsessions from delusions, is challenging, growing evidence indicates that OC symptoms can be reliably identified in a substantial proportion of patients by instruments valid for typical OCD such as the Yale–Brown Obsessive-Compulsive Scale (Y-BOCS; Goodman *et al.* 1989). Thus, examining psychometric properties of Y-BOCS in assessing severity of OCS in patients with schizophrenia, de Haan *et al.* (2006) found good internal consistency and inter-rater reliability of the scale, supporting its utility in schizophrenia patients. Furthermore, explicitly evaluating insight into OCS in a sample of hospitalized schizo-obsessive patients, using the Brown Assessment of Beliefs Scale (Eisen *et al.* 1998), Poyurovsky *et al.* (2007) found that a majority of patients (48 of 57 [85%]) exhibited good or fair insight into OCS. The proportion of patients with poor insight in this study (15%) is within the range 10–36% observed in "pure" OCD (Catapano *et al.* 2001; Matsunaga *et al.* 2002), and corresponds to the 12% revealed in the large-scale Brown Longitudinal OCD study (Pinto *et al.* 2006). Overall, these findings strongly support the premise that OCS in schizophrenia is an identifiable dimension of psychopathology independent of core schizophrenia symptoms. Remarkably, insight into OCS positively correlated with global awareness of schizophrenia; however, there was a lack of association between insight into OCS and awareness of delusions (Poyurovsky *et al.* 2007). This is consistent with our clinical experience with the schizo-obsessive subgroup, indicating that it is not uncommon that, while the patients refer to OCS

as senseless and distressful (i.e., ego-dystonic), they may be fully convinced of the "true" nature of their delusional ideas (e.g., persecution, and so ego-syntonic). Longitudinal evaluation of the temporal inter-relationship between insight into OCS and awareness of schizophrenia during the course of illness is imperative, since the degree of insight may fluctuate and some schizo-obsessive individuals with good or fair insight develop delusional transformation of OCS, particularly during psychotic exacerbations. Such prospective assessment, in turn, would contribute to a better recognition of OCS in schizophrenia throughout the entire course of illness.

Studies examining clinical characteristics of schizo-obsessive patients are consistent in revealing a striking similarity of primary OCS in schizo-obsessive individuals and "pure" OCD patients (Eisen *et al.* 1997; Tibbo *et al.* 2000; Poyurovsky *et al.* 2001; Ohta *et al.* 2003; Ongür and Goff 2005; Pinto *et al.* 2006; Rajkumar *et al.* 2008). Like their OCD counterparts, the majority of schizo-obsessive patients have both obsessions and compulsions, with only a few patients exhibiting mono-symptomatic OCS. There is also consistency regarding the most frequently observed OC symptoms (aggressive, contamination and somatic obsessions; cleaning/washing, counting, ordering/arranging and hoarding compulsions). The severity of OCS in schizo-obsessive patients, measured by the Y-BOCS, ranges from moderate to severe (Y-BOCS scores of 16–40), thus supporting their clinical significance. These findings and lack of intercorrelation in the severity of OCS and core schizophrenia symptoms in a majority of reports lends additional support to the independent nature of OCS and their clinical significance in schizo-obsessive patients.

On the basis of the inter-relationship between OCS and schizophrenia symptoms, the following complex psychopathological phenotypes were identified: (1) "classic" ego-dystonic obsessions and/or compulsions unrelated to the content of delusions and hallucinations, and (2) OCS related to the content of delusions and hallucinations in addition to "classic" ego-dystonic OCD symptoms. Box 6.1 illustrates these two phenotypes.

In addition to these psychopathological schizo-obsessive phenotypes, there is an alternative phenotype characterized by complete interference of OCS with delusions, hallucinations, and formal thought disorders, associated with lack of insight and absence of typical OCD symptoms throughout the entire

Box 6.1 Case examples of the two phenotypes with differing inter-relationship of obsessive-compulsive symptoms and schizophrenic symptoms

Obsessive-compulsive symptoms independent of schizophrenia symptoms

A 24-year-old unmarried man was admitted to a psychiatric hospital for a first acute psychotic episode characterized by delusions of persecution, auditory hallucinations, and bizarre behavior. Eight months earlier, the patient complained that his neighbors were watching him and were trying to hypnotize him. He also heard voices "making fun of him." These psychotic symptoms were associated with a substantial social decline and functional impairment. A DSM-IV diagnosis of schizophrenic disorder, paranoid type was established. According to both the patient and his parents, since age 15, he had constantly worried that he would hurt his parents, and to neutralize these thoughts, he touched his nose repeatedly. He also had an irresistible urge to count steps while walking and to keep all school belongings in symmetry. He recognized that his worries and rituals were excessive and unreasonable. At age 18, OCD was diagnosed. His OCD symptoms were unnoticed during the current psychotic episode owing to the severe and pervasive nature of the paranoid delusions, but they became detectable after resolution of psychosis.

Obsessive-compulsive symptoms overlapping with positive schizophrenia symptoms

A 50-year-old single woman had an 18-year history of DSM-IV schizophrenic disorder, paranoid type, characterized by delusions of persecution, auditory hallucinations, and formal thought disorders. Negative symptoms included flat affect and significant decline in social interests. At age 35, three years after her first schizophrenic episode, she complained of intrusive, distressful, and time-consuming thoughts that she was cursing God. She was convinced that other people knew about these thoughts and were able to "read her mind." She had a constant need for reassurance and repeatedly asked others if she deserved punishment. In addition, the patient had typical compulsions (repeated checking of electrical appliances and counting floor tiles) unrelated to schizophrenia symptoms. She was aware of the unreasonable nature of these acts but was unable to resist performing them. The obsessive thoughts of cursing God were exacerbated during psychotic episodes and diminished in remission, when she gained partial insight into their intrusive nature. By contrast, her compulsive non-schizophrenia-related behavior did not surface during acute psychotic episodes but became prominent during remission.

course of the illness (Porto *et al.* 1997; Poyurovsky *et al.* 2003).

Considering the substantial overlap between OCS and positive schizophrenic symptoms and the diagnostic pitfalls in identification of OCS in schizophrenia, Bottas *et al.* (2005) suggested that the following guidelines might assist in identification of OCS in the presence of psychosis:

- in general, OCS in schizophrenia are phenomenologically similar to DSM-IV "pure" OCD
- a repetitious behavior should be considered a compulsion if it occurs in response to an obsession but not delusion
- recurrent intrusive ego-dystonic thoughts should not be considered obsessions if they are related exclusively to delusional themes; reassessment of these "questionable obsessions" may be necessary after resolution of acute psychotic symptoms
- primary obsessional slowness may be mistaken for prodromal schizophrenia or thought disorder;

such patients may be unable to articulate any obsessions and may exhibit no compulsions.

Overall, from the phenomenological perspective, a schizo-obsessive phenotype most likely represents a heterogeneous group of psychopathological expressions with a complex inter-relationship between OCS and schizophrenia symptoms. Differences in symptom profiles, with distinct "proximity" of OCS to psychotic dimension, may imply differences in pathophysiology or etiology; they could reflect differences between OCD as a comorbid disorder or as an additional psychopathological dimension of schizophrenia.

Effect of obsessive-compulsive symptoms on schizophrenia symptom severity

Reports are inconsistent with respect to the effect of OCS on the severity of schizophrenia symptoms, with some studies, primarily in recent-onset psychosis, showing lower severity of delusions and formal thought disorders (Poyurovsky *et al.* 1999a; Tibbo *et al.* 2000; de Haan *et al.* 2006) and others showing higher severity of schizophrenia symptoms predominantly in chronic schizo-obsessive patients (Lysaker *et al.* 2000; Ongür and Goff 2005). The majority of studies, however, did not reveal any differences in the severity of positive schizophrenia symptoms between schizophrenia patients with and without OCD (Poyurovsky *et al.* 2001; Ohta *et al.* 2003; Byerly *et al.* 2005; de Haan *et al.* 2005). These discrepancies may be accounted for by the cross-sectional design of the studies and the inclusion of diverse patient populations (e.g., recent onset, chronic). It is conceivable that OCS exert a "moderating" effect on the expression of some positive schizophrenia symptoms only during the initial stages of schizophrenia. Consistently, more severe negative symptomatology has been observed in patients with chronic schizophrenia and OCD (Fenton and McGlashan 1986; Lysaker *et al.* 2000). Since negative, but not positive, symptoms are associated with a greater likelihood of cognitive impairment and poor clinical outcome, it is not surprising that schizo-obsessive patients are generally characterized by poorer prognosis, lower functioning, and more pronounced neurocognitive deficits (Fenton and McGlashan 1986; Berman *et al.* 1995; Lysaker *et al.* 2000, 2002; Poyurovsky *et al.* 2001).

The first systematic review and meta-analysis (23 and 18 studies, respectively) aimed to clarify the effect of OCS/OCD on the severity of schizophrenia symptoms has recently been completed (Cunill *et al.* 2009). The presence of OCS in schizo-obsessive patients was associated with higher global symptoms as compared with schizophrenia patients: standardized mean difference, 0.39 (95% confidence interval [CI], 0.14–0.64); positive dimension, 0.28 (95% CI, 0.00–0.56); and negative dimension, 0.36 (95% CI, 0.11–0.62). However, the magnitude of association was modest at best, especially for positive and negative dimensions, and the sensitivity analysis showed a loss of association when the studies with the largest effect sizes were withdrawn. Moreover, when a categorical definition of OCD was used, no effect of OCD on the severity of schizophrenia symptoms was found. A substantial heterogeneity arising from different study designs and sample characteristics is a major limitation of this meta-analysis. In addition, longitudinal prospective evaluation of a putative modifying effect of OCS on the severity of schizophrenia symptoms is clearly warranted.

Clinical course

Evaluation of temporal inter-relationships between OCS and schizophrenia symptoms has neurobiological, prognostic, and treatment implications. Devulapalli *et al.* (2008) conducted a meta-analysis of the results from eight studies reporting age at onset of OCS and schizophrenia symptoms in schizo-obsessive patients. Analysis of age at onset of the two disorders revealed that roughly half of the patients (71 of 148) were diagnosed with OCD prior to schizophrenia, whereas 45 (30.4%) were diagnosed with schizophrenic symptoms first and the remaining 32 (21.6%) with both disorders concurrently. When comparing the percentages of patients diagnosed with OCD first to those diagnosed with schizophrenia, statistical significance was reached when a fixed effects model was used ($p = 0.04$). All studies reported a lower age of OCD onset (mean, 21.2 years) than the age of schizophrenia onset (mean, 24.9 years); however, there were no statistically significant differences between the mean ages of onset in the individual studies, primarily because of insufficient power.

The finding that OCS precedes schizophrenic symptoms in a substantial proportion of schizo-obsessive patients indicates that at least some of them were diagnosed with "pure" OCD prior to schizophrenia and treated with serotonin reuptake inhibitors (SRIs) (Poyurovsky *et al.* 2008a). It is plausible that the use of SRIs, while ameliorating OCS, may accelerate the emergence of the first psychotic symptoms of schizophrenia. Prospective identification of predictors of transition from OCD to schizo-obsessive disorder has apparent diagnostic and treatment implications.

Additional OCD spectrum disorders

Obsessive-compulsive disorder is a highly comorbid condition, of which major depressive disorder and anxiety disorders are the most frequently diagnosed comorbidities (Nestadt *et al.* 2001; Ruscio *et al.* 2010). It has also been strongly associated with somatoform disorders, body dysmorphic disorder (BDD), hypochondriasis, chronic tic disorders, and eating disorders (McElroy *et al.* 1994; Bartz and Hollander 2006). It has been suggested that some of these comorbid conditions (e.g., BDD and tic disorders) may share common etiologic pathways with OCD, while others (e.g., major depressive disorder) may represent secondary syndromes (McElroy *et al.*

1994; Nestadt *et al.* 2001). Indeed, considerable overlap has been found in the clinical presentation, familial inheritance, basal ganglia dysfunction, and pharmacotherapy of BDD, tic disorders, and OCD, which supports the existence of a putative OCD spectrum (Bartz and Hollander 2006). If OCS represent a separate psychopathological dimension in schizophrenia, it is plausible that, similar to "pure" OCD, there is a preferential aggregation of OCD spectrum disorders in schizo-obsessive patients but not in their non-OCD schizophrenia counterparts. The results of such comparative evaluation of comorbid disorders in what appeared to be the largest sample of schizo-obsessive patients to date (100) have been reported by Poyurovsky *et al.* (2006a). Using the SCID for axis I disorders (SCID-I) and stepwise logistic regression to analyze differences in comorbid disorders between the two schizophrenia groups with and without OCD, compelling evidence of differentiation with respect to OCD spectrum disorders has been found. Hence, the schizo-obsessive group had a substantially higher rate of BDD (schizo-obsessive, 8 of 100 patients; schziophrenia, 0 of 100 patients; $p = 0.039$) and chronic tic disorders (schizo-obsessive, 16 of 100 patients; schizophrenia, 4 of 100 patients; odds ratio 4.57; $p = 0.018$). There was also a higher rate of comorbid eating disorders; however, the difference was no longer significant after adjustment for a between-group difference in age at onset of schizophrenia. Overall, combining OCD spectrum disorders (BDD, tic disorders, eating disorders, hypochondriasis) yielded a robust between-group difference in the number of patients with OCD spectrum disorder (schizo-obsessive, 30/100 patients; schizophrenia, 8/100 patients; odds ratio 4.35; $p = 0.001$). Since no significant between-group difference in the rate of major depressive disorder, anxiety disorders, and substance use disorders was revealed, it is likely that there is a specific elevation in the rate of OCD spectrum disorders in the schizo-obsessive group rather than an elevation of psychopathology in general. From the clinical perspective, the finding of an aggregation of OCD spectrum disorders in schizo-obsessive patients justifies a systematic search for and assessment of these comorbidities in schizophrenia patients. Conversely, since the presence of OCD spectrum disorders increases the odds of OCD in schizophrenia patients, targeting these additional syndromes may improve identification of an obsessive-compulsive component in schizophrenia.

Occurrence of OCD in specific schizophrenia populations

Childhood-onset and adolescent schizophrenia

Early-onset forms of disorders are an avenue to the understanding of underlying mechanisms of disease in general medicine. Molecular genetic discoveries in human diseases as diverse as breast cancer, Alzheimer's disease, and insulin-dependent diabetes mellitus have been tied to subsets of patients with an earlier age of onset of illness. There is increasing evidence indicating that both childhood- and adolescent-onset schizophrenia lie on the clinical and neurobiological continuum with the adult-onset disorder (Nicolson *et al.* 2000). Data suggesting clinical continuity of early-and adult-onset schizo-obsessive disorder is currently emerging. Hence, the Colorado Childhood-Onset Schizophrenia Research Program, focusing on genetic factors, physiological correlates, and treatment of children who develop schizophrenia or schizoaffective disorder prior to their 13th birthday, examined the prevalence of comorbid disorders (Ross *et al.* 2006). Using a structured clinical interview, the authors assessed 83 children (mean age, 9.9 ± 2.5 years) and found that 99% of the sample had at least one lifetime comorbid axis I diagnosis (Ross *et al.* 2006). The most common comorbid diagnoses were attention-deficit hyperactivity disorder (84%), affective disorders (34%), and anxiety disorders (55%). The occurrence of OCD was identified in 13% (3/83) of girls and 23% (14/83) of boys, resulting in total lifetime rate of 20%, a remarkably similar finding to that found in adult-onset schizophrenia. The fact that more boys than girls with schizophrenia had comorbid OCD is noteworthy, since it is conceivable that schizo-obsessive boys have an earlier age at onset of OCD similar to their counterparts with "pure" OCD. Notably, the rate of pharmacological treatment for comorbid syndromes in this study was low, less than 25%, suggesting that focusing on treatment of schizophrenia and disregarding comorbid conditions may contribute to poor outcomes for schizophrenia patients with comorbid disorders (Bermanzohn *et al.* 2000). The lack of empirically supported guidelines for treatment of comorbid conditions in schizophrenia, however, may also play a role.

Preliminary findings concerning the rate of occurrence of DSM-IV OCD in adolescent schizophrenia appears to be akin to that found in childhood- and adult-onset forms. Nechmad *et al.* (2003) revealed that of 50 hospitalized adolescents with schizophrenia and schizoaffective disorder (32 boys, 18 girls; mean age 17.0 ± 2.1 years; mean age at schizophrenia onset 14.8 ± 2.2 years), 13 (26.0%) also met the DSM-IV criteria for OCD. Compared with the non-OCD schizophrenia patients, the schizo-obsessive adolescents in this study had negative symptoms that were significantly more severe, and there was a positive correlation between the severity of negative symptoms and OCS. In addition, despite the similar ages at onset of schizophrenia, a higher, although statistically non-significant, percentage of schizo-obsessive patients than of non-OCD schizophrenia patients required re-hospitalization (53.8% and 37.8%, respectively). These findings suggest that the interaction of OCD and more severe schizophrenic symptoms (e.g., negative symptoms) creates a poorer prognosis for adolescent schizophrenia patients with OCD that is similar to that seen in their adult counterparts.

The same authors went on to conduct a systematic phenomenological characterization of the two carefully matched groups of adolescent schizophrenia patients with and without OCD (22 patients each; age 13–18 years; number of hospitalizations 1 to 3) (Faragian *et al.* 2008; Poyurovsky *et al.* 2008a). Within the schizo-obsessive group, the majority of patients (20/22, 90.9%) had both obsessions and compulsions of moderate to severe severity that preceded or co-occurred with the onset of schizophrenia. Like adults, the majority of the adolescent schizo-obsessive patients (86.3%) exhibited good or fair insight into OCD, as assessed by the Brown Assessment of Beliefs Scale. The effect size of the correlation between insight into OCD and awareness of schizophrenia in the schizo-obsessive group was negligible ($r = 0.15$, $p = 0.52$); and there were no correlations between Y-BOCS subscale scores and positive, negative, or disorganized dimension scores ($r = 0.07$–0.29; $p > 0.1$). Overall, these findings indicate that OCS in adolescent schizo-obsessive patients, akin to adults, are distinct and distinguishable from core schizophrenia symptoms. Box 6.2 gives a case example of an adolescent schizophrenia patient with OCS.

Remarkably, in this study, age at onset of schizophrenia, as determined by the emergence of first psychotic symptoms, was significantly earlier in the schizo-obsessive group than in the non-OCD schizophrenia group (12.4 ± 2.9 years vs. 14.9 ± 2.3 years; $p = 0.002$). Earlier age at onset of schizophrenia symptoms in the adolescent schizo-obsessive group is noteworthy since it may indicate an accentuated neurodevelopmental origin of the schizo-obsessive subgroup. Early-onset subtypes of schizophrenia and

---

Box 6.2 Case example: an adolescent schizophrenia patient with obsessive-compulsive symptoms

Ms. S, a 16-year-old girl, was admitted to a psychiatric hospital following her first acute psychotic episode characterized by psychomotor agitation, delusions of reference and persecution, and auditory hallucinations. Three months prior to admission, she complained that her classmates were talking about her, reading her mind, and deliberately confusing her by sending "hypnotized messages." She also heard voices that made derogatory comments about her appearance. An abrupt change in behavior that tended towards delinquency and a substantial decline in school achievements accompanied these psychotic symptoms. A DSM-IV diagnosis of schizophrenic disorder, paranoid type, was established. According to both the patient and her parents, since age 12, she constantly performed cleaning and washing rituals for fear of contracting "a dirty disease." She also had an irresistible urge to check her school belongings and keep them in a special "magic" order. She had a constant need for reassurance and repeatedly asked her parents if she had performed her rituals in "just the right" order. She recognized that her worries and rituals were unreasonable and excessive but was unable to control them. At age 14, two years prior to her first psychotic episode, DSM-IV OCD was diagnosed and treatment with an antiobsessive agent, fluvoxamine (up to 200 mg/day), was initiated. Retrospective analysis of the course of illness revealed that initial psychotic symptoms developed during fluvoxamine administration. The positive schizophrenia symptoms beneficially responded to monotherapy with antipsychotic risperidone (3 mg/day). The OCS were present during the prodromal phase of schizophrenia, were unnoticed during the current acute psychotic episode, and became identifiable after resolution of psychosis. After resolution of the acute psychosis, fluvoxamine (100 mg/day) was resumed as an adjunctive medication to an ongoing regimen of risperidone (2 mg/day). Six months of combined risperidone–fluvoxamine treatment was associated with a remission of positive schizophrenia symptoms and a gradual decline of OCS severity.

OCD have been suggested as valuable endophenotypes in the search for pathogenetic mechanisms of both conditions (Jablensky 2006; Sobin *et al.* 2000). Finally, compared with schizophrenia patients, a significantly higher percentage of adolescent schizo-obsessive patients had SCID-detectable OCD spectrum disorders, primarily tic disorders, (51.2% vs. 5.9%, $p < 0.01$), but not mood, anxiety, or substance use disorders. These findings corroborate preferential aggregation of OCD spectrum disorders found in adult schizo-obsessive patients.

Although far from being conclusive, the results of phenomenological characterization of adolescent schizo-obsessive patients imply that the presence of OCD modifies some clinical characteristics of schizophrenia, and that the pattern of this modifying effect is comparable with that revealed in adult schizo-obsessive patients. This, in turn, lends support to the assumption that, akin to "pure" schizophrenia, there is a clinical continuity between adolescent and adult forms of schizophrenia associated with OCD. Further studies are needed to evaluate the neurobiological (genetic, imaging, neurocognitive) foundation for a putative phenomenological continuity between adolescent and adult forms of schizo-obsessive subset of schizophrenia.

Elderly schizophrenia

Clinical significance of obsessive–compulsive phenomena in adolescent and adult schizophrenia, along with evidence indicating that symptoms of both schizophrenia and OCD persist into senescence in a substantial proportion of patients (Skoog and Skoog 1999), prompted explicit evaluation of rate of occurrence of OCD in elderly schizophrenia patients. Fifty elderly patients consecutively hospitalized for acute exacerbation of DSM-IV schizophrenia or schizoaffective disorder were assessed using SCID and appropriate rating scales (Poyurovsky *et al.* 2006b). Of the 50 participants, eight (16%) also met DSM-IV criteria for OCD. Schizophrenia patients with and without OCD did not differ significantly in demographic and clinical variables. In four of the eight in the schizo-obsessive group, OCD first appeared in the third decade, preceded the onset of schizophrenia and persisted into senescence. In the remaining schizo-obsessive patients, OCD mean age of onset was 52.6 ± 5.2 years, roughly 15 years after the onset of schizophrenia. Since in all patients OCD preceded administration

of atypical antipsychotic agents, their role in OCD occurrence was negligible. Instead, the authors hypothesized that the late onset of OCD was related to a complex interaction of chronic course of schizophrenia, aging, and unknown OCD-predisposing factors associated putatively with basal ganglia pathology. Notably, late-onset OCD has been reported in association with brain pathology, such as stroke, Parkinson's disease, and dementias, which may superimpose schizophrenia in elderly individuals (Voon *et al.* 2006). Clinical impact of OCD in elderly schizophrenia is supported by an increased rate of readmissions (Prince *et al.* 2008) and by a reduced quality of well-being (Wetherell *et al.* 2003) in elderly schizo-obsessive patients compared with individuals with "pure" schizophrenia. Identification of this potentially treatable condition is imperative to provide adequate care of elderly schizophrenia patients.

Schizotypal personality disorder in OCD patients

Schizotypal personality disorder (SPD) shares common phenomenological, biological, genetic, and treatment response characteristics with schizophrenia (Siever and Davis 2004). Intercorrelation between schizotypal and OC dimensions has been consistently found in non-clinical samples of students selected on the basis of self-report scales of schizotypy (Dinn *et al.* 2002), as well as in the treatment-seeking OCD population (Rossi and Daneluzzo 2002). Nevertheless, the rate of occurrence of SPD in OCD is yet to be clarified. The observed rates vary substantially (0–50%) (Table 6.3). This may be explained by differences in the definition of schizotypal features (categorical versus dimensional), method of evaluation (structured interview versus chart review), and the patient population studied. Despite their methodological differences, studies are consistent in demonstrating that OCD patients with associated SPD exhibit a more deteriorative course and poorer prognosis than those with "pure" OCD (Baer *et al.* 1990; Eisen and Rasmussen 1993; Ravizza *et al.* 1995). None of these studies, however, was prospective.

The clinical validity of the OCD–schizotypy association is supported by the revealed differences in demographic and clinical characteristics of OCD patients with and without schizotypal features (Eisen and Rasmussen 1993; Matsunaga *et al.* 2000; Sobin *et al.* 2000). Specifically, early age of onset, male gender,

Table 6.3 Rate of occurrence of schizotypal personality disorder in patients with obsessive-compulsive disorder

Authors	Study sample	Study design and diagnostic criteria	Prevalence of schizotypal personality disorder in OCD	Comments
Jenike et al. (1986)	43 OCD patients	Chart review, DSM-III for SPD	33%	OCD–SPD patients had poorer prognosis
Rasmussen and Tsuang (1986)	44 OCD patients	Semistructured interview	0%	
Baer et al. (1990)	96 OCD patients	SCID for DSM-III personality disorders	5%	SPD a predictor of poor outcome in OCD
Black et al. (1993)	32 OCD patients; 33 controls	SCID for DSM-III personality disorders	18.8% OCD; 3% controls	OCD patients also had more cluster C personality disorders
Eisen and Rasmussen (1993)	475 OCD patients	Semistructured interview, DSM-IIIR criteria for OCD and SPD	3%	A majority of OCD–SPD patients were men and had a deteriorative course
Sobin et al. (2000)	119 OCD patients	Self-rated scale for schizotypy	50%	OCD patients with schizotypy had earlier age of onset, more comorbid diagnoses, and learning disability
Samuels et al. (2000)	72 OCD probands and 72 controls; plus their first-degree relatives	Direct interview	0% OCD; 1.4% control probands	
Matsunaga et al. (2000)	94 OCD patients	SCID for personality disorders	23% men 4% women	

SPD, schizotypal personality disorder; SCID, Structured Clinical Interview for DSM-Patient Edition; DSM, *Diagnostic and Statistical Manual of Mental Disorders.*

counting compulsions, and a history of specific phobia substantially increased the odds of schizotypy in patients with lifetime OCD. In addition, more schizotypal OCD patients than their "pure" OCD counterparts appeared to be unmarried and unemployed. Explicitly evaluating two groups of OCD patients with and without SPD (15 patients and 31 patients, respectively), Poyurovsky et al. (2008b) identified poorer insight, higher negative schizophrenia symptom scores, and lower general functioning scores in the schizotypal OCD group. Interestingly, not only did schizotypal OCD patients exhibit poor insight into OCD symptoms, a substantial proportion (approximately 20%) also developed delusional transformation of obsessions. Overall, schizotypal OCD patients seem to have marital, occupational, and general functioning deficits akin to individuals with schizophrenia-spectrum disorders. This study is noteworthy in that that family information regarding OCD and schizophrenia-spectrum disorders

in 131 first-degree relatives of the two OCD groups, with and without SPD, was obtained. As expected, there was a substantial aggregation of OCD cases in the relatives of both groups (13% in each), supporting a well-established familial transmission of the disorder (Pauls 2008). In contrast, 33% of the schizotypal OCD patients had at least one first-degree relative with schizophrenia-spectrum disorders while only 3% did so in the "pure" OCD group ($\chi^2 = 5.48$; $p = 0.019$). The fact that the schizotypal OCD group had a family load of schizophrenia-spectrum disorders indicates that, in a subset of patients, OCD and schizophrenia-spectrum disorders co-transmit in families. From the clinical perspective, detection of schizophrenia-spectrum disorders in first-degree relatives may contribute to better identification of schizotypal personality disorder in OCD patients.

Compelling evidence indicates that the presence of SPD predicts poor response to standard pharmacological (selective SRIs [SSRIs]) and behavioral intervention in OCD patients and seems to be a predictor of response to a low dose of adjunctive antipsychotic agents (McDougle *et al.* 1990). Overall, a category of OCD with schizotypal features seems to have clinical and predictive validity and probably etiological specificity. However, well-designed controlled comparative studies evaluating clinical characteristics and neurobiological and neurocognitive markers in OCD patients with and without schizotypal features are warranted to provide a comprehensive characterization of an OCD–SPD subgroup and its differentiation from the schizo-obsessive subgroup of schizophrenia.

Treatment of schizophrenia with obsessive-compulsive symptoms

Although there is growing recognition of the occurrence of OCS in schizophrenia, research addressing treatment interventions in this difficult-to-treat patient population is still in the initial stages. Well-designed large-scale controlled studies in schizo-obsessive patients are lacking.

Addition of serotonin reuptake inhibitors

The independent nature of OCS in a vast majority of schizo-obsessive individuals, and their clinical similarity with "pure" OCD, prompted evaluation of the adjunctive antiobsessive agents in antipsychotic-treated schizo-obsessive patients. Fluvoxamine added to a stable regimen of first-generation antipsychotic drugs (FGAs) (14 patients; 100–200 mg/day for eight weeks) accounted for a greater reduction in Y-BOCS total score ($p = 0.02$) and compulsion subscale ($p < 0.05$) as compared with schizo-obsessive patients randomized to continue previous antipsychotic therapy (16 patients) (Reznik and Sirota 2000) An additional and clinically meaningful advantage of adjunctive fluvoxamine was an improvement in OCD-related pathological slowness and doubt. Clinical utility of the drug was supported by the results of an open-label study of fluvoxamine addition to FGAs (up to 150 mg/day for 12 weeks) among 10 inpatients with clinically stable DSM-IV schizophrenic disorder and comorbid OCD (Poyurovsky *et al.* 1999b).There was a significant improvement in an obsessive component of OCD ($p < 0.02$) in addition to a modest improvement of both positive and negative schizophrenia symptoms. This study draws attention to fluvoxamine's potential to exacerbate psychosis and increase aggressiveness in schizo-obsessive patients with prior indications of impulsivity and aggressive behavior. It is plausible that patients with clinically significant aggressiveness may be at higher risk of psychotic exacerbation treatment with adjunctive fluvoxamine and probably other SSRIs.

Adjunctive clomipramine, a tricyclic antidepressant and a non-selective SRI, was also evaluated as a putative therapeutic option. A small placebo-controlled crossover study and a number of case reports revealed that clomipramine (dose range from 50 to 300 mg/day) was associated with beneficial effect on OCS, reduction of anxiety accompanied by compulsive rituals, and improvement of positive and negative schizophrenia symptoms in some schizo-obsessive patients (Zohar *et al.* 1993; Berman *et al.* 1995; Poyurovsky and Weizman 1998). However, a lack of therapeutic effect of clomipramine and exacerbation of psychosis were also reported (Margetis 2008). In addition, the anticholinergic properties of clomipramine, as well as its cardiovascular side effects and associated weight gain, limit its utility in schizophrenia patients, particularly those who are treated with low-potency FGAs, anticholinergic agents, or clozapine.

Overall, the fact that a sizeable proportion of schizo-obsessive patients does not respond or is intolerant to an SRI addition indicates that OCS in schizophrenia is not readily amenable to antiobsessional agents. No predictors of response and long-term treatment outcomes have yet been established. An additional pitfall of the SRI–antipsychotic drug combination is the potential for clinically significant pharmacokinetic drug interactions. Indeed, elevated plasma concentrations of haloperidol and clozapine five- to tenfold with adjunctive fluvoxamine and roughly twofold with adjunctive fluoxetine and paroxetine have been reported (Hiemke *et al.* 1994). This, in turn, may increase the likelihood of antipsychotic drug-induced side effects (e.g., extrapyramidal side effects, decreased seizure threshold).

Monotherapy with atypical antipsychotic agents

Monotherapy with FGAs appears to be ineffective in schizo-obsessive patients presumably because of their limited serotonergic properties (Green *et al.* 2003). The bulk of reports to date indicates that SGAs with their serotonin/dopamine antagonism may induce de novo or aggravate preexisting OCS in schizophrenia patients (described below). Yet there is growing evidence indicating that monotherapy with certain SGAs may alleviate preexisting OCS in schizophrenia patients, pointing toward a bi-directional effect of SGAs on OCS in schizophrenia. To address this issue, van Nimwegen et al. (2008) conducted a large-scale randomized comparative study of olanzapine (59 patients) and risperidone (63 patients) in young patients with recent-onset schizophrenia–spectrum disorders. The primary outcome measure was the mean baseline-to-endpoint change in total score on the Y-BOCS. By the end of a six-week trial, olanzapine (mean dose 11.3 mg) but not risperidone (mean dose 3.0 mg) was associated with a meaningful decrease in a severity of OCS (2.2 vs. 0.3; $z = -2.651$; $p < 0.01$). In contrast, although not statistically significant, more patients who initially scored 0 on the Y-BOCS in the risperidone group than in the olanzapine group developed OCS (eight vs. two). This study collaborates earlier reports suggesting that in some schizo-obsessive patients monotherapy with olanzapine may improve both schizophrenic and OC dimensions of psychopathology without running a risk of OCS exacerbation (Poyurovsky et al. 2000) It also raises an intriguing question of differential effects of SGAs on OCS in schizophrenia. From the pharmacological perspective, olanzapine possesses a lower affinity for the serotonin $5-HT_{2A}$ receptor than risperidone (affinity constant 4 ± 0.4 nmol/l for olanzapine and 0.6 ± 0.2 nmol/l for risperidone) and higher affinity for the $5-HT_{2C}$ receptor (11 ± 1 nmol/l for olanzapine and 26 ± 5 nmol/l for for risperidone) (Bymaster 1996). A signal attenuation animal model of OCD supports the relevance of $5-HT_{2C}$ rather than $5-HT_{2A}$ receptor blockade in the orbitofrontal cortex for the antiobsessive effect (Flaisher-Grinberg et al. 2008). Conceivably, olanzapine's lower $5-HT_{2A}$ receptor antagonism may be associated with a lower propensity to induce or exacerbate schizophrenia-related OCS, while its marked $5-HT_{2C}$ receptor blockade accounts for the OCS-ameliorating effect. A differential drug effect on glutamatergic neurotransmission, implicated in the pathogenesis of both schizophrenia and OCD, may also be relevant. Indeed, olanzapine but not risperidone restores the deficit in prepulse inhibition, a model of sensorimotor gating deficits observed in both disorders, induced by N-methyl-D-aspartate (NMDA) receptor inhibitors (Geyer et al. 2001).

Apparently, SGAs are not alike in their effect on schizophrenia-related OCS. "Fine tuning" of the underlying neurotransmitter systems, primarily serotoninergic and dopaminergic, seems to be essential in the OCS-improving rather than the OCS-provoking effect of an antipsychotic drug. In this respect, interesting results of a preliminary investigation of aripiprazole, a SGA with unique pharmacological properties, in schizo-obsessive patients have been reported (Glick et al. 2008). Aripiprazole is distinguished from the majority of SGAs by its partial dopamine agonism coupled with a low $5-HT_2$ to D_2 receptor affinity ratio and a low $5-HT_{1A}$ receptor occupancy (Mamo et al. 2007). Aripiprazole's distinctive receptor pharmacology suggests that it may be of therapeutic value in schizo-obsessive patients without potentially inducing or exacerbating OCS. In a six-week, small open-label, flexible-dose trial, monotherapy with aripiprazole (10–30 mg/day) resulted in a meaningful clinical improvement of OCS in schizophrenia patients who were partially responsive to a prior exposure to either FGAs or SGAs. Six of the seven study completers showed a decrease of roughly 35% from baseline on the Y-BOCS, combined with an improvement of schizophrenia symptoms. It is obvious that even modest improvement of functioning as a result of an improvement in an OCS component, as revealed in this study, may be clinically meaningful for this challenging subset of schizophrenia patients.

An additional avenue in psychopharmacology research for schizo-obsessive disorder focuses on alternative underlying mechanisms shared by the two disorders. Recent findings implicate abnormalities in glutamatergic neurotransmission, in addition to dopaminergic and serotonergic pathways. Specifically, in schizophrenia, characteristic symptoms and cognitive deficits have been produced in remitted schizophrenia patients by the NMDA receptor antagonist ketamine, and agents that stimulate glutamatergic neurotransmission appeared to have antipsychotic properties (Krystal et al. 2005). In OCD, elevated levels of a combined measure of glutamate and glutamine in brain regions relevant to OCD were found by magnetic resonance spectroscopy (Whiteside et al. 2006), as was an increase in glutamate in cerebrospinal fluid (Chakrabarty et al. 2005). Preliminary data indicate a beneficial effect of agents with marked antiglutamatergic properties (memantine, riluzole) in patients with treatment-resistant OCD (Poyurovsky et al. 2005; Pittenger et al. 2006). These findings premised a pilot study of lamotrigine, an anticonvulsant with marked downstream effects on neuronal function including inhibition of glutamate release. In an eight-week, open-label trial, lamotrigine (25 mg/day for one week, 50 mg for two weeks, 100 mg for two weeks, 200 mg for three weeks) was added to ongoing psychotropic drug regimens in 11 schizophrenia patients with clinically significant OCS (Poyurovsky et al. 2010). The Y-BOCS score of the nine patients completing the trial decreased significantly from baseline to week eight (22.9 ± 6.1 vs. 17.4 ± 3.6; $t = 2.33$; $p = 0.033$), and five (55.5%) patients were deemed responders ($\geq$ 35% decrease in a total Y-BOCS score). The OCS-attenuating effect of lamotrigine was not accompanied by improvement of schizophrenia symptoms, supporting evidence for a lack of effectiveness of lamotrigine for schizophrenia symptoms revealed in two recent large-scale studies of lamotrigine addition among schizophrenia patients with residual psychotic symptoms (Goff et al. 2007). In contrast, depressive symptoms, assessed with the Calgary Depression Rating Scale, improved significantly (6.4 ± 1.5 vs. 4.0 ± 2.5; $t = 3.19$; $p = 0.013$), and this change was positively correlated with OCS improvement ($r = 0.69$; $p = 0.04$). Intriguingly, all responders in this small study were patients with schizoaffective disorder, bipolar or depressive type, who had depressive symptoms at trial entry. Lamotrigine was found efficacious in relieving depressive symptoms and maintaining euthymia in patients with bipolar disorder (Ketter and Calabrese 2002). Hence, it is plausible that lamotrigine's beneficial effect on depressive symptoms accounted for a secondary improvement of OCS. Explicit evaluation of lamotrigine's effect on OCS in schizophrenia patients without depressive psychopathology would clarify whether lamotrigine exerts specific antiobsessive properties in those schizo-obsessive patients who have marked affective symptoms.

Overall, progress has been made during the last decade in the pursuit of effective pharmacotherapy for a schizo-obsessive subgroup, and preliminary signs of efficacy have been seen. These signs, however, may well represent an observer- and/or patient-expectancy effect, which is not uncommon in uncontrolled pilot studies. Large-scale randomized controlled trials are desperately needed to substantiate initial encouraging results. The following questions have yet to be answered: Who are the candidates for monotherapy with an SGA among schizo-obsessive individuals, and who would benefit from the addition of antiobsessive agents? At what stage of schizophrenic illness should antiobsessive agents be initiated? What are the short- and the long-term risks and benefits of antipsychotic–SRI combinations in schizo-obsessive patients? How should antipsychotic-induced OCS in schizophrenia patients be dealt with?

Presently in the absence of evidence-based data, the following recommendations may be considered when treating schizo-obsessive patients.

1. Monotherapy with SGAs is a first-line treatment for schizo-obsessive patients. Preliminary reports indicate that olanzapine and aripiprazole exert beneficial effect on both schizophrenia and OCS in some patients. Data regarding therapeutic efficacy of other SGAs (quetiapine, ziprasidone, risperidone) in schizo-obsessive patients are still lacking. A therapeutic benefit should be weighed against a side effect profile for each atypical antipsychotic.
2. Addition of an SSRI to a SGA is the next step when there is insufficient response to monotherapy with an SGA. The OCS in schizophrenia may be considered a target for an antiobsessive drug intervention only when the severity of OCS reaches a threshold for clinical significance, and the clinical features are similar to typical OCD. Antiobsessive agents should be administered only in stabilized patients who are being treated with antipsychotic drugs. In addition, schizo-obsessive patients with a history of impulsivity and aggressiveness may be at higher risk of psychotic exacerbation during adjunctive fluvoxamine and potentially other SSRI treatments. Careful evaluation of the potential risks and benefits of adjunctive pharmacotherapy in schizo-obsessive patients is a prerequisite for successful pharmacotherapy.
3. Lack of response to the first SGA/SSRI combination may justify switching to an alternative SGA/SSRI or clomipramine combination.
4. Since monotherapy with FGAs appears to be of limited value in schizo-obsessive patients, the FGA/SSRI combination may be a reasonable next step prior to initiation of treatment with clozapine. For steps 2–4, pharmacokinetic interactions and potential side effects of the combination should be closely monitored. The SSRIs with minimal drug–drug interactions, such as citalopram and

sertraline, may be preferable as adjunctive agents; however, data regarding their clinical utility in schizo-obsessive individuals are still lacking.

5. Clozapine monotherapy should be reserved for treatment-resistant schizo-obsessive patients. Although the majority of case reports have dealt with de novo emergence or exacerbation of OCS in schizophrenia, there are some preliminary data indicating that clozapine in a relatively low dose range (75–300 mg) may exert beneficial effect at least in some schizo-obsessive individuals (Bermanzohn et al. 1997; Tibbo and Gendemann 1999). Until findings from controlled studies regarding clozapine's beneficial effect in schizo-obsessive individuals are available, slow up-titration of clozapine and close monitoring of its potential OCS-improving versus OCS-provoking effect in schizophrenia patients is recommended.

6. Lack of therapeutic effect of clozapine monotherapy justifies a trial of a clozapine–SSRI combination. The SSRI should be added to clozapine with caution, and those which are devoid of clinically significant drug–drug interactions (citalopram or sertraline) seem to be safer.

7. Cognitive-behavioral therapy addressing an OCS component may contribute to an integrative treatment approach in schizo-obsessive patients (Peasley-Miklus et al. 2005).

8. Electroconvulsive therapy is the last resort when pharmacotherapy fails (Lavin and Halligan 1996). A beneficial effect of deep brain stimulation in a highly treatment-resistant schizophrenia patient with OCS has also been reported (Plewnia et al. 2008).

Antipsychotic drug-induced obsessive-compulsive symptoms

The complex nature of interactions between the primary schizophrenic disorder, comorbid OCS, and antipsychotic drug treatment is highlighted by the phenomenon of antipsychotic-induced OCS. There is increasing awareness among researchers and clinicians that SGAs have a potential to induce de novo or exacerbate preexisting OCS in schizophrenia patients, while being efficacious as adjunctive treatment in treatment-resistant OCD (the latter aspect of the "antipsychotic-OCS paradox" is beyond the scope of this review). The causal relationship between atypical antipsychotics and OCS is supported by the dose-dependent nature of the SGA–OCS interaction and the abatement of OCS on withdrawal of atypical agents, followed by their reappearance on reintroduction of the offending agent. Findings that OCS may also be induced by SGAs in patients with bipolar disorder, mental retardation, delusional disorder, and psychotic depression indicates that this is a drug-specific effect in susceptible patients rather than an illness-related effect. An additional argument favoring the potential of SGAs to induce OCS is that the majority of reported patients experience de novo emergence of OCS (de Haan et al. 2002; Lykouras et al. 2003; Poyurovsky et al. 2004; Mahendran et al. 2007; Mukhopadhaya et al. 2009).

The magnitude of the problem is supported by its substantial incidence rate and the fact that drug-induced OCS were reported in association with virtually all SGAs (clozapine, olanzapine, risperidone, quetiapine, aripiprazole). When a strict definition of DSM-IV OCD was employed, an incidence of 3% (9 of 303 patients) was detected (Mahendran et al. 2007). However, relaxing criteria from OCD to OCS accounted for a substantially higher incidence rate. Hence, Lim et al. (2007) using a structured interview and the Y-BOCS screened 209 SGA-treated patients with schizophrenia and schizoaffective disorder and found OCS in 44 (21.1%) of the participants; in 26 (12.4%) of them OCS was considered related to the antipsychotic drug. Estimates of de novo OCS as high as 20% and 24% in clozapine-treated schizophrenia patients have also been reported (Ertugrul et al. 2005; Mukhopadhaya et al. 2009). Whether clozapine is associated with a particular OCS-provoking potential is yet to be clarified since data concerning the propensity of each specific antipsychotic agent to induce OCS in schizophrenia patients are limited. In the only comparative prospective six-week study addressing the potential of olanzapine and risperidone to induce/exacerbate OCS in 113 patients with recent-onset schizophrenia, de Haan et al. (2002) found no differences between the two antipsychotic drugs. There was an indication that the duration of olanzapine, but not risperidone, treatment correlated with the severity of OCS. With the exception of this study, a limiting factor in all reports is their cross-sectional and retrospective design.

The diagnosis of antipsychotic-drug-induced OCS in patients with schizophrenia poses a challenge. Based on the available literature and in the absence of evidence-based data, the following characteristics of

OCS induced by SGAs may be useful to the clinician in suspected cases:

1. Most of the reported drug-induced cases of OCS occur in men, indicating their possible predominance in susceptibility.
2. Schizophrenia patients with preexisting OCS may be at particular risk of drug-induced exacerbation of OCS; however a majority of reports deals with the de novo emergence of OCS.
3. Drug-induced OCS are characterized by a predominance of compulsions over obsessions, supporting the view that the diagnosis of OCS in schizophrenia should be validated primarily by the presence of compulsions (Eisen *et al.* 1997). The content of OCS is typical for OCD and readily distinguishable from schizophrenic delusions. In addition, most affected patients show insight into the nature of the OCS.
4. In a majority of the patients with olanzapine- or risperidone-induced OCS, symptoms appeared early, within initial weeks of treatment. By contrast, clozapine-treated patients could be divided by time of onset of OCS into two groups: early (up to 12 weeks) and delayed (15–96 weeks).
5. A wide range of doses was associated with the OCS-provoking effect of olanzapine (5–25 mg/day), compared with relatively high doses (> 3 mg/day) for risperidone. Indeed, lower risperidone doses (< 2 mg/day) were consistently credited with the beneficial adjunctive effect of the drug in "pure" OCD (Bloch *et al.* 2006). Two dose levels associated with OCS induction by clozapine were identified: low (150–250 mg/day) in early-onset OCS, and high (350–900 mg/day) in delayed-onset.

As for management of SGA-induced OCS, three major therapeutic approaches have been used: dose reduction or discontinuation of the drug, addition of SSRIs, or both. Discontinuation/reduction was reported in a majority of the risperidone- and olanzapine-treated patients, whereas adjunctive SRIs were the preferred option in clozapine-induced OCS. A switch to an antipsychotic with potentially lower OCS-induced potential is an additional treatment option. Assuming that this effect is accounted for at least in part by a marked 5-HT_{1A} antagonism, switch to amisulpiride, a highly selective D_2/D_3 receptor antagonist with a negligible 5-HT_{2A} receptor antagonistic effect may be a promising option (Kim *et al.* 2008).

Conclusions

Schizophrenia and OCD are distinct clinical entities. Nevertheless they coexist in a substantial proportion of patients and form a putative schizophrenia–OCD axis of separate but partially overlapping disorders. Intensive research since the mid-1990s has provided ample evidence indicating that OCS are an identifiable, common, and clinically significant dimension of psychopathology in schizophrenia patients. In a considerable proportion of patients, OCS are detectable prior to the onset of schizophrenia or during the first psychotic episode, supporting the notion that OCS is not a sequel to schizophrenia-related factors. Moreover, OCS are present across the lifespan in adolescent, adult, and elderly schizophrenia patients, exerting a modifying, generally deteriorating, effect on severity of symptoms, course of illness, and prognosis of schizophrenia. However, additional cross-sectional and follow-up studies of sufficient sample sizes are necessary to address state- and course-dependent inter-relationships between OCS and schizophrenic symptoms.

Application of both categorical and dimensional definitions of obsessive-compulsive phenomena, as well as a comprehensive description of independent and psychotic-related OCS, is necessary to address their association with a primary schizophrenic disorder. Overall, considering the diagnostic drawbacks in the discrimination between obsessive-compulsive and psychotic phenomena, it seems that, until more studies on the nature and course of OCD symptoms in schizophrenia are available, the diagnosis of schizo-obsessive disorder should be confined only to those patients who meet full DSM-IV criteria of both schizophrenia and OCD. Noteworthy, Eisen *et al.* (1997) have suggested that the diagnosis of OCD comorbidity in schizophrenia patients should be based on the presence of compulsions that seem to be a phenomenon which is less delusion dependent. If OCS are related to the content of delusions or formal thought disorders, the presence of additional typical OCS that meet DSM-IV criteria of OCD would be required to establish the diagnosis of schizo-obsessive disorder. Patients who exhibit OCS exclusively restricted to positive schizophrenia symptoms and present only during acute psychotic episode (e.g., compulsive hand washing resulting from command hallucinations; or obsessive preoccupation with "feelings of discontinuation of normal flow of thoughts") should not currently be considered schizo-obsessive until more studies are available on the nature of this phenomenon and its relatedness to the schizo-obsessive spectrum of disorders. In contrast, patients who fail to recognize OCS as senseless and unreasonable and do not meet the criteria of schizophrenia can be referred to as OCD "with poor insight" (DSM-IV; American Psychiatric Association 1994) or OCD with psychotic features (Insel and Akiskal 1986). Finally, patients who meet full DSM-IV criteria of both OCD and SPD can be referred to as having schizotypal OCD.

An important step towards delineation of specific subgroups within a putative schizophrenia–OCD axis may be the use of endophenotypic markers relevant to both disorders, such as those designed to reflect central psychophysiological inhibition (i.e., prepulse inhibition, antisaccade task, certain neurocognitive tasks). These endophenotypes may help to reveal quantitative differences that presumably correlate with the degree of association between the two disorders. Furthermore, since endophenotypes represent stable and heritable traits, their assessment in relatives of probands with isolated and comorbid forms of disorders may contribute to their phenomenological distinction. Structural and functional brain imaging techniques may be of particular importance in delineating pure and comorbid forms of disorders on a schizophrenia–OCD axis. Overall, comprehensive phenotyping of homogeneous subgroups on an schizophrenia–OCD axis may eventually contribute to the identification of common and unique neurobiological and environmental factors that contribute to the development of schizophrenia, OCD, and their comorbid forms, and will facilitate a search for effective treatments for the schizo-obsessive subgroup of schizophrenia.

References

American Psychiatric Association (1994). *Diagnostic and Statistical Manual of Mental Disorders*, 4th edn. Washington, DC: American Psychiatric Press.

Appelbaum PS, Robbins PC, Roth LH (1999). Dimensional approach to delusions: comparison across types and diagnoses. *Am J Psychiatry* 156: 1938–1943.

Baer L, Jenike MA, Ricciardi JN II, *et al.* (1990). Standardized assessment of personality disorders in obsessive-compulsive disorder. *Arch Gen Psychiatry* 47: 826–830.

Bartz JA, Hollander E (2006). Is obsessive-compulsive disorder an anxiety disorder? *Prog Neuropsychopharmacol Biol Psychiatry* 30: 338–352.

Baylé FJ, Krebs MO, Epelbaum C, Levy D, Hardy P (2001). Clinical features of panic attacks in schizophrenia. *Eur Psychiatry* 16: 349–353.

Berman I, Kalinowski A, Berman S, Lengua J, Green AI (1995). Obsessive-compulsive symptoms in chronic schizophrenia. *Compr Psychiatry* 36: 6–10.

Bermanzohn PC, Porto L, Arlow PB, *et al.* (1997). Are some neuroleptic-refractory symptoms of schizophrenia really obsessions? *CNS Spectr* 2: 51–57.

Bermanzohn PC, Porto L, Arlow PB, *et al.* (2000). Hierarchical diagnosis in chronic schizophrenia: a clinical study of co-occurring syndromes. *Schizophr Bull* 26: 517–525.

Black DW, Noyes R, Jr, Pfohl B, Goldstein RB, Blum N (1993). Personality disorder in obsessive-compulsive volunteers, well comparison subjects, and their first-degree relatives. *Am J Psychiatry* 150: 1226–1232.

Bland RC, Newman SC, Orn H (1987). Schizophrenia: lifetime co-morbidity in a community sample. *Acta Psychiatr Scand* 75: 383–391.

Bloch MH, Landeros-Weisenberger A, Kelmendi B, *et al.* (2006). A systematic review: antipsychotic augmentation with treatment refractory obsessive-compulsive disorder. *Mol Psychiatry* 11: 622–632.

Bottas A, Cooke RG, Richter MA (2005). Comorbidity and pathophysiology of obsessive-compulsive disorder in schizophrenia: is there evidence for a schizo-obsessive subtype of schizophrenia? *J Psychiatry Neurosci* 30: 187–193.

Byerly M, Goodman W, Acholonu W, Bugno R, Rush AJ (2005). Obsessive-compulsive symptoms in schizophrenia: frequency and clinical features. *Schizophr Res* 76: 309–316.

Bymaster FP (1996). Radioreceptor binding profile of the atypical antipsychotic olanzapine. *Neuropsychopharmacology* 14: 87–96.

Cassano GB, Pini S, Saettoni M, Rucci P, Dell'Osso L (1998). Occurrence and clinical correlates of psychiatric comorbidity in patients with psychotic disorders. *J Clin Psychiatry* 59: 60–68.

Catapano F, Sperandeo R, Perris F, Lanzaro M, Maj M (2001). Insight and resistance in patients with obsessive-compulsive disorder. *Psychopathology* 34: 62–68.

Chakrabarty K, Bhattacharyya S, Christopher R, Khanna S (2005). Glutamatergic dysfunction in OCD. *Neuropsychopharmacology* 30: 1735–1740.

Cosoff SJ, Hafner RJ (1998). The prevalence of comorbid anxiety in schizophrenia, schizoaffective disorder and bipolar disorder. *Aust N Z J Psychiatry* 32: 67–72.

Craig T, Hwang MY, Bromet EJ (2002). Obsessive-compulsive and panic symptoms in patients with first-admission psychosis. *Am J Psychiatry* **159**: 592–598.

Cunill R, Castells X, Simeon D (2009). Relationships between obsessive-compulsive symptomatology and severity of psychosis in schizophrenia: a systematic review and meta-analysis. *J Clin Psychiatry* **70**: 70–82.

de Haan L, Beuk N, Hoogenboom B, Dingemans P, Linszen D (2002). Obsessive-compulsive symptoms during treatment with olanzapine and risperidone: a prospective study of 113 patients with recent-onset schizophrenia or related disorders. *J Clin Psychiatry* **63**: 104–107.

de Haan L, Hoogenboom B, Beuk N, van Amelsvoort T, Linszen D (2005). Obsessive-compulsive symptoms and positive, negative, and depressive symptoms in patients with recent-onset schizophrenic disorders. *Can J Psychiatry* **50**: 519–24.

de Haan L, Hoogeboom B, Beuk N, *et al.* (2006). Reliability and validity of the Yale–Brown Obsessive-Compulsive Scale in schizophrenia patients. *Psychopharmacol Bull* **39**: 25–30.

Devulapalli KK, Welge JA, Nasrallah HA (2008). Temporal sequence of clinical manifestation in schizophrenia with co-morbid OCD: review and meta-analysis. *Psychiatry Res* **161**: 105–108.

Dinn WM, Harris CL, Aycicegi A, Greene P, Andover MS (2002). Positive and negative schizotypy in a student sample: neurocognitive and clinical correlates. *Schizophr Res* **56**: 171–185.

Dominguez RA, Backman KE, Lugo SC (1999). Demographics, prevalence, and clinical features of the schizo-obsessive subtype of schizophrenia. *CNS Spectr* **4**: 50–56.

Eisen JL, Rasmussen SA (1993). Obsessive-compulsive disorder with psychotic features. *J Clin Psychiatry* **54**: 373–379.

Eisen JL, Beer DA, Pato MT, Venditto TA, Rasmussen SA (1997). Obsessive-compulsive disorder in patients with schizophrenia and schizoaffective disorder. *Am J Psychiatry* **154**: 271–273.

Eisen JL, Phillips KA, Baer L, *et al.* (1998). The Brown Assessment of Beliefs Scale: reliability and validity. *Am J Psychiatry* **155**: 102–108.

Emsley RA, Roberts MC, Rataemane S, *et al.* (2002). Ethnicity and treatment response in schizophrenia: a comparison of 3 ethnic groups. *J Clin Psychiatry* **63**: 9–14.

Ertugrul A, Anil Yagcioglu AE, Eni N, Yazici KM (2005). Obsessive-compulsive symptoms in clozapine-treated schizophrenic patients. *Psychiatry Clin Neurosci* **59**: 219–22.

Fabisch K, Fabisch H, Langs G, Huber HP, Zapotoczky HG (2001). Incidence of obsessive-compulsive phenomena in the course of acute schizophrenia and schizoaffective disorder. *Eur Psychiatry* **16**: 336–341.

Faragian S, Kurs R, Poyurovsky M (2008). Insight into obsessive-compulsive symptoms and awareness of illness in adolescent schizophrenia patients with and without OCD. *Child Psychiatry Hum Dev* **39**: 39–48.

Fenton WS, McGlashan TH (1986). The prognostic significance of obsessive-compulsive symptoms in schizophrenia. *Am J Psychiatry* **143**: 437–441.

Flaisher-Grinberg S, Klavir O, Joel D (2008). The role of 5-HT$_{2A}$ and 5-HT$_{2C}$ receptors in the signal attenuation rat model of obsessive-compulsive disorder. *Int J Neuropsychopharmacol* **14**: 1–15.

Geyer MA, Krebs-Thomson K, Braff DL, Swerdlow NR (2001). Pharmacological studies of prepulse inhibition models of sensorimotor gating deficits in schizophrenia: a decade in review. *Psychopharmacol* **156**: 117–154.

Glick ID, Poyurovsky M, Ivanova O, Koran LM (2008). Aripiprazole in schizophrenia patients with comorbid obsessive-compulsive symptoms. *J Clin Psychiatry* **69**: 1856–1859.

Goff DC, Keefe R, Citrome L, *et al.* (2007). Lamotrigine as add-on therapy in schizophrenia: results of 2 placebo-controlled trials. *J Clin Psychopharmacol* **27**: 582–589.

Goodman WK, Price LH, Rasmussen SA, *et al.* (1989). The Yale–Brown Obsessive-Compulsive Scale. I. Development, use, and reliability. *Arch Gen Psychiatry* **46**: 1006–1011.

Goodwin RD, Amador XF, Malaspina D, *et al.* (2003). Anxiety and substance use comorbidity among inpatients with schizophrenia. *Schizophr Res* **61**: 89–95.

Green AI, Canuso CM, Brenner MJ, Wojcik JD (2003). Detection and management of comorbidity in patients with schizophrenia. *Psychiatr Clin N Am* **26**: 115–139.

Hiemke C, Weigmann H, Härtter S, *et al.* (1994). Elevated levels of clozapine in serum after addition of fluvoxamine. *J Clin Psychopharmacol* **14**: 279–281.

Higuchi H, Kamata M, Yoshimoto M, Shimizu T, Hishikawa Y (1999). Panic attacks in patients with chronic schizophrenia: A complication of long-term neuroleptic treatment. *Psychiatry Clin Neurosci* **53**: 91–94.

Hoch P, Polatin P (1949). Pseudoneurotic forms of schizophrenia. *Psychiatry Q* **23**: 248–276.

Insel TR, Akiskal HS (1986). OCD with psychotic features: a phenomenological analysis. *Am J Psychiatry* **143**: 1527–1533.

Jablensky A (2006). Subtyping schizophrenia: implications for genetic research. *Mol Psychiatry* **11**: 815–836.

Jenike MA, Baer L, Minichiello WE, Schwartz CE, Carey RJ Jr. (1986). Concomitant obsessive-compulsive disorder and schizotypal personality disorder. *Am J Psychiatry* **143**: 530–532.

Karno M, Golding JM, Sorenson SB, Burnam MA (1988). The epidemiology of obsessive-compulsive disorder in five US communities. *Arch Gen Psychiatry* **45**: 1094–1099.

Kayahan B, Ozturk O, Veznedaroglu B, Eraslan D (2005). Obsessive-compulsive symptoms in schizophrenia: prevalance and clinical correlates. *Psychiatry Clin Neurosci* **59**: 291–295.

Ketter TA, Calabrese JR (2002). Stabilization of mood from below versus above baseline in bipolar disorder: a new nomenclature. *J Clin Psychiatry* **63**: 146–151.

Kim S-WS, Il-Seon KJ-M, Yang S-J, *et al.* (2008). Amisulpride improves obsessive-compulsive symptoms in schizophrenia patients taking atypical antipsychotics: an open-label switch study. *J Clin Psychopharmacol* **28**: 349–352.

Krüger S, Bräunig P, Höffler J, *et al.* (2000). Prevalence of obsessive-compulsive disorder in schizophrenia and significance of motor symptoms. *J Neuropsychiatry Clin Neurosci* **12**: 16–24.

Krystal JH, Perry EB Jr, Gueorguieva R, *et al.* (2005). Comparative and interactive human psychopharmacologic effects of ketamine and amphetamine: implications for glutamatergic and dopaminergic model psychoses and cognitive function. *Arch Gen Psychiatry* **62**: 985–994.

Lavin MR, Halligan P (1996). ECT for comorbid obsessive-compulsive disorder and schizophrenia. *Am J Psychiatry* **153**: 1652–1653.

Lim M, Park DY, Kwon JS, Joo YH, Hong KS (2007). Prevalence and clinical characteristics of obsessive-compulsive symptoms associated with atypical antipsychotics. *J Clin Psychopharmacol* **27**: 712–713.

Lykouras L, Alevizos B, Michalopoulou P, Rabavilas A (2003). Obsessive–compulsive symptoms induced by atypical antipsychotics. A review of the reported cases. *Progr Neuropsychopharmacol Biol Psychiatry* **27**: 333–346.

Lysaker PH, Marks KA, Picone JB, *et al.* (2000). Obsessive and compulsive symptoms in schizophrenia. Clinical and neurocognitive correlates. *J Nerv Ment Dis* **188**: 78–83.

Lysaker PH, Bryson GJ, Marks KA, Greig TC, Bell MD (2002). Association of obsessions and compulsions in schizophrenia with neurocognition and negative symptoms. *J Neuropsychiatry Clin Neurosci* **14**: 449–453.

Mahendran R, Liew E, Subramaniam M (2007). De novo emergence of obsessive-compulsive symptoms with atypical antipsychotics in Asian patients with schizophrenia or schizo-affective disorder: a retrospective cross-sectional study. *J Clin Psychiatry* **68**: 542–545.

Mamo D, Graff A, Mizrahi R, *et al.* (2007). Differential effects of Aripiprazole on D_2, $5-HT_2$, and $5-HT_{1A}$ receptor occupancy in patients with schizophrenia: a triple tracer PET study. *Am J Psychiatry* **164**: 1411–1417.

Margetis B (2008). Aggravation of schizophrenia by clomipramine in a patient with comorbid obsessive-compulsive disorder. *Psychopharmacol Bull* **41**: 9–11.

Matsunaga H, Kiriike N, Matsui T, *et al.* (2000). Gender differences in social and interpersonal features and personality disorders among Japanese patients with obsessive-compulsive disorder. *Compr Psychiatry* **41**: 266–272.

Matsunaga H, Kiriike N, Matsui T, *et al.* (2002). Obsessive-compulsive disorder with poor insight. *Compr Psychiatry* **43**: 150–157.

McDougle CJ, Goodman WK, Price LH, *et al.* (1990). Neuroleptic addition in fluvoxamine-refractory obsessive-compulsive disorder. *Am J Psychiatry* **147**: 652–654.

McElroy, SL, Phillips, KA, Keck, P (1994). Obsessive-compulsive spectrum disorders. *J Clin Psychiatry* **55** (Suppl 10): 33–51.

Meghani SR, Penick EC, Nickel EJ, *et al.* (1998). Schizophrenia patients with and without OCD. In *Proceedings of the 151st Annual Meeting of the American Psychiatric Association*, Toronto.

Mukhopadhaya K, Krishnaiah R, Taye T, *et al.* (2009). Obsessive-compulsive disorder in UK clozapine-treated schizophrenia and schizoaffective disorder: a cause for clinical concern. *J Psychopharmacol* **23**: 6–13.

Mullins S, Spence SA (2003). Re-examining thought insertion. Semi-structured literature review and conceptual analysis. *Br J Psychiatry* **182**: 293–298.

Nechmad A, Ratzoni G, Poyurovsky M, *et al.* (2003). Obsessive-compulsive disorder in adolescent schizophrenia patients. *Am J Psychiatry* **160**: 1002–1004.

Nestadt G, Samuels J, Riddle MA, *et al.* (2001). The relationship between obsessive-compulsive disorder and anxiety and affective disorders: results from the Johns Hopkins OCD Family Study. *Psychol Med* **31**: 481–487.

Nicolson R, Lenane M, Hamburger SD, *et al.* (2000). Lessons from childhood-onset schizophrenia. *Brain Res Brain Res Rev* **31**: 147–156.

Niehaus DJ, Koen L, Muller J, *et al.* (2005). Obsessive compulsive disorder: prevalence in Xhosa-speaking schizophrenia patients. *S Afr Med J* **95**: 120–122.

Ohta M, Kokai M, Morita Y (2003). Features of obsessive-compulsive disorder in patients primarily diagnosed with schizophrenia. *Psychiatry Clin Neurosci* **57**: 67–74.

Ongür D, Goff DC (2005). Obsessive-compulsive symptoms in schizophrenia: associated clinical features, cognitive function and medication status. *Schizophr Res* **75**: 349–362.

Pallanti S, Quercioli L, Hollander E (2004). Social anxiety in outpatients with schizophrenia: a relevant cause of disability. *Am J Psychiatry* **161**: 53–58.

Pauls DL (2008). The genetics of obsessive compulsive disorder: a review of the evidence. *Am J Med Genet C: Semin Med Genet* **148**: 133–139.

Pinto A, Mancebo MC, Eisen JL, Pagano ME, Rasmussen SA (2006). The Brown Longitudinal Obsessive Compulsive Study: clinical features and symptoms of the sample at intake. *J Clin Psychiatry* **67**: 703–711.

Pittenger C, Krystal JH, Coric V (2006). Glutamate-modulating drugs as novel pharmacotherapeutic agents in the treatment of obsessive-compulsive disorder. *Neurotherapeutics* **3**: 69–81.

Peasley-Miklus C, Massie E, Baslett G, Carmin C (2005). Treating obsessive-compulsive disorder and schizophrenia: The case of Sam. *Cogn Behav Pract* **12**: 379–383.

Plewnia C, Schober F, Rilk A, et al. (2008). Sustained improvement of obsessive-compulsive disorder by deep brain stimulation in a woman with residual schizophrenia. *Int J Neuropsychopharmacol* **13**: 1–3.

Porto L, Bermanzohn PC, Pollack S (1997). A profile of obsessive-compulsive symptoms in schizophrenia. *CNS Spectr* **2**: 21–25.

Poyurovsky M, Weizman A (1998). Intravenous clomipramine for a schizophrenic patient with obsessive-compulsive symptoms. *Am J Psychiatry* **155**: 1993.

Poyurovsky M, Fuchs K, Weizman A (1999a). Obsessive-compulsive symptoms in patients with first episode schizophrenia. *Am J Psychiatry* **156**: 1998–2000.

Poyurovsky M, Isakov V, Hromnikov S, et al. (1999b). Fluvoxamine treatment of obsessive-compulsive symptoms in schizophrenic patients: an add-on open study. *Int Clin Psychopharmacol* **14**: 95–100.

Poyurovsky M, Dorfman-Etrog P, Hermesh H, et al. (2000). Beneficial effect of olanzapine in schizophrenic patients with obsessive-compulsive symptoms. *Int Clin Psychopharmacol* **15**: 169–173.

Poyurovsky M, Hromnikov S, Isakov V, et al. (2001). Obsessive-compulsive disorder in chronic institutionalized schizophrenic patients. *Psychiatry Res* **102**: 49–57.

Poyurovsky M, Kriss V, Weisman G, et al. (2003). Comparison of clinical characteristics and comorbidity in schizophrenia patients with and without obsessive-compulsive disorder: schizophrenic and OC symptoms in schizophrenia. *J Clin Psychiatry* **64**: 1300–1307.

Poyurovsky M, Weizman A, Weizman R, (2004). Obsessive-compulsive disorder in schizophrenia: clinical characteristics and treatment. *CNS Drugs* **18**: 989–1010.

Poyurovsky M, Weizman R, Weizman A, Koran L (2005). Memantine for treatment-resistant OCD. *Am J Psychiatry* **162**: 2191–2192.

Poyurovsky M, Fuchs C, Faragian S, et al. (2006a). Preferential aggregation of obsessive-compulsive spectrum disorders in schizophrenia patients with obsessive-compulsive disorder. *Can J Psychiatry* **51**: 746–754.

Poyurovsky M, Bergman J, Weizman R (2006b). Obsessive-compulsive disorder in elderly schizophrenia patients. *J Psychiatry Res* **40**: 189–191.

Poyurovsky M, Faragian S, Kleinman-Balush V, et al. (2007). Awareness of illness and insight into obsessive-compulsive symptoms in schizophrenia patients with obsessive-compulsive disorder. *J Nerv Ment Dis* **195**: 765–768.

Poyurovsky M, Faragian S, Shabeta A, Kosov A (2008a). Comparison of clinical characteristics, co-morbidity and pharmacotherapy in adolescent schizophrenia patients with and without obsessive-compulsive disorder. *Psychiatry Res* **159**: 133–139.

Poyurovsky M, Faragian S, Pashinian A, et al. (2008b). Clinical characteristics of schizotypal-related obsessive-compulsive disorder. *Psychiatry Res* **159**: 254–258.

Poyurovsky M, Glick I, Koran LM (2010). Lamotrigine augmentation in schizoprhenia and schizo-affective patients with obsessive-compulsive symptoms. *J Psychopharmacol* **24**: 861–866.

Prince JD, Akincigil A, Kalay E, et al. (2008). Psychiatric rehospitalization among elderly persons in the United States. *Psychiatr Serv* **59**: 1038–1045.

Rajkumar RP, Reddy YC, Kandavel T (2008). Clinical profile of "schizo-obsessive" disorder: a comparative study. *Compr Psychiatry* **49**: 262–268.

Rasmussen SA, Tsuang MT (1986). Clinical characteristics and family history in DSM-III obsessive-compulsive disorder. *Am J Psychiatry* **143**: 317–322.

Ravizza L, Barzega G, Bellino S, Bogetto F, Maina G (1995). Predictors of drug treatment response in obsessive-compulsive disorder. *J Clin Psychiatry* **56**: 368–373.

Regier DA, Narrow WE, Rae DS (1990). The epidemiology of anxiety disorders: the Epidemiologic Catchment Area (ECA) experience. *J Psychiatry Res* **24**(Suppl 2): 3–14.

Reznik I, Sirota P (2000). Obsessive and compulsive symptoms in schizophrenia: a randomized controlled trial with fluvoxamine and neuroleptics. *J Clin Psychopharmacol* **20**: 410–416.

Rosen I (1956). The clinical significance of obsessions in schizophrenia. *J Mental Sci* **103**: 773–785.

Ross RG, Heinlein S, Tregellas H (2006). High rates of comorbidity are found in childhood-onset schizophrenia. *Schizophr Res* **88**: 90–95.

Rossi A, Daneluzzo E (2002). Schizotypal dimensions in normals and schizophrenic patients: a comparison with other clinical samples. *Schizophr Res* **54**: 67–75.

Ruscio AM, Stein DJ, Chiu WT, Kessler RC (2010). The epidemiology of obsessive-compulsive disorder in the National Comorbidity Survey Replication. *Mol Psychiatry* **15**: 53–63.

Samuels J, Nestadt G, Bienvenu OJ, *et al.* (2000). Personality disorders and normal personality dimensions in obsessive-compulsive disorder. *Br J Psychiatry* **177**: 457–462.

Siever LJ, Davis KL (2004). The pathophysiology of schizophrenia disorders: perspectives from the spectrum. *Am J Psychiatry* **161**: 398–413.

Sim K, Chua TH, Chan YH, Mahendran R, Chong SA (2006). Psychiatric comorbidity in first episode schizophrenia: a 2 year, longitudinal outcome study. *J Psychiatry Res* **40**: 656–663.

Skoog G, Skoog I (1999). A 40-year follow-up of patients with obsessive-compulsive disorder *Arch Gen Psychiatry* **56**: 121–127.

Sobin C, Blundell ML, Weiller F, *et al.* (2000). Evidence of a schizotypy subtype in OCD. *J Psychiatr Res* **34**: 15–24.

Strakowski SM, Tohen M, Stoll AL, *et al.* (1993). Comorbidity in psychosis at first hospitalization. *Am J Psychiatry* **150**: 752–757.

Stengel EA (1945). A study of some clinical aspects of the relationship between obsessional neurosis and psychotic reaction types. *J Mental Sci* **91**: 166–187.

Tibbo P, Gendemann K (1999). Improvement of obsessions and compulsions with clozapine in an individual with schizophrenia. *Can J Psychiatry* **44**: 1049–1050.

Tibbo P, Kroetsch M, Chue P, Warneke L (2000). Obsessive-compulsive disorder in schizophrenia. *J Psychiatr Res* **34**: 139–146.

van Nimwegen L, de Haan L, van Beveren N, *et al.* (2008). Obsessive-compulsive symptoms in a randomized, double-blind study with olanzapine or risperidone in young patients with early psychosis. *J Clin Psychopharmacol* **28**: 214–218.

Voon V, Hassan K, Zurowski M, *et al.* (2006). Prevalence of repetitive and reward-seeking behaviors in Parkinson disease. *Neurology* **67**: 1254–1257.

Weissman MM, Bland RC, Canino GJ, *et al.* (1994). The cross national epidemiology of obsessive compulsive disorder. The Cross National Collaborative Group. *J Clin Psychiatry* **55**(Suppl): 5–10.

Wetherell JL, Palmer BW, Thorp SR, *et al.* (2003). Anxiety symptoms and quality of life in middle-aged and older outpatients with schizophrenia and schizoaffective disorder. *J Clin Psychiatry* **64**: 1476–82.

Whiteside SP, Port JD, Deacon BJ, Abramowitz JS (2006). A magnetic resonance spectroscopy investigation of obsessive-compulsive disorder and anxiety. *Psychiatry Res* **146**: 137–147.

Zohar J, Kaplan Z, Benjamin J (1993). Clomipramine treatment of obsessive compulsive symptomatology in schizophrenic patients. *J Clin Psychiatry* **54**: 385–388.

Medication management of obsessive-compulsive disorder in children and adolescents

Andrew R. Gilbert

Introduction

Obsessive-compulsive disorder (OCD) is a severe and potentially disabling psychiatric disorder with a substantial prevalence (1–2%) in childhood and adolescence (Flament *et al.* 1988). Childhood-onset OCD, characterized by onset prior to 18 years of age, can lead to severe morbidity and, despite the existence of effective therapies, there is often a delay between symptom onset and treatment. Although its pathophysiology remains to be fully elucidated, evidence suggests that pediatric OCD likely results from a complex interaction between multiple genetic and non-genetic factors. Meanwhile, evidence continues to emerge supporting the treatment efficacy of serotonin reuptake inhibitors (SRIs), augmentation strategies affecting other neurotransmitter systems, cognitive-behavioral therapy (CBT), as well as the combination of pharmacotherapy and psychotherapy.

The primary aim of this chapter is to review the pharmacological management of pediatric OCD. It is organized into the following sections: (1) the constellation of symptoms that are typically seen in youth with OCD, including the assessment of symptoms; (2) our current understanding of the pathophysiology of OCD, including biological theories and various neurotransmitter systems implicated in the disorder; (3) specific medications used in the treatment of pediatric OCD; (4) treatment approaches to youth with OCD and comorbid disorders; and (5) safe initiation and management of medications. The chapter concludes with a list of "clinical pearls" derived from this discussion.

Clinical description/assessment

Consistent with other pediatric conditions, OCD in childhood and adolescence has distinct yet overlapping features with the adult-onset type. It is a clinically heterogeneous disorder and has substantial comorbidity with other neuropsychiatric disorders, which may affect the course and treatment of OCD.

Obsessive-compulsive disorder is an anxiety disorder characterized by obsessions (intrusive, unwanted thoughts/images) and/or compulsions (repetitive behaviors or mental activities that an individual feels driven to perform) that are time consuming and distressing and interfere with normal functioning (American Psychiatric Association 1994; Leonard *et al.* 2005; Geller 2006). Obsessions (such as thoughts about contamination) are generally considered anxiety provoking while compulsions (such as frequent hand washing) are anxiety neutralizing. Adult OCD patients will often recognize that their obsessions are irrational but, irrespective of this insight, will continue to experience anxiety/discomfort and engage in compulsions. Youth with OCD, however, depending upon cognitive and developmental factors, may have limited insight.

The mean age of onset of childhood-onset OCD ranges from 7.5 to 12.5 years, while the age at assessment is generally two to three years after onset (Geller *et al.* 1998). Pediatric OCD has substantial comorbidity with other psychiatric disorders, with rates of comorbid psychiatric diagnoses of up to 50% in children (Flament *et al.* 1988). Common comorbid conditions include attention-deficit hyperactivity disorder (ADHD), other anxiety disorders, mood disorders, and tic disorders. Pediatric OCD has a 3:2 male to female ratio. It appears that a substantial number of cases of childhood-onset OCD can either remit or become subclinical over time (Stewart *et al.* 2004). An early age of onset, increased illness duration, inpatient treatment, and symptom dimensions such as sexual, religious or hoarding obsessions can lead to a longer course. Comorbid psychiatric disorders and poor initial treatment response can negatively impact upon prognosis.

A multidimensional model of OCD has been developed that describes the disorder as characterized by distinct but overlapping features, called "symptom dimensions" (Mataix-Cols et al. 2005). Factor analytic studies of adults have consistently identified at least four temporally stable symptom dimensions: contamination/washing, symmetry/ordering, checking, and hoarding. In adults, these symptom dimensions have been found to correlate meaningfully with various genetic and neuro-imaging variables as well as treatment response and comorbid conditions (Mataix-Cols et al. 2005; Rosario-Campos et al. 2006). Recent studies have recognized similar symptom dimensions in youth with OCD, suggesting that these symptoms may be apparent early in the course of illness and may remain stable throughout childhood and adolescence (Stewart et al. 2007; Mataix-Cols et al. 2008) and may be related to treatment response (Grados and Riddle 2008).

A unique feature of pediatric OCD is an acute-onset "subtype" that frequently follows streptococcal infections (Allen et al. 1995; Murphy and Pichichero 2002; Arnold and Richter 2001; Snider et al. 2005). Pediatric autoimmune neuropsychiatric disorder associated with streptococcal infections (PANDAS) is characterized by the sudden onset of OCD and/or tic disorder symptoms, often accompanied by motoric hyperactivity, including choreiform movements. The symptoms follow a "saw tooth" course and a temporal relationship between severity and infection. A diagnosis of PANDAS requires symptoms to emerge prior to adolescence and at least two episodes of temporal relationships between symptom onset/exacerbations and documented group A beta-hemolytic streptococcal infections. Until evidence-based treatment parameters have been established for management of PANDAS, patients are best managed by treating both OCD and infections according to standard protocols.

The Children's Yale–Brown Obsessive Compulsive Scale (CY-BOCS) is a reliable and valid instrument for assessment of OCD symptom severity in youth (Scahill et al. 1997). Mild cases of OCD are characterized by CY-BOCS scores of 8–15, moderate OCD by CY-BOCS scores of 16–23, and severe OCD by CY-BOCS scores ≥ 24.

Pathophysiological model

A neurobiological model of OCD has evolved over the past several decades, advanced by findings from neuroimaging, genetics, and epidemiological and treatment studies (Modell et al. 1989; Swedo et al. 1989; Baxter et al. 1996; Schwartz 1998;Mataix-Cols et al. 2005). In general, this theory implicates specific fronto-subcortical abnormalities in the etiopathogenesis of adult and pediatric OCD, suggesting potential imbalances on molecular, cellular, and both structural and functional circuitry levels. Studies strongly implicate an imbalance in the direct and indirect cortico-striato-thalamic (CST) pathways, with a net effect of excess tone in the direct relative to the indirect circuit. Studies in adults and children have consistently supported abnormal activity and/or structure in the orbitofrontal cortex as well as the caudate. Along with the recent emergence of cognitive and affective neuroscience research, there has been growth in neuroscientific studies of OCD and adaptations to this original model (Mataix-Cols and van der Heuvel 2006). It appears that other neural regions, such as executive and cognitive (dorsolateral prefrontal cortex) and limbic, regulatory and cognitive (dorsal anterior cingulate) are likely important contributors to the pathophysiology of OCD (Ursu et al. 2003; Fitzgerald et al. 2005; Lawrence et al. 2006).

A greater understanding of the roles of several neurotransmitters in OCD has recently emerged. Because of the efficacy of serotonin-specific medications in the treatment of OCD, a serotonin hypothesis of OCD had previously dominated biological models of OCD. However, recognition of the significance of glutamate and dopamine in the pathophysiology of OCD has developed through treatment, imaging, and genetics studies (Rosenberg et al. 2000; Arnold et al. 2006).

Serotonin

The efficacy of the highly serotonergic tricyclic antidepressant clomipramine as a treatment for OCD strongly influenced a serotonin hypothesis of OCD (Aouizerate et al. 2005). Indeed, clomipramine and other serotonin-specific agents, such as the selective SRIs (SSRIs), have proven effective in treating OCD in both adults and youth (Flament et al. 1985a, 1985b; Leonard et al. 1988, 1989; March et al. 1998). It has been postulated that OCD is associated with an imbalance in serotonergic modulation of the direct and indirect circuits and this could potentially be restored with SRI treatment (Modell *et al.* 1989). Candidate gene studies have implicated various serotonin receptors in the pathogenesis of OCD (Hanna *et al.* 1998; Walitza *et al.* 2002; Meira-Lima *et al.* 2004; Levitan *et al.* 2006). However, since the response rate to SRIs is less than 50%, the effectiveness of SRIs in some patients with OCD does not necessarily mean that there is serotonergic dysfunction in this disorder. Furthermore, clinical reports of treatment of adult OCD consistently suggest that doses of SSRIs are substantially higher than necessary to completely occupy the 5-HT transporter in most brain regions.

Dopamine

Dopamine is likely an important neurotransmitter involved in the pathophysiology of OCD (Perani *et al.* 2008). Since serotonin is an important modulator of dopaminergic activity, the serotonin hypothesis of OCD suggested a failure of the serotonergic system in regulating dopaminergic control of fronto-striatal circuits. In fact, the improved efficacy of SSRIs at higher dosages may result from their impact upon dopaminergic systems at these higher dosages. Effective treatment of treatment-refractory OCD using augmentation of SSRIs with dopaminergic agents also supports a dopaminergic role in the disorder. Furthermore, several comorbid conditions, including tic disorders, are linked to dopaminergic dysfunction and this, therefore, supports a dopaminergic role in OCD.

Glutamate

Recent findings from neuroimaging and genetics studies have strongly implicated glutamate in the pathophysiology of OCD. Since glutamate plays a key role in modulating activity in cortical pyramidal neurons, essential components of CST circuitry, a role in OCD is likely. Furthermore, recent evidence of abnormal glutamate levels in CST components in youth with OCD (Rosenberg *et al.* 2000) further support its role. Finally, several genetics studies have found abnormalities in the glutamate transporter and the gene *GRIN2B*, encoding the 2b subunit of the *N*-methyl-D-aspartate (NMDA) glutamatergic receptor, in OCD (Arnold *et al.* 2006; Arnold *et al.* 2004; Hanna *et al.* 2005) and one report revealed evidence of elevated glutamate levels in cerebrospinal fluid in adult OCD subjects (Chakrabarty *et al.* 2005). Taken together, these findings have led to recent treatment studies using glutamate-related

medications (Coric *et al.* 2005; Lafleur *et al.* 2006; Pittenger *et al.* 2006; Grant *et al.* 2007; Bloch *et al.* 2008a, 2008b; Wilhelm *et al.* 2008).

Drug treatments

Serotonin reuptake inhibitors

Consistent with adult studies, pharmacotherapy studies of pediatric OCD have established the efficacy of clomipramine and several SSRIs (DeVeaugh-Geiss *et al.* 1989; Riddle *et al.* 1990, 1992; Geller *et al.* 2001). A meta-analysis of pediatric OCD pharmacotherapy randomized controlled trials (RCT) reported an approximate 30–40% reduction in symptom severity attributable to SRI use, with an effect size of 0.46 (95% confidence interval [CI], 0.37–0.55) (Geller *et al.* 2003a). Another recent meta-analysis, which only included controlled treatment trials in pediatric OCD, reported that the only effective treatments for pediatric OCD were pharmacotherapy with SRIs (effect size, 0.48; 95% CI, 0.36–0.61) or clomipramine (effect size, 0.85; 95% CI, 0.32–1.39), and CBT (effect size, 1.45; 95% CI, 0.68–2.22) (Watson and Rees 2008).

Clomipramine

The efficacy of clomipramine, the first medication studied in this population, supported serotonin specificity in effective treatment of OCD. Flament *et al.* (1985b) carried out a 10-week, double-blind, placebo-controlled, crossover study in 23 pediatric OCD subjects; they found that clomipramine (in doses of 3 mg/kg) was significantly more effective than placebo in reducing OCD symptom severity. A 12-week, double-blind, crossover, comparison study of clomipramine (highly serotonergic) and desiprimine (not serotonergic) was carried out in 48 youths with OCD; clomipramine significantly reduced OCD symptom severity compared with desiprimine (Leonard *et al.* 1988). DeVeaugh-Geiss *et al.* 1990 carried out an eight-week, multicenter, double-blind, parallel, comparison study and found that clomimprimine was superior to placebo in 60 pediatric OCD subjects.

Selective serotonin reuptake inhibitors

A large body of evidence supports the efficacy of several SSRIs in the treatment of pediatric OCD, making SSRIs the first-line pharmacotherapuetic treatment of choice. In RCTs, fluoxetine, fluvoxamine, and

Table 7.1 Dosages of SRIs usually administered to youth with obsessive-compulsive disorder

Medication	Starting dosage (mg/day)	Dosage range (mg/day)
Selective serotonin reuptake inhibitor		
Citalopram	5–10	10–60
Escitalopram	5–10	10–40
Fluoxetine*	5–10	10–80
Fluvoxamine*	12.5–50	50–300
Paroxetine	5–10	10–60
Sertraline*	12.5–25	50–250
Tricyclic antidepressant		
Clomipramine*	12.5–25	50–200

* FDA approved medications for treatment of children and adolescents with OCD.

sertraline have been shown to be superior to placebo in youths with OCD (March *et al.* 1998; Geller *et al.* 2001; Riddle *et al.* 2001; Liebowitz *et al.* 2002; Pediatric OCD Treatment Study Team 2004). All three drugs are FDA approved for use in children of the following ages: sertraline for six years and older; fluoxetine and fluvoxamine in those eight years and older. Several recent open studies have supported the efficacy of other SSRIs, including citalopram (Thomsen 1997; Mukaddes *et al.* 2003) and paroxetine (Rosenberg *et al.* 1999). The Pediatric OCD Treatment Study (POTS) trial, a large, 12-week, multicenter, masked RCT, reported significant advantages to treatment with combination CBT/sertraline ($p = 0.001$), CBT alone ($p = 0.003$), or sertraline alone ($p = 0.006$) compared with placebo (Pediatric OCD Treatment Study Team 2004). The target dose of the sertraline in this study was 200 mg/day. The CBT-alone and sertraline-alone groups did not differ significantly from each other. The rate of clinical remission (CY-BOCS ≤ 10) in the combined treatment group was significantly greater than in the sertraline-alone group ($p = 0.03$) and placebo ($p < 0.001$) but not the CBT alone group.

A recent review of treatment for pediatric OCD supported the POTS findings, reporting that CBT is an effective treatment and may lead to better outcomes when combined with medication than achieved with medication alone (O'Kearney *et al.* 2006). Another meta-analysis of all FDA-registered placebo-controlled clinical trials for pediatric OCD (total of six studies) found a moderate but significant advantage of drug over placebo (Bridge *et al.* 2007). The pooled rates of response were 52% in SSRI-treated participants and 32% in those receiving placebo, resulting in a number needed to treat of six. A meta-analysis of randomized placebo-controlled pediatric OCD studies that examined the use of fluoxetine, sertraline, paroxetine, and fluvoxamine reported a combined effect size of 0.46 (95% CI, 0.37–0.55) (Geller *et al.* 2003a). These important treatment studies have led to reviews and practice guidelines to recommend CBT (including exposure and response prevention [ERP]) and/or SSRIs as first-line treatment for children and adolescents with OCD. There is no evidence in pediatric OCD for greater efficacy using one SSRI compared with another (Geller *et al.* 2003a) and there have been no direct head-to-head studies comparing SSRIs. The only comparison study carried out has been the POTS study (Pediatric OCD Treatment Study Team 2004; Reinblatt and Riddle 2006). Currently the FDA has approved fluoxetine, fluvoxamine, sertraline, and clomipramine to treat youth with OCD (Table 7.1).

Adjunctive treatments

Augmentation of an SSRI with an atypical antipsychotic drug for treatment-resistant OCD in adults has been studied and is an accepted treatment approach (Bloch *et al.* 2006). Only two open-label studies, however, have examined this augmentation strategy in youth with OCD despite evidence that it takes place relatively frequently (Fitzgerald *et al.* 1999; Thomsen 2004). In an open trial of four pediatric subjects with treatment-refractory OCD symptoms, Fitzgerald *et al.* (1999) reported effective risperidone augmentation of SRIs. In an open 12-week trial of adjunctive risperidone (≤ 2 mg/day) in 17 adolescents with OCD, Thomsen (2004) reported significant reduction of Y-BOCS scores. In a more recent case report, a 13-year-old adolescent male with treatment-refractory OCD had a substantial reduction in CY-BOCS scores following addition of low-dose aripiprazole, then sertraline, in combination with CBT (Storch *et al.* 2008). He experienced no adverse side effects such as weight gain, which are frequently associated with the use of atypical antipsychotics. It will be important to carry out RCTs of such augmentation strategies in treating children and adolescents with OCD in order to assess their efficacy.

Medication augmentation strategies should generally be used for situations when patients have not responded to established effective interventions and continue to experience substantial OCD symptoms. It is reasonable to consider "treatment resistance" as the failure of at least two SSRIs or one SSRI and clomipramine as well as the failure of CBT. Medication trials should be at least 10 weeks of each at the maximum recommended/tolerated doses with no change for a preceding three weeks. Adequate trials of CBT are considered to be eight to ten total sessions or five to six exposure sessions.

New directions

As noted, glutamate has been strongly implicated in the pathophysiology of OCD. A recent open-label trial of riluzole, a glutamate antagonist, in children with treatment-resistant OCD reported reduction of symptom severity (> 46%) in four of six subjects (Grant *et al.* 2007). There were no reported adverse side effects. Another recent study of adults with OCD supported the use of augmentation of behavior therapy with D-cycloserine, a partial agonist of the NMDA receptor (Wilhelm *et al.* 2008). Clearly, future studies, including RCTs and larger samples of children and adolescents, are needed to advance the use of glutamate-related treatment of youth with OCD.

Treatment of OCD with comorbid disorders

As mentioned above and in earlier chapters, pediatric OCD has substantial comorbidity with other neuropsychiatric disorders (Geller 2006). Recent studies have found that comorbid conditions can significantly affect severity, course, and treatment of youth with OCD (Leonard *et al.* 1993; Geller *et al.* 2003b 2007; Masi *et al.* 2007; Storch *et al.* 2007; Ivarsson and Melin 2008; Walitza *et al.* 2008). Ginsburg *et al.* 2008 recently reviewed predictors of SRI treatment in studies of children and adolescents with OCD and found that youth with comorbid tics and possibly externalizing disorders, specifically oppositional defiant disorder and conduct disorder, may be less likely to respond to medication alone. Another recent study examining the impact of comorbid tic disorders on treatment found that patients with comorbid tics had lower scores on the CY-BOCS following treatment with medication (sertraline) alone (March *et al.* 2007). Interestingly, tics did not impact upon the efficacy of CBT and combined treatment compared with placebo. The authors concluded that, consistent with findings from the original POTS study, patients with or without a comorbid tic disorder have a greater likelihood of symptom improvement with either CBT or combined treatment compared with medication alone (March *et al.* 2007). Another study found that youth with OCD and comorbid tics were more likely to be SRI non-responders than those without comorbid tics (Masi *et al.* 2005). Pediatric OCD and bipolar disorder comorbidity may also be associated with a poor response to treatment (Masi *et al.* 2007). Masi *et al.* found that comorbid bipolar disorder was associated with earlier onset and greater severity and functional impairment of OCD symptoms, as well as more frequent hoarding obsessions and compulsions, and poorer response to treatment.

Disentangling symptoms of comorbid disorders from the symptoms of OCD is clearly important in effectively managing youth with OCD. Once identified, comorbid conditions should be treated with pharmacological and/or psychotherapeutic evidence-based techniques as indicated by current practice parameters. Fortunately, SSRIs have minimal interactions with effective treatments for ADHD (stimulants), tic disorders (neuroleptics, α_2-adrenoceptor agonists), and bipolar disorder (lithium, anticonvulsants, neuroleptics). Mood stabilization with appropriate medications should be achieved prior to use of SSRIs in patients with comorbid bipolar disorder.

Management of pharmacological treatments

Initiation and maintenance of treatment

Typical starting and maintenance dosages of SRIs used for treatment of pediatric OCD are listed in Table 7.1. If clomipramine is the chosen medication, baseline electrocardiograph and vital statistics (including orthostatic blood pressure) should be collected. Electrocardiography should be repeated at the 2 mg/kg dose stage and with dosage increments up to 5 mg/kg or within therapeutic range. Blood concentration monitoring should follow medication changes, with serum concentrations not exceeding 150–250 μg/l.

Following initiation of the SRI, weekly or biweekly pharmacotherapy appointments are indicated for the first month of a new trial. Regular communication by phone can be made available during the initial month of treatment and/or until stabilization is achieved. The frequency of pharmacological management appointments can gradually be spread out to monthly and bimonthly meetings after the first month and can move to biannual meetings after the first six months (unless there are substantial challenges to achievement of stabilization). Following stabilization of symptoms, treatment is generally continued for approximately 6–12 months. A medication-free trial ("drug holiday") may be indicated during the first low-stress period after approximately six months to one year of continual treatment (Pine 2002). If a patient experiences two to three relapses of moderate severity, then longer-term treatment of symptoms should be considered.

Side effects

Several adverse effects may impact upon efficacy, especially via reduced compliance, including neuropsychiatric conditions, such as akathisia, activation, mania and amotivation, and somatic side effects such as gastrointestinal disturbances and sexual dysfunction (Murphy et al. 2008). Akathisia, activation, and mania can be difficult to distinguish. Most activation will occur within the initial two weeks of treatment and is frequently dose dependent, responding to a reduced dose. All patients with a history of mania and/or a family history of mania should be managed

with caution, especially during the initial stages of treatment and during any dosage changes. Manic symptoms that appear to be induced by SRI use should be treated no differently than sudden onset of mania in suspected bipolar disorder; therefore, a reduction and/or discontinuation of the SRI is indicated. Gastrointestinal side effects, which are frequently transient, are often dose dependent and respond well to a reduction in dose and/or taking the medications following a meal. Sexual side effects include loss of interest and arousal as well as anorgasmia. Unfortunately, there are limited data regarding management of SSRI sexual side effects in adolescents (Scharko 2004; Scharko and Reimer 2004). Clomiprimine may produce anticholinergic side effects, such as dry mouth, blurred vision, and constipation. These side effects are frequently transient. Antihistaminic side effects may include weight gain and fatigue. Clinically insignificant elevations in heart rate and blood pressure may also occur with clomipramine.

Suicide

Recent evidence that SSRIs may increase the risk of spontaneously reported suicidal adverse events highlights the importance of safe management of these medications while treating youth with OCD. A recent meta-analysis examining SSRIs and suicidal ideation/behavior (Bridge et al. 2007) reported that pooled absolute rates of suicidal ideation and suicide attempt from all FDA-registered placebo-controlled trials for pediatric OCD treatment were 1% in SSRI-treated participants and 0.3% in those receiving placebo; the number needed to harm was 200. Most of these suicidal adverse events were increases in suicidal ideation, with relatively few attempts and no completions. The report found that for every youth with OCD who experienced a suicidal adverse event, 33 experienced a clinical response. Therefore, Bridge et al. (2007) have suggested that benefits from SSRIs are greater than the risk of a suicidal event in this patient population.

Conclusions

Pharmacotherapy for pediatric OCD can be an effective treatment approach to this common and potentially disabling condition. In moderate to severe OCD, treatment with medication is an appropriate choice. Because of the substantial psychiatric comorbidity and its potential impact upon course and treatment response, a thorough psychiatric evaluation and

---

Box 7.1 Clinical pearls

A thorough psychiatric evaluation is important, with emphasis on comorbid disorders as these can impact upon treatment and course.

A thorough medical history is also important, with particular emphasis on temporal relationships between symptoms and streptococcal infections.

Although medications (SRIs) alone and CBT alone do not appear to differ enough to rank one above the other in terms of treatment efficacy, CBT is generally recommended for mild cases of OCD (CY-BOCS 8–15).

Medications (SRIs), in combination with CBT, are indicated for moderate (CY-BOCS 16–23) to severe (CY-BOCS ≥ 24) OCD.

Because of a better side effect profile, SSRIs are considered first-line pharmacological treatment over clomipramine.

Collaboration with therapists in your community who have training in ERP and CBT, especially with youth, will go a long way towards helping your patients.

It may take up to 12 weeks of SRI treatment for benefits to occur.

Following stabilization, treatment is generally continued for approximately 6–12 months.

---

appropriate management of comorbid conditions are both very important. Although the course of pediatric OCD remains to be fully elucidated, an estimated 41% of patients with full OCD will have persistent symptoms and 60% with full or subthreshold OCD will have persistent symptoms (Stewart *et al.* 2004). As noted, factors that have a negative impact upon prognosis include an early age of onset, long symptom duration, comorbid psychiatric illnesses, and a poor initial treatment response (Stewart *et al.* 2004). In general, most drug trials consider a 25% decrease in symptom severity, as measured by the CY-BOCS, as indicative of a positive treatment response. As noted above, treatment studies have found that pharmacotherapy may lead to an approximate 30–50% reduction in OCD symptoms (Bridge *et al.* 2007). Monitoring of symptom severity, using the CY-BOCS, is an important component of treatment in light of the uncertain clinical trajectory and course of pediatric OCD patients (Stewart *et al.* 2004). Box 7.1 summarizes the discussion of this chapter into the "clinical pearls".

References

Allen AJ, Leonard HL, Swedo SE (1995). Case study: a new infection-triggered, autoimmune subtype of pediatric OCD and Tourette's syndrome. *J Am Acad Child Adolesc Psychiatry.* **34**: 307–311.

American Psychiatric Association (1994). *Diagnostic and Statistical Manual of Mental Disorders*, 4th edn. Washington, DC: American Psychiatric Press.

Aouizerate B, Guehl D, Cuny E, *et al.* (2005). Updated overview of the putative role of the serotoninergic system in obsessive-compulsive disorder. *Neuropsychiatr Dis Treat* **1**: 231–243.

Arnold PD, Richter MA (2001). Is obsessive-compulsive disorder an autoimmune disease? *Cmaj* **165**: 1353–1358.

Arnold PD, Rosenberg DR, Mundo E, *et al.* (2004). Association of a glutamate (NMDA) subunit receptor gene (*GRIN2B*) with obsessive-compulsive disorder: a preliminary study. *Psychopharmacology (Berl).* **174**: 530–538.

Arnold PD, Sicard T, Burroughs E, Richter MA, Kennedy JL (2006). Glutamate transporter gene *SLC1A1* associated with obsessive-compulsive disorder. *Arch Gen Psychiatry* **63**: 769–776.

Baxter LR, Jr., Saxena S, Brody AL, *et al.* (1996). Brain mediation of obsessive-compulsive disorder symptoms: evidence from functional brain imaging studies in the human and nonhuman primate. *Semin Clin Neuropsychiatry* **1**: 32–47.

Bloch MH, Landeros-Weisenberger A, Kelmendi B, *et al.* (2006). A systematic review: antipsychotic augmentation with treatment refractory obsessive-compulsive disorder. *Mol Psychiatry* **11**: 622–632.

Bloch MH, Landeros-Weisenberger A, Rosario MC, Pittenger C, Leckman JF (2008a). Meta-analysis of the symptom structure of obsessive-compulsive disorder. *Am J Psychiatry* **165**: 1532–1542.

Bloch MH, Landeros-Weisenberger A, Sen S, *et al.* (2008b). Association of the serotonin transporter polymorphism and obsessive-compulsive disorder: systematic review. *Am J Med Genet B Neuropsychiatr Genet* **147B**: 850–858.

Bridge JA, Iyengar S, Salary CB, *et al.* (2007). Clinical response and risk for reported suicidal ideation and suicide attempts in pediatric antidepressant treatment: a meta-analysis of randomized controlled trials. *JAMA* **297**: 1683–1696.

Chakrabarty K, Bhattacharyya S, Christopher R, Khanna S (2005). Glutamatergic dysfunction in OCD. *Neuropsychopharmacology* **30**: 1735–1740.

Coric V, Taskiran S, Pittenger C, *et al.* (2005). Riluzole augmentation in treatment-resistant obsessive-compulsive disorder: an open-label trial. *Biol Psychiatry* 1 **58**: 424–428.

DeVeaugh-Geiss J, Landau P, Katz R (1989). Preliminary results from a multicenter trial of clomipramine in obsessive-compulsive disorder. *Psychopharmacol Bull* **25**: 36–40.

DeVeaugh-Geiss J, Katz R, Landau P, Goodman W, Rasmussen S (1990). Clinical predictors of treatment response in obsessive compulsive disorder: exploratory analyses from multicenter trials of clomipramine. *Psychopharmacol Bull* **26**: 54–59.

Fitzgerald KD, Stewart CM, Tawile V, Rosenberg DR (1999). Risperidone augmentation of serotonin reuptake inhibitor treatment of pediatric obsessive compulsive disorder. *J Child Adolesc Psychopharmacol* **9**: 115–123.

Fitzgerald KD, Welsh RC, Gehring WJ, *et al.* (2005). Error-related hyperactivity of the anterior cingulate cortex in obsessive-compulsive disorder. *Biol Psychiatry* 1 **57**: 287–294.

Flament MF, Rapoport JL, Berg CJ, *et al.* (1985a). Clomipramine treatment of childhood obsessive-compulsive disorder. A double-blind controlled study. *Arch Gen Psychiatry* **42**: 977–983.

Flament MF, Rapoport JL, Kilts C (1985b). A controlled trial of clomipramine in childhood obsessive compulsive disorder. *Psychopharmacol Bull* **21**: 150–152.

Flament MF, Whitaker A, Rapoport JL, *et al.* (1988). Obsessive compulsive disorder in adolescence: an epidemiological study. *J Am Acad Child Adolesc Psychiatry* **27**: 764–771.

Geller DA (2006). Obsessive-compulsive and spectrum disorders in children and adolescents. *Psychiatr Clin N Am* **29**: 353–370.

Geller DA, Biederman J, Jones J, *et al.* (1998). Obsessive-compulsive disorder in children and adolescents: a review. *Harv Rev Psychiatry* **5**: 260–273.

Geller DA, Hoog SL, Heiligenstein JH, *et al.* (2001). Fluoxetine treatment for obsessive-compulsive disorder in children and adolescents: a placebo-controlled clinical trial. *J Am Acad Child Adolesc Psychiatry* **40**: 773–779.

Geller DA, Biederman J, Stewart SE, *et al.* (2003a). Which SSRI? A meta-analysis of pharmacotherapy trials in pediatric obsessive-compulsive disorder. *Am J Psychiatry* **160**: 1919–1928.

Geller DA, Biederman J, Stewart SE, *et al.* (2003b). Impact of comorbidity on treatment response to paroxetine in pediatric obsessive-compulsive disorder: is the use of exclusion criteria empirically supported in randomized clinical trials? *J Child Adolesc Psychopharmacol* **13**(Suppl 1): S19–S29.

Geller DA, Petty C, Vivas F, *et al.* (2007). Further evidence for co-segregation between pediatric obsessive compulsive disorder and attention deficit hyperactivity disorder: a familial risk analysis. *Biol Psychiatry* **61**: 1388–1394.

Ginsburg GS, Kingery JN, Drake KL, Grados MA (2008). Predictors of treatment response in pediatric obsessive-compulsive disorder. *J Am Acad Child Adolesc Psychiatry* **47**: 868–878.

Grados M, Riddle MA (2008). Do all obsessive-compulsive disorder subtypes respond to medication? *Int Rev Psychiatry* **20**: 189–193.

Grant P, Lougee L, Hirschtritt M, Swedo SE (2007). An open-label trial of riluzole, a glutamate antagonist, in children with treatment-resistant obsessive-compulsive disorder. *J Child Adolesc Psychopharmacol* **17**: 761–767.

Hanna GL, Himle JA, Curtis GC, *et al.* (1998). Serotonin transporter and seasonal variation in blood serotonin in families with obsessive-compulsive disorder. *Neuropsychopharmacology* **18**: 102–111.

Hanna GL, Himle JA, Curtis GC, Gillespie BW (2005). A family study of obsessive-compulsive disorder with pediatric probands. *Am J Med Genet B Neuropsychiatr Genet* **134**: 13–19.

Ivarsson T, Melin K (2008). Autism spectrum traits in children and adolescents with obsessive-compulsive disorder (OCD). *J Anxiety Disord* **22**: 969–978.

Lafleur DL, Pittenger C, Kelmendi B, *et al.* (2006). N-Acetylcysteine augmentation in serotonin reuptake inhibitor refractory obsessive-compulsive disorder. *Psychopharmacology (Berl)* **184**: 254–256.

Lawrence NS, Wooderson S, Mataix-Cols D, *et al.* (2006). Decision making and set shifting impairments are associated with distinct symptom dimensions in obsessive-compulsive disorder. *Neuropsychology* **20**: 409–419.

Leonard HL, Swedo S, Rapoport JL, Coffey M, Cheslow D (1988). Treatment of childhood obsessive compulsive disorder with clomipramine and desmethylimipramine: a double-blind crossover comparison. *Psychopharmacol Bull* **24**: 93–95.

Leonard HL, Swedo SE, Rapoport JL, *et al.* (1989). Treatment of obsessive-compulsive disorder with clomipramine and desipramine in children and adolescents. A double-blind crossover comparison. *Arch Gen Psychiatry* **46**: 1088–1092.

Leonard HL, Swedo SE, Lenane MC, *et al.* (1993). A 2- to 7-year follow-up study of 54 obsessive-compulsive children and adolescents. *Arch Gen Psychiatry* **50**: 429–439.

Leonard HL, Ale CM, Freeman JB, Garcia AM, Ng JS (2005). Obsessive-compulsive disorder. *Child Adolesc Psychiatr Clin N Am* **14**: 727–743, viii.

Levitan RD, Kaplan AS, Masellis M, *et al.* (2006). The serotonin-1Dbeta receptor gene and severity of obsessive-compulsive disorder in women with bulimia nervosa. *Eur Neuropsychopharmacol* **16**: 1–6.

Liebowitz MR, Turner SM, Piacentini J, *et al.* (2002). Fluoxetine in children and adolescents with OCD: a placebo-controlled trial. *J Am Acad Child Adolesc Psychiatry* **41**: 1431–1438.

March JS, Biederman J, Wolkow R, *et al.* (1998). Sertraline in children and adolescents with obsessive-compulsive disorder: a multicenter randomized controlled trial. *JAMA* **280**: 1752–1756.

March JS, Franklin ME, Leonard H, *et al.* (2007). Tics moderate treatment outcome with sertraline but not cognitive-behavior therapy in pediatric obsessive-compulsive disorder. *Biol Psychiatry* **61**: 344–347.

Masi G, Millepiedi S, Mucci M, *et al.* (2005). A naturalistic study of referred children and adolescents with obsessive-compulsive disorder. *J Am Acad Child Adolesc Psychiatry* **44**: 673–681.

Masi G, Perugi G, Millepiedi S, *et al.* (2007). Bipolar co-morbidity in pediatric obsessive-compulsive disorder: clinical and treatment implications. *J Child Adolesc Psychopharmacol* **17**: 475–486.

Mataix-Cols D, van den Heuvel OA (2006). Common and distinct neural correlates of obsessive-compulsive and related disorders. *Psychiatr Clin N Am* **29**: 391–410, viii.

Mataix-Cols D, Rosario-Campos MC, Leckman JF (2005). A multidimensional model of obsessive-compulsive disorder. *Am J Psychiatry* **162**: 228–238.

Mataix-Cols D, Nakatani E, Micali N, Heyman I (2008). Structure of obsessive-compulsive symptoms in pediatric OCD. *J Am Acad Child Adolesc Psychiatry* **47**: 773–778.

Meira-Lima I, Shavitt RG, Miguita K, *et al.* (2004). Association analysis of the catechol-*O*-methyltransferase (COMT), serotonin transporter (5-HTT) and serotonin 2A receptor (5HT$_{2A}$) gene polymorphisms with obsessive-compulsive disorder. *Genes Brain Behav* **3**: 75–79.

Modell JG, Mountz JM, Curtis GC, Greden JF (1989). Neurophysiologic dysfunction in basal ganglia/limbic striatal and thalamocortical circuits as a pathogenetic mechanism of obsessive-compulsive disorder. *J Neuropsychiatry Clin Neurosci* **1**: 27–36.

Mukaddes NM, Abali O, Kaynak N (2003). Citalopram treatment of children and adolescents with obsessive-compulsive disorder: a preliminary report. *Psychiatry Clin Neurosci* **57**: 405–408.

Murphy ML, Pichichero ME (2002). Prospective identification and treatment of children with pediatric autoimmune neuropsychiatric disorder associated with group A streptococcal infection (PANDAS). *Arch Pediatr Adolesc Med* **156**: 356–361.

Murphy TK, Segarra A, Storch EA, Goodman WK (2008). SSRI adverse events: how to monitor and manage. *Int Rev Psychiatry* **20**: 203–208.

O'Kearney RT, Anstey KJ, von Sanden C (2006). Behavioural and cognitive behavioural therapy for obsessive compulsive disorder in children and adolescents. *Cochrane Database Syst Rev* (4):CD004856.

Pediatric OCD Treatment Study Team (2004). Cognitive–behavioral therapy, sertraline, and their combination for children and adolescents with obsessive–compulsive disorder: the Pediatric OCD Treatment Study (POTS) randomized controlled trial. *JAMA* **292**: 1969–1976.

Perani D, Garibotto V, Gorini A, *et al.* (2008). In vivo PET study of 5HT(2A) serotonin and D(2) dopamine dysfunction in drug-naive obsessive-compulsive disorder. *Neuroimage* **42**: 306–314.

Pine DS (2002). Treating children and adolescents with selective serotonin reuptake inhibitors: how long is appropriate? *J Child Adolesc Psychopharmacol* **12**: 189–203.

Pittenger C, Krystal JH, Coric V (2006). Glutamate-modulating drugs as novel pharmacotherapeutic agents in the treatment of obsessive-compulsive disorder. *Neurotherapeutics* **3**: 69–81.

Reinblatt SP, Riddle MA (2006). Selective serotonin reuptake inhibitor-induced apathy: a pediatric case series. *J Child Adolesc Psychopharmacol* **16**: 227–233.

Riddle MA, Hardin MT, King R, Scahill L, Woolston JL (1990). Fluoxetine treatment of children and adolescents with Tourette's and obsessive compulsive disorders: preliminary clinical experience. *J Am Acad Child Adolesc Psychiatry* **29**: 45–48.

Riddle MA, Scahill L, King RA, *et al.* (1992). Double-blind, crossover trial of fluoxetine and placebo in children and adolescents with obsessive-compulsive disorder. *J Am Acad Child Adolesc Psychiatry* **31**: 1062–1069.

Riddle MA, Reeve EA, Yaryura-Tobias JA, *et al.* (2001). Fluvoxamine for children and adolescents with obsessive-compulsive disorder: a randomized, controlled, multicenter trial. *J Am Acad Child Adolesc Psychiatry* **40**: 222–229.

Rosario-Campos MC, Miguel EC, Quatrano S, *et al.* (2006). The Dimensional Yale–Brown Obsessive-Compulsive Scale (DY-BOCS): an instrument for assessing obsessive-compulsive symptom dimensions. *Mol Psychiatry* **11**: 495–504.

Rosenberg DR, Stewart CM, Fitzgerald KD, Tawile V, Carroll E (1999). Paroxetine open-label treatment of pediatric outpatients with obsessive-compulsive disorder. *J Am Acad Child Adolesc Psychiatry* **38**: 1180–1185.

Rosenberg DR, MacMaster FP, Keshavan MS, *et al.* (2000). Decrease in caudate glutamatergic concentrations in pediatric obsessive- compulsive disorder patients taking paroxetine. *J Am Acad Child Adolesc Psychiatry* **39**: 1096–1103.

Scahill L, Riddle MA, McSwiggin-Hardin M, *et al.* (1997). Children's Yale–Brown Obsessive Compulsive Scale: reliability and validity. *J Am Acad Child Adolesc Psychiatry* **36**: 844–852.

Scharko AM (2004). Selective serotonin reuptake inhibitor-induced sexual dysfunction in adolescents: a review. *J Am Acad Child Adolesc Psychiatry* **43**: 1071–1079.

Scharko AM, Reiner WG (2004). SSRI-induced sexual dysfunction in adolescents. *J Am Acad Child Adolesc Psychiatry* **43**: 1067–1068.

Schwartz JM (1998). Neuroanatomical aspects of cognitive-behavioural therapy response in obsessive-compulsive disorder. An evolving perspective on brain and behaviour. *Br J Psychiatry Suppl* **35**: 38–44.

Snider LA, Lougee L, Slattery M, Grant P, Swedo SE (2005). Antibiotic prophylaxis with azithromycin or penicillin for childhood-onset neuropsychiatric disorders. *Biol Psychiatry* **57**: 788–792.

Stewart SE, Geller DA, Jenike M, *et al.* (2004). Long-term outcome of pediatric obsessive-compulsive disorder: a meta-analysis and qualitative review of the literature. *Acta Psychiatr Scand* **110**: 4–13.

Stewart SE, Rosario MC, Brown TA, *et al.* (2007). Principal components analysis of obsessive-compulsive disorder symptoms in children and adolescents. *Biol Psychiatry* **61**: 285–291.

Storch EA, Lack CW, Merlo LJ, *et al.* (2007). Clinical features of children and adolescents with obsessive-compulsive disorder and hoarding symptoms. *Compr Psychiatry* **48**: 313–318.

Storch EA, Lehmkuhl H, Geffken GR, Touchton A, Murphy TK (2008). Aripiprazole augmentation of incomplete treatment response in an adolescent male with obsessive-compulsive disorder. *Depress Anxiety* **25**: 172–174.

Swedo SE, Rapoport JL, Leonard H, Lenane M, Cheslow D (1989). Obsessive-compulsive disorder in children and adolescents. Clinical phenomenology of 70 consecutive cases. *Arch Gen Psychiatry* **46**: 335–341.

Thomsen PH (1997). Child and adolescent obsessive-compulsive disorder treated with citalopram: findings from an open trial of 23 cases. *J Child Adolesc Psychopharmacol* **7**: 157–166.

Thomsen PH (2004). Risperidone augmentation in the treatment of severe adolescent OCD in SSRI-refractory cases: a case-series. *Ann Clin Psychiatry* **16**: 201–207.

Ursu S, Stenger VA, Shear MK, Jones MR, Carter CS (2003). Overactive action monitoring in obsessive-compulsive disorder: evidence from functional magnetic resonance imaging. *Psychol Sci* **14**: 347–353.

Walitza S, Wewetzer C, Warnke A, *et al.* (2002). 5-HT$_{2A}$ promoter polymorphism: Z438G/A in children and adolescents with obsessive-compulsive disorders. *Mol Psychiatry* **7**: 1054–1057.

Walitza S, Zellmann H, Irblich B, *et al.* (2008). Children and adolescents with obsessive-compulsive disorder and comorbid attention-deficit/hyperactivity disorder: preliminary results of a prospective follow-up study. *J Neural Transm* **115**: 187–190.

Watson HJ, Rees CS (2008). Meta-analysis of randomized, controlled treatment trials for pediatric obsessive-compulsive disorder. *J Child Psychol Psychiatry* **49**: 489–498.

Wilhelm S, Buhlmann U, Tolin DF, *et al.* (2008). Augmentation of behavior therapy with D-cycloserine for obsessive-compulsive disorder. *Am J Psychiatry* **165**: 335–341; quiz 409.

Exposure and response prevention treatment for obsessive-compulsive disorder

Fugen Neziroglu, Beth Forhman, and Sony Khemlani-Patel

Introduction

Behavior therapy, specifically exposure and response prevention (ERP), has been utilized to treat obsessive-compulsive disorder (OCD) from the late 1960s to the present, with promising results. This chapter will cover the theoretical model of ERP, its application to comorbid conditions, and adjunct therapies, such as cognitive therapy (CT) and acceptance and commitment therapy (ACT).

Theoretical basis of exposure and response prevention therapy

The roots of ERP are in learning theory and it is considered to be a form of counter-conditioning and extinction. In 1958, Wolpe utilized systematic desensitization to cause the waning of anxiety reactions by coupling relaxation with anxiety-exacerbating situations. Mowrer (1947) described a two-factor theory of fear and avoidance behavior in anxiety disorders, suggesting that fear develops based upon classical conditioning and is sustained through operant conditioning. Dollard and Miller (1950) applied this theory to the development of OCD. Through classical conditioning, a neutral stimulus that is paired with an unconditional stimulus acquires the same properties as the unconditional stimulus and thus elicits anxiety. New responses need to be learnt to decrease the anxiety in the presence of the conditioned (neutral) stimulus. These learned responses are designated as "avoidance or escape responses" (Dollard and Miller 1950) as they remove anxiety and, therefore, are negatively reinforcing.

The procedures of ERP were originally derived from animal experiments. Fixated or stereotyped behaviors in animals, which are analogous to human compulsive behaviors, are difficult to remove. Maier (1949) discovered that the "guidance technique" could be effective in preventing a rat from carrying out a fixed behavior by guiding it manually toward the previously avoided situation. Baum (1965, 1969a, 1969b) taught rats avoidance behaviors and then prevented their response, resulting in the extinguishing of avoidance behaviors. When an aversive stimulus is not paired with a conditioned stimulus, rats do not avoid the stimulus because they learn that avoiding the stimulus is not useful. Thus fear is extinguished when it is not functional to avoid the stimulus. In 1966, ERP was introduced as the first effective psychological treatment for OCD, when Meyer exposed two patients who had OCD to anxiety-evoking stimuli and, with constant supervision, prevented them from engaging in compulsions. One patient had a hand washing ritual and the other contended with obsessions. Both patients remained improved at the end of a two-year follow-up.

Exposure therapy was developed with the objective of assisting patients to challenge their obsessive fears, anxieties, doubts, and worries emanating from situations, traumatic memories, or objects. There are two mechanisms of exposure programs, in vivo and imaginal exposure. According to Folette and Smith (2005), "imaginal exposure" is the repeated visualization of images or actions or repeated recounting of memories; "in vivo exposure" is the repeated confrontation with the feared objects or situations." There is a consensus that imaginal exposure has benefit for patients who are obsessive compulsive.

Foa and Kozak (1996) reported that imaginal exposure had significant clinical efficacy for OCD patients whose obsessional fears centered on disastrous and apocalyptic consequences. According to these authors,

Clinical Obsessive-Compulsive Disorders in Adults and Children, ed. Robert Hudak and Darin D. Dougherty.
Published by Cambridge University Press. Copyright © Cambridge University Press 2011.

imaginal exposure is extremely useful when in vivo exposures are not possible. Additionally, patients who have a propensity to engage in widespread mental rituals as avoidance strategies during in vivo exposures can also benefit from imaginal exposure. Finally, the clinical utility of imaginal exposure can be expanded through the use of homework, whereby exposure scenarios can be recorded and patients can listen to the audiotapes sandwiched between sessions.

The role of relational frame theory

Apart from learning theory, another major contributing theory that is utilized in our understanding of numerous disorders is relational frame theory. It is a psychological theory of language and cognition that was proposed by by Hayes *et al.* (2001). It is rooted in "functional contextualism," which is viewed as a continuation of B. F. Skinner's work on "radical behaviorism." The theory proposes that the use of specific language constructs exacerbates the experience of pain, causing "cognitive fusion." According to Hayes *et al.* (2001), individuals become part of their "verbal representations, assessments and rationales." These verbal representations are now viewed as real circumstances and negative events to avoid at all costs. The individual's account of an aversive event may have some of the meaning of that event. According to Hayes *et al.*, when a survivor of trauma discusses a traumatic event, the feelings that were present during the trauma may be present during the description of the event. For example, if a person is merged with the belief that something is terribly wrong with them, they will shun circumstances that evoke that idea. The evasions of those circumstances strengthen the power of the eluded event because they reinforce the verbal assessment process.

Relational frame theory (Hayes *et al.* 2001) highlights the role of language and its impact on human emotions and cognitions, and how it potentially results in the suffering of human beings. Animals require a direct experience with an object for learning to occur; they learn about events that predict the onset of something (e.g., Show a cookie, say "cookie" and the dog salivates). By comparison, a child can learn that touching a hot stove will burn without having direct experience with a hot stove. Our ability to use language allows us to learn about things by being told even though we may never have experienced a particular event. Humans can also learn after the fact; in other words, they are taught once an event has occurred whereas other animals need to have the event precede the onset of the response. This bi-directionality is the most important defining feature of human language and cognition and explains why evaluative or classical conditioning can occur and why arbitrary associations can be made.

Another important feature of human language and cognition involves the emergence of complex networks of related events. The ability to think relationally allows us not only to make predictions, similar to other animals via classical conditioning, but also to generate various other relations. Relational responding is established during early language training by teaching relational frames (e.g., learning things that are "similar"; learning temporal and causal relations, "before and after," "if/then;" learning comparative and evaluative, "better than," "bigger than," etc.). Relational frame theory seeks to explain the generative nature of language and cognitions. It draws from both classical (Pavlovian) and operant (Skinnerian) conditioning to explain various thoughts and emotions.

The ACT approach is based on relational frame theory and will be described later in this chapter. This approach may be especially useful in increasing tolerance of unpleasant emotions and decreasing overvalued ideation, thereby increasing patients' willingness to participate in ERP.

The role of neurotransmitter changes in brain

In addition to conditioning and relational responding, which helps to explain the etiology of OCD and the efficacy of ERP, there are two other frameworks that suggest ERP may be effective by modifying the neurobiology of the individual. Neziroglu *et al.* (1990) reported sertonoergic activity changes in eight patients who received daily 90 minutes of ERP for three weeks without any medication. They found that platelet plasma serotonin decreased and imipramine binding site number and binding affinity increased after intensive behavior therapy. At the follow-up at four weeks, plasma serotonin values returned to baseline, whereas the binding site number and binding affinity remained the same as at the end of treatment. These results suggest that ERP may modify biochemistry of OCD individuals. In 1992, Baxter *et al.* found that metabolic rates in the caudate nucleus decreased significantly compared with pretreatment rates in responders to behavior therapy and fluoxetine. Schwartz and colleague (1996) replicated these findings, also

Table 8.1 Summary of early exposure and response prevention (ERP) studies for obsessive-compulsive disorder

Authors	Treatment	Participants	Results
Meyer (1966)	ERP	15 (single subject)	10 much improved; 5 moderately improved
Mills *et al.* (1973)	ERP; 11–14 days	5	All significantly improved
Boulgouris and Bakiakos (1973)	ERP; average of 11 sessions	3	All improved
Boersman *et al.* (1976)	ERP; average of 11 sessions	13	54% had no symptoms; 23% improved; 23% no change
Rabavilas *et al.* (1976)	ERP; average of 11 sessions	12	50% improved; 33% slightly improved; 17% no change
Kirk (1983)	ERP; 5–10+ sessions	36	58% much improved; 17% moderately improved; 8% no change
Foa *et al.* (1983)	ERP; average of 11.5 daily sessions	50	58% much improved; 38% improved; 4% failures
Foa *et al.* (1983)	ERP; 10–20 daily 2 hour sessions	72	43% much improved; 44% improved; 13% failures
Hoogduin and Duivenvoorden (1988)	ERP; 10 sessions in 20 weeks	60	78% improved; 20% no change
Keijsers *et al.* (1994)	ERP; 18 sessions in 2 months	40	60% improved; 40% no change
Bolton *et al.* (1995)	ERP; open time period	15	At follow-up, 52% symptom free; 48% still had symptoms

demonstrating significant changes in right caudate glucose metabolic activity. Nakatani and colleagues (2003) randomly assigned OCD patients to either 12 weeks of behavioral therapy or 200 mg fluvoxamine. Based on pre- and post-treatment functional neuroimaging, both groups demonstrated significant bilateral elevation in regional cerebral blood flow in the basal ganglia. More recently, Saxena and colleagues (2009) found that only four weeks of daily behavior therapy resulted in significant declines in bilateral thalamic activity and significant increases in right dorsal anterior cingulate cortex activity in 10 OCD patients compared with controls.

Exposure and response prevention treatment for OCD

A number of researchers tested the efficacy of ERP treatments for OCD, after the initial efforts of Meyer (1966). During the 1960s through 2000, a number of investigations proved the efficacy of ERP. Early on, some of the research designs were not randomized

and controlled. It should be noted that a 50% reduction in symptoms is considered as successful treatment, while a 30% reduction in symptoms is considered a failure. There have been a number of reviews of these studies, for example Abel (1993), Foa *et al.* (1998), and Neziroglu *et al.* (2006), who review studies done pre-1995 as well as the advances made up to 2006. Table 8.1 lists some early studies.

Comparison of exposure and response prevention with cognitive-behavioral therapy

Early series of studies found that ERP was more effective than relaxation training (Rachman *et al.* 1971, 1973; Hodgson *et al.* 1972; Marks *et al.* 1975 *et al.*).

Other CBT techniques have been tried for ERP, including thought stopping. Hachman and McLean (1975) treated 10 OCD patients in a crossover design of four weeks each of thought stopping and ERP. Nine patients improved, five mostly with ERP and four mostly with thought stopping. Neziroglu and Neuman

(1990) compared rational emotive therapy, ERP, and thought stopping in OCD patients with pure obsessions. They found that ERP and rational emotive therapy were equally effective, but thought stopping was ineffective in addressing obsessional symptoms.

In a study by Abramowitz (1997), ERP was found to be more effective than relaxation and correspondingly as effective as CT, although other controlled studies have indicated a minor advantage for ERP over CT.

In a comparison with anxiety management techniques, ERP was seen as having a significantly greater impact on obsessive-compulsive symptoms (OCS) (Lindsay *et al.* 1997). Patients receiving anxiety management did not show any change in OCS, while patients receiving ERP evidenced major improvement.

Whittal *et al.* (2005) compared 12 weeks of ERP with 12 weeks of CBT, with patients randomly assigned to either group. Fifty-nine patients completed treatment and there was no significant difference in scores on the Yale–Brown Obsessive Compulsive Scale (Y-BOCS) at either end of treatment or after a three-month follow-up. Since there is overlap between the two techniques, it is difficult to draw definitive conclusions as to whether one treatment is clearly superior to the other.

Van Oppen *et al.* (2005) examined the long-term efficacy of CT alone, in vivo exposure alone, and CBT (either CT or ERP) in combination with fluvoxamine in the treatment of OCD. Out of 122 patients, follow-up data was collected from 102 patients and indicated that 54% of the patients no longer met the criteria for OCD, although there was no difference between the three treatment groups. It should be noted that patients who evidenced attrition had more severe OCD complaints and OCSs than patients who completed the study.

Simpson *et al.* (2008a) found that motivational interviewing evidenced potential for enhancing treatment outcomes with ERP. A manual was developed and six patients with moderate to severe OCD were treated, with five evidencing improvement in their Y-BOCS scores and an increase in their quality of life, with three patients attaining a post-treatment Y-BOCS score of less than 12.

Simpson, *et al.* (2008b) also conducted a randomized, controlled trial at two academic outpatient clinics with 108 adult OCD patients to compare the effects of augmenting serotonin reuptake inhibitors (SRIs) with ERP versus stress management training. Participants had a Y-BOCS score greater than 16 and were given a therapeutic SRI dose for at least 12 weeks prior to entry. The design consisted of 17 sessions of either ERP or stress management training twice a week while continuing SRI pharmacotherapy. It was found that ERP was superior to stress management training in reducing OCSs. At week eight, significantly more patients receiving ERP than patients receiving stress management training had a decrease in OCS severity by at least 25%.

Many studies since the 1970s have assessed the benefit of adding CT to ERP, with mixed results. Some studies have found that both treatments are equally effective (Emmelkamp *et al.* 1988; Emmelkamp and Beens 1991). In the first randomized controlled study comparing ERP with CT, both techniques were equally effective, with CT demonstrating more changes in faulty belief measurements (van Oppen *et al.* 1995). Overall, CT has been thought of as particularly useful in certain situations, especially to reduce patient dropout rates (Abramowitz *et al.* 2005a), to address high overvalued ideation, and to address depressive symptomatology (Neziroglu *et al.* 2006).

Comparison of exposure and response prevention with drug treatment

Only a few early studies compared efficacy of behavior therapy, medications, and a combination of both. Marks *et al.* (1980) examined the impact of clomipramine with and without ERP and found that the combination was more effective in OCD patients who were depressed but medications had no impact on the OCSs alone. Similar results were found by other studies (Mavissakalian *et al.* 1985). One other study found that both clomipramine and ERP were equally effective, but those who received ERP continued to improve at a three-year follow-up, while those on medication did not (Solyom and Sookman 1977). Mawson *et al.* (1982) conducted a study with 40 OCD patients who received either placebo or clomipramine, combined with either 15 hours or 30 hours of ERP, with a two-year follow-up. At the end of treatment, all patients improved, but those who received 30 hours of ERP demonstrated greater reductions in rituals. The two-year follow-up did not differ significantly from the results at the end of treatment. Marks and colleagues (1988) treated 37 OCD patients with ERP for 17 weeks, with homework assignments or not, and therapist-aided exposure. Half of the patients were treated with clomipramine but its administration did not add significantly to the exposure. A literature review by Foa *et al.* (1998) found that ERP evidenced greater efficacy than the selective SRIs (SSRIs). However, when methodological disparity was controlled, ERP was found to have a comparable influence to the SSRIs and clomipramine.

Hembree *et al.* (2003) assessed long-term outcome by randomly assigning 62 OCD patients to one of three groups: ERP alone, serotonergic (fluvoxamine or clomipramine) medications alone, or a combination of both. At 17 months post-treatment, there was no difference in OCS severity among the three groups. However, when remaining on a medication for the whole period was taken into account, differences occurred and this suggested that long-term outcome of ERP may be superior to that of serotonergic drugs after their discontinuation, in contrast to the situation with continued medications. Patients who continued medications had equal benefits to ERP. Simpson *et al.* (2004) conducted a similar randomized clinical trial comparing ERP alone, clomipramine alone, or the combination. They found that that ERP alone and ERP plus medications led to lower relapse rates. They also found that responders receiving ERP with or without medications were significantly better after treatment discontinuation that those receiving medication only.

In an important study by Foa and colleagues (2005), 122 adult OCD patients were treated in a double-blind, randomized, placebo-controlled trial comparing ERP, clomipramine, their combination (ERP added to clomipramine), and pill placebo at one center that had expertise in pharmacotherapy, another with expertise in ERP, and the third with expertise in both arenas. The design consisted of ERP for four weeks, followed by eight weekly maintenance sessions, and/or clomipramine given for 12 weeks. The results at the twelfth week indicated that the effects of all active treatments were superior to placebo. The effect of ERP did not differ from ERP plus clomipramine, and both were superior to clomipramine only.

A more recent study investigated whether ERP augments SSRIs for the treatment of OCD (Simpson *et al.* 2008b). All participants were taking a stable therapeutic dose of an SSRI and received 17 sessions of either ERP or stress management. The results indicated that ERP was superior to stress management: significantly more patients receiving ERP than stress management had a decrease of at least 25% in symptom severity. The authors concluded, however, that 17 sessions was not sufficient.

Recently, D-cycloserine, a glutamatergic partial *N*-methyl-D-aspartate (NMDA) agonist, which has been known to reduce fear in patients and animals, has been investigated for OCD. Kushner *et al.* (2007) conducted a study in which D-cycloserine was given to patients with OCD two hours before ERP. Their conclusion was that the drug reduced the number of exposure sessions and therapy attrition. After only four sessions of ERP, the group receiving D-cycloserine reported significantly greater decreases in distress associated with obsessions compared with the placebo group. It should be noted that the placebo group achieved the same results after the provision of additional sessions.

In a study by Storch *et al.* (2007), 24 adults with OCD were randomly assigned to one of two groups; each received 12 ERP sessions, with either D-cycloserine or a placebo administered four hours prior to every session. The beginning session consisted of developing a ritual hierarchy and psychoeducation about OCD. Session two consisted of a practice exposure. Sessions 3–12 consisted of ERP exercises. There were no statistically significant differences in outcome among the two groups. The benefits of D-cycloserine were possibly lost through the time interval between administration of the drug and initiation of treatment.

Long-term effects of exposure and response prevention therapy

Foa and Goldstein (1978) conducted a single-subject study with a three-year follow-up of 21 OCD patients treated with ERP. At the end of treatment, 85% had no symptoms, 10% were much improved, and 5% experienced no change. At the three-year follow-up, 79% had no symptoms, 10% improved, and 11% experienced no change. This confirmed the effectiveness of ERP.

Catts and McConaghy (1975) treated six OCD patients with ERP in a single-subject design with a two-year follow-up. At the end of treatment, 17% had no symptoms, 17% were much improved, and 66% improved. At the two-year follow-up, 50% of the patients had no symptoms and 50% were much improved. In one study, patients were followed for six years after receiving three or six weeks of ERP plus clomipramine or placebo for 36 weeks (O'Sullivan *et al.* 1991). Patients remained significantly improved and the best predictor of long-term improvement was improvement at the end of the treatment period. Those taking clomipramine were no better off then those who had discontinued.

For a review of the numerous studies showing long-term efficacy see Baer and Minichiello (1990) and Yaryura-Tobias and Neziroglu (1997).

Intensive versus weekly exposure and response prevention therapy

Initially, most ERP took place weekly with daily exposure guided by a therapist, an approach that was found to be effective. A comparison by Abramowitz et al. in 2003 suggested that intensive ERP and twice-weekly ERP had similar outcomes. However, patients with severe OCSs that severely compromise their functioning need and benefit from intensive, daily treatment (Huppert and Foa 2005). For these patients, the therapist provides help in contending with daily difficulties and providing much needed motivation to participate fully in ERP. Most challenging and difficult cases of OCD require intensive treatment, particularly if the following issues are prevalent: difficulty enduring discomfort, poor motivation, a depressed mood, and a family structure that resists change.

Instruments utilized to detect the severity of OCSs include the Y-BOCS (Goodman et al. 1989) and the Obsessive Compulsive Inventory-Revised (OCI-R; Foa et al. 2002).

Clinical interviews with patients and their families help to determine the necessity for intensive versus weekly therapy. Intensive therapy is recommended in a number of situations, including (1) impairment in multiple domains of life (i.e., the inability to work, symptoms resulting in a temporary leave of absence from work, social avoidance, marital or family discord); (2) symptoms leading to patients being homebound; (3) significant family discord; (4) symptoms impacting other family members, especially children, or placing family members in a particularly unhealthy situation; (5) partial response to previous weekly CBT; (6) compulsive behaviors placing patients in danger, such as using bleach to decontaminate; (7) comorbid conditions that are moderate to severe; 8) high overvalued ideation; and (9) patients being unable to complete and generalize gains to the home environment despite numerous attempts. Aside from symptom severity, practical reasons often determine treatment intensity. Patients often request significant improvement before a major life event or family life cycle event

(such as an impending marriage, new job, or beginning academic career). Chapter 13 discusses intensive therapy in greater detail.

Efficacy of exposure and response prevention therapy in subtypes of OCD

Subtypes of OCD have been delineated in terms of their symptoms: prevalent obsessions and compulsions (i.e., contamination/cleaning, harm/checking, hoarding/symmetry, religious/sexual, and somatic/hypochondriacal). In reviewing the research, washing/cleaning compulsions, overt compulsions, and symmetry/ordering/arranging compulsions respond favorably to ERP, while sexual obsessions, religious obsessions, hoarding, and pure obsessions do not respond as well (Mataix-Cols et al. 2002; Abramowitz et al. 2008; Brakoulias and Starcevic 2008; et al. et al. Seishin 2008).

The substance of obsessions and compulsions in OCD is extremely varied and this diversity prompted the development of research related to examining OCD through factor and cluster analysis (Leckman et al. 1997; Abramowitz et al. 2003, 2005b; et al. Lee et al. 2005a; Bagley et al. 2009 et al.).

In 2003, an obsession model was developed that categorized obsessions into *autogenous obsessions* and *reactive obsessions* (Lee et al. 2005b). According to Lee and Telch (2005), autogenous obsessions are unacceptable and unrealistic thoughts, images, or impulses that tend to be perceived as threatening (i.e., sexual, aggressive, blasphemous, or repulsive thoughts, images, or impulses). These thoughts, images, or impulses can occur without a source of activation or by a thought that is emblematically related. Quite the reverse, reactive obsessions are prompted by external signals and cues, are somewhat realistic, and generate anxiety based upon the negative consequence that will follow. Reactive obsessions, according to Lee and Telch (2005), consist of "thoughts, concerns or doubts about contamination, mistakes, accidents, asymmetry or disarray." Lee and Kwon (2003) described differential emotional and cognitive appraisals and responses to autogenous obsessions versus reactive obsessions, including thought-control and behavioral control strategies, respectively.

Currently, OCD is viewed as a heterogeneous class of disorders that may comprise overlapping subtypes (McKay and Neziroglu 2009). The development of valid phenotypic and methodological approaches are necessary (McKay and Neziroglu 2009; Seishin 2008) as treatment is not customized to symptom subtypes (Brakoulias, and Starcevic 2008). Much research has been conducted to identify subtypes and treatment outcome; in fact a special issue has been devoted to this in *Behavior Therapy* (volume 36(4) in 2005).

Efficacy of exposure and response prevention therapy in obsessive-compulsive spectrum disorders

Obsessions and compulsions can appear in a variety of disorders, making differential diagnosis difficult. Careful assessment and clinical interviews, and/or background clinical history, can clarify whether the symptoms are indicative of OCD alone, of another closely related disorder, or of comorbidity. As a general rule, standard ERP strategies can be applied if comorbid OCD or OCSs are present. The following section will discuss management of OCSs when present in other disorders.

Body dysmorphic disorder (BDD), hypochondriasis, eating disorders, trichotillomania, and Tourette's syndrome are typically included in the obsessive-compulsive spectrum disorders (Hollander 1993; Hollander and Wong 1995; Yaryura-Tobias and Neziroglu 1997). Since OCD and these disorders are typically comorbid, CBT strategies are often employed for multiple issues concurrently.

Overvalued ideation is often higher in BDD and hypochondriasis (McKay *et al.* 1997; Neziroglu *et al.* 2000), requiring careful decisions about when to conduct ERP. Multiple sessions of CT may need to be employed first. Patients with BDD can also experience significant comorbid depression, suicidal ideation, or other comorbidity that necessitates separate intervention previous to ERP for the BDD symptoms. Assessment of motivation and readiness for change are also necessary for hypochondriasis and BDD. Many similarities exist between these two disorders in terms of depression and high levels of overvalued ideation compared with OCD (Neziroglu and Khemlani-Patel 2005). Patients with BDD who are actively pursuing cosmetic/dermatological procedures may benefit from therapist involvement in those consultation appointments to clarify recommendations made by the cosmetic surgeon to prevent misinterpretation. Because of high distress and impairment, patients often require multiple sessions a week as well as home visits. Rates for comorbidity between OCD and BDD range from 16% (Bienvenu *et al.* 2000) to 37% (Hollander *et al.* 1993).

Hypochondriasis and OCD share many common symptoms (Fallon *et al.* 1992; Neziroglu *et al.* 2000); therefore, the two conditions can often be misdiagnosed by clinicians. Patients with hypochondriasis typically misinterpret bodily sensations as symptoms of a serious illness whereas individuals with somatic obsessions are concerned with contracting a particular disease. Both disorders, however, display thoughts that are difficult to resist, intrusive, and lead to increased anxiety (Warwick and Salkovskis 1990). The cognitive distortions in hypochondriasis include a misinterpretation of ambiguous stimuli or evaluating situations as more threatening than they really are (Salkovskis and Warwick 2001). Both patients with hypochondriasis and those with OCD display intolerance for uncertainty, inflated sense of responsibility, and over-appraisal of threat (Salkovskis and Warwick 2001; Starcevic 2001). These similarities suggest that hypochondriasis should be placed with the spectrum disorders. However, patients with hypochondriasis present with higher overvalued ideation than OCD, which may require additional CT, more than typically used for OCD. Patients with hypochondriasis may also be less compliant with their psychotropic medications because of fear of side effects or misperceptions about the negative impact of the medication on their bodies. Similar to BDD, patients with hypochondriasis often seek medical procedures, rather than psychological treatment, as a solution to their distress.

Tourette's syndrome has similarities to OCD in that it is also an impulse control disorder. However, a distinction must be made between OCD compulsions, which are viewed as intentional, and tics, which are seen as involuntary. However, most clinicians view patients with Tourette's syndrome as having some ability to moderate their symptoms through habit reversal (Steingard and Dillon-Stout 1992; Yaryura-Tobias and Neziroglu 1997; Wilhelm *et al.* 2003).

OCD and Tourette's syndrome are highly comorbid, especially subthreshold OCSs in Tourette's syndrome. Researchers have found that when the OCD is present in Tourette's syndrome, symmetry, touching, self-injurious behaviors, and aggressive and violent obsessions are found more frequently (George *et al.* 1993; Holzer, *et al.* 1994; Cath *et al.* 2000, 2001).

Differential diagnosis can be difficult especially for complex tics, which more closely resemble compulsive behaviors, and when touching, tapping, or the "right" feeling is present. Differential diagnosis can be made by assessing for intrusive thoughts associated with the behaviors. The complex tics can be addressed by using ERP (Verdellen *et al.* 2004; Wetterneck and Woods 2006) in addition to standard habit reversal techniques.

Trichotillomania is not as readily included in the OC spectrum because of differences in function of the repetitive behavior, cognitions, and affect (Stanley and Cohen 1999). Others argue that OC spectrum disorders fall on a continuum of compulsivity versus impulsivity (Hollander and Cohen 1996). Approximately 15 to 27% of patients with trichotillomania have coexisting OCD (Christenson *et al.* 1991).

Effective treatment for trichotillomania is habit reversal training (Azrin and Nunn 1973). It is a CBT-based technique consisting of numerous techniques, including self-monitoring, building awareness of the behavior, and developing competing responses. It also includes components of ERP, including placing individuals in vulnerable hair pulling situations and practicing refraining from the behavior. For example, a patient who often pulls while reading may practice reading in session while practicing resisting any urges to pull.

Efficacy of exposure and response prevention therapy in hoarding

Factor analysis research (Leckman *et al.* 1997; Miguel *et al.* 2005) and cluster analysis research has suggested that hoarding is a distinct subtype of OCD (*et al.* Calamari *et al.* 1999; Hasler *et al.* 2005). There are many distinct differences between hoarding and OCD, including age of onset (hoarding has a later onset), different comorbid conditions, higher overvalued ideation, and lower overall functioning (Saxena *et al.* 2002; Steketee and Frost 2003; Neziroglu *et al.* 2004; Steketee and Frost 2007). Treatment for hoarding incorporates the addition of training in organization, time management, and decision-making skills. Family intervention appears more necessary for hoarding than other OCD symptoms. Cognitive therapy in preparation for the ERP is necessary for hoarding in almost all circumstances, whereas patients with good insight in other OCD symptoms do not always require intensive CT prior to initiating ERP. Patients with hoarding, however, are more secretive, fearful, and shameful about symptoms, and are more guarded about treatment.

Treatment-resistant and treatment-refractory OCD

The most consistent predictor of outcome for behavior therapy in OCD is compliance with ERP (Mataix-Cols *et al.* 2002). Treatment non-compliance, or treatment resistance, encompasses a range of behaviors, including inconsistent homework completion, frequent session cancellation, and resistance to completing in-session ERP. Non-compliance is a complex issue with various contributing factors, including comorbid disorders (personality disorders, substance abuse, and mood disorders), high overvalued ideation, and low tolerance for discomfort.

Treatment refractory, however, typically refers to patients who have participated in empirically validated treatment for OCD and yet do not have significant symptom reduction on standardized measures of OCD, such as the Y-BOCS or the Padua Inventory.

A number of researchers have suggested standardized methods to assess for resistance or refractory to treatment. Rauch *et al.* (1996) suggested that re-examining the dosage, duration, and response to all of the treatments offered. They also suggested re-examining the diagnosis itself, as well as comorbid conditions that might impact outcome. Many other researchers have suggested a stepwise approach to the evaluation of treatment response, with an evaluation of the actual amount of ERP and the actual techniques employed, since behavior therapy can include ineffective treatments for OCD, such as systematic desensitization or relaxation. Suggested amounts of ERP range from 13 to 24 hours of ERP to determine treatment failure (Rauch *et al.* 1996).

Neurosurgical options should only be considered for patients with chronic, debilitating, and very severe OCD and after a thorough evaluation of the above-mentioned factors. Non-destructive neurosurgical procedure options include deep brain stimulation and transcranial magnetic stimulation. Current destructive neurosurgical procedure options include anterior cingulotomy, anterior capsulotomy, subcaudate tractotomy, and limbic leucotomy (Rauch *et al.* 1996). These treatment approaches were developed based upon brain imaging studies that correlated an association between obsessions and compulsions and dysfunctions of pathways in specific regions of the brain (Baxter *et al.* 1992; Rauch *et al.* 1994). There are significant limitations to these procedures, including a lack of randomized, controlled studies, the small number of patients who have undergone these procedures, the lack of an accurate means of identifying patients who would benefit from these treatments, and the limited experience of surgeons that have performed these procedures (see Ch. 2 for greater details).

Complications hindering exposure and response prevention therapy

There are a number of key variables that hinder ERP and become obstacles to effective treatment, including depression and other comorbid diagnoses, high overvalued ideation, lack of education regarding the diagnosis or treatment, comorbid personality disorders, and unrealistic patient expectations. Family variables can also be an impediment to ERP, including parenting style, parental reactions to the disorder, and psychiatric diagnoses of other family members. Equally important, but not given enough attention, are therapeutic factors, consisting of therapist style, anxiety in the therapeutic environment, therapist frustration and/or burnout, and the pacing of sessions and homework.

Overvalued ideation

Overvalued ideation denotes the intensity or strength in a conviction or belief. It refers to the correctness, strength, reasonableness, or sensibility of a belief. These ideas tend to be fixed and possibly amenable to modification only if confronted and challenged. This term differs greatly from "poor insight," which is a specifier used in the *Diagnostic and Statistical Manual of Mental Disorders* (DSM).

Overvalued ideation is on a continuum between rationality and delusions (Kozak and Foa 1994). Those patients with OCD and severe overvalued ideation can almost seem delusional, but it should be remembered that they present differently to schizophrenia patients (Huppert and Foa 2005).

Wernicke (1906) stated that overvalued ideation resides in misattribution through a deficit in insight that is governed in affect and added that they are drawn from the periphery and resistant to change or modification. Jaspers (1913) viewed overvalued ideation as being bound to personality, challengeable, isolated and transient.

High overvalued ideation is very widespread in the obsessive-compulsive spectrum disorders, particularly BDD, hypochondriasis, and hoarding (McKay *et al.* 1997, 2000, 2010; Neziroglu and Khemlani-Patel 2005).

Overvalued ideation as a symptom dimension is extremely significant because of its predictive value in treatment (Neziroglu *et al.* 2001). Patients are extremely reluctant to participate in ERP when their belief system is strong. It can effectively be assessed through the following instruments: Y-BOCS, the Brown Assessment of Beliefs Scale (Eisen *et al.* 1998), and the Overvalued Ideation Scale (Neziroglu *et al.* 2001). Cognitive restructuring may be a valuable tool in addressing overvalued ideation.

Estimations of poor insight in patients with OCD range from 15 to 36% (Kishore *et al.* 2004). A high overvalued ideation impacts treatment and course of illness.

Depression

When depression is present in OCD, it is often secondary to the OCD. In fact, it usually develops after OCD symptoms, suggesting it is a result of the distress associated with the OCD (Rasmussen and Eisen 1992; Welner *et al.* 1976). Major depression is seen in 25–30% of OCD patients (Steketee *et al.* 2000), with lifetime rates much higher. Comorbid depression in OCD is a significant contributor to poor quality of life, suggesting that targeting depressive symptoms is a crucial treatment component (Masellis *et al.* 2003). Individuals without comorbid depression appear to have lower severity ERP post-treatment scores (Abramowitz *et al.* 2000).

When a true comorbid depression is present with OCD, it may need to be addressed prior to the OCD with CT and behavioral activation, and/or appropriate medications. Comorbid depression impacts compliance with ERP homework assignments as well as between-session habituation. Patients with OCD without comorbid depression have better post-treatment and follow-up scores on severity measures (Abramowitz *et al.* 2000).

Comorbid depression has been viewed as a variable that influences treatment outcome. Approximately one third of patients who have OCD have a comorbid diagnosis of depression (Rasmussen and Tsuang 1986; Rasmussen and Eisen, 1992; Phillips *et al.* 1993; Perugi *et al.* 1997; Antony *et al.* 1998; Neziroglu *et al.* 1999, 2006). Patients with comorbid severe depression do not experience between- or within-session habituation during ERP (Foa 1979). If the initial assessment indicates moderate to severe comorbid depression, it is imperative to target those symptoms either exclusively for a number of sessions or concurrently with the OC spectrum disorder. Traditional CBT assignments to increase participation in pleasurable activities, behavioral activation, and a psychopharmacological consult for antidepressant medication may be necessary (Neziroglu and Yaryura-Tobias 1993).

Comorbid disorders

The existence of comorbidity can significantly impact the effectiveness of ERP and affect patient motivation and follow through. It is essential to address the disorder that is generating the greatest amount of concern for the patient. Symptoms that are prohibiting attendance or involvement in therapy must be dealt with prior to ERP treatment.

Personality

Numerous studies have found high rates of axis II personality disorders comorbid with OCD (Samuels et al. 2000), with high rates of cluster C anxious personality disorders, specifically, obsessive-compulsive personality disorder (Bejerot et al. 2000) and avoidant personality disorder (Samuels et al. 2000), Early studies found that incidence of schizotypal personality disorder coexisting with OCD is around 8%, whereas schizotypal features are higher (28%; Stanley et al. 1990). McKay and Neziroglu (1996) suggested using social skills training along with ERP to achieve a more profound impact on the OCD.

Other personality characteristics have also been associated with OCD, including neuroticism (Samuels et al. 2000). One study using the five factor model of personality for OCD found that lower scores on openness to ideas was associated with greater obsession severity (as measured by the Y-BOCS), whereas lower openness to actions was associated with greater compulsive severity, suggesting that openness may be a nonspecific vulnerability in OCD etiology (Rector et al. 2005).

Disgust reaction with and without anxiety

Studies suggest that in addition to anxiety and fear, disgust may play an important role in OCD. A review of the neurocircuitry of OCD and disgust highlight several similarities in their neural bases. Analysis of literature on functional neuroimaging studies revealed increases in neural activity unique to disgust (Husted et al. 2006). Based on this review of research, it was concluded that significant activity occurs in the insular cortex and cortico–striato–thalamic–cortical circuitry when disgust is elicited, which is contrary to increased activity in the amygdala during emotions such as fear and anxiety. Functional imaging in OCD patients presenting with contamination fear shows an elevation in neural activity in the same areas (Phillips et al. 2000). In fact, OCD participants showed an even higher level of activation than healthy controls in the insula, the parahippocampal cortex, and inferior frontal gyrus (Phillips et al. 2000) and left insula, right supramarginal gyrus, left caudate nucleus, and right thalamus (Schienle et al. 2005a, 2005b) when exposed to disgust-inducing pictures. The contamination and disease-avoidance evolutionary importance for disgust as an emotion, together with overlapping neural activity in patients presenting with contamination fear OCD, suggests a strong potential connection of disgust and OCD.

More recent studies continue to provide evidence of heightened neural activity from disgust reactions in OCD patients. Lawrence et al. (2007) examined neural responses to facial expressions of disgust in OCD patients with washing symptoms. They showed enhanced responses to facial disgust expressions in the left inferior frontal gyrus (ventrolateral, prefrontal cortex, Brodmann area 47). These findings were consistent with other similar studies examining neural activation in response to disgust in OCD patients (Sprengelmeyer et al. 1998; Shapira et al. 2003; Schienle et al. 2005a, 2005b).

In conjunction with neurological similarities between disgust and OCD, increased disgust sensitivity has been examined as a major etiological factor in OCD. Charash and McKay (2002) examined the relationship between disgust and OCD and showed a significant correlation between disgust sensitivity and obsessive thoughts on the Cleaning and Checking Scales of the Maudsley Obsessive-Compulsive Inventory. To determine which domains of disgust sensitivity are related to which kinds of OCD symptom, Tolin et al. (2006) examined disgust sensitivity and OCSs in a non-clinical sample. They gathered data on disgust sensitivity, OCSs, trait anxiety, and depression symptoms using self-report measures, which included the Disgust Sensitivity (DS) scale, the OCI-R, the Self-Rated Anxiety Scale, and the Center for Epidemiological Studies – Depression Scale. Similar to previous findings, when controlling for anxiety and depression, several correlations between disgust sensitivity and OCD symptoms remained significant. When examining relationships between DS and OCI-R subscales, OCI-R Washing and DS Hygiene Subscales were significantly correlated and found to have the clearest relationship.

Findings from Olatunji et al. (2004) were consistent with previous research in that they found a significant relationship between disgust and contamination fear. Their study was replicated using a US sample of 292 undergraduates and a Dutch sample of 260 students to examine similarities and differences of disgust and contamination fears across cultures (Sawchuk et al. 2006). The US sample reported higher disgust sensitivity overall, with the largest between-group differences occurring on the Sex and Sympathetic Magic domains. Culture differences, therefore, should be considered when examining the role of disgust in contamination fears. The authors hypothesized that social influence and culture shaping may be a considerable factor in the development of disgust sensitivity.

Interactions between anxiety and disgust have also been investigated in contamination-based OCD. Two studies by Cisler et al. (2007) generated robust findings for the interaction of anxiety sensitivity and disgust sensitivity as a predictor of contamination fears in a non-clinical sample. Both anxiety sensitivity and disgust sensitivity independently predicted contamination fears. The additive effects of anxiety sensitivity and disgust sensitivity were qualified by an interaction between the two constructs. In explaining their findings, the authors described how maladaptive contamination fears may develop through this interaction. They hypothesized that a fear of responding with disgust may heighten the aversive subjective experience of feeling disgust, which then leads to contamination fears accompanied by heightened avoidance, compensatory behaviors, and negative appraisals.

In addition to self-report investigations, a good portion of literature supports disgust-mediated behavioral avoidance in contamination-based OCD. Tsao and McKay (2004) examined the role of disgust in individuals with contamination fear subtype of OCD using behavioral avoidance tests (BATs). The test areas included food, animals, body products, body envelope violations, death, and sympathetic magic. The high and low trait-anxious did not significantly differ on any BAT outcome variable. Increased disgust sensitivity for the contamination fearful group, however, was evident through significant differences on performance in food, animal, body envelope, and sympathetic magic BATs. Furthermore, animal and magic BATs

discriminated significantly between the high trait-anxious group and the contamination fearful group, suggesting that responses were governed by disgust reactions and not solely generalized anxiety in these particular areas. The authors concluded that the findings of this study may suggest that behavioral avoidance in this subtype of OCD could be caused by severe disgust reactions and not simply by irrational fears of germs and/or other harmful agents.

To further investigate behavioral avoidance in contamination-based OCD, Olatunji et al. (2007) used a college student sample divided into groups representing participants with high OCD contamination concerns and low concerns based on scores from the Vancouver Obsessional Compulsive Inventory. Disgust sensitivity was measured using the DS and BATs. Following administration of questionnaires, participants watched a disgust-eliciting video clip and then underwent eight disgust-related BATs consistent with previous literature. In the BATs assessment, the group with high OCD contamination concerns had significantly more refusals to comply than the group with low concerns on all tasks with the exception of the envelope violations task. They were also significantly less willing to approach the repugnant stimuli of these tasks.

A mediational analysis based on Baron and Kenny's model of mediation revealed that behavioral avoidance of BATs was mediated by disgust sensitivity in the group with high OCD contamination concerns, although only partial mediation was found for body products and hygiene tasks (Olatunji et al. 2007). This is consistent with other findings in similar studies, suggesting that other factors such as health anxiety fears may be involved. Another important finding of this study is that fear and disgust ratings on the Brief Psychiatric Rating Scale were highly correlated, suggesting a potential co-occurrence of fear and disgust emotions in behavioral avoidance of disgusting stimuli.

Deacon and Olatunji (2007) further clarified the role of disgust sensitivity as a predictor of behavioral avoidance in contamination fear. Participants were assigned to high and low contamination fearful groups based upon scores on the Padua Inventory. Measures of disgust (DS scale), anxiety (Beck Anxiety Inventory), depression (Beck Depression Inventory), and threat overestimation (Contamination Cognitions Scale) were completed. Three contamination-based BATs were used (used comb, cookie on the floor, and bedpan with toilet water) as measures of behavioral avoidance. When gender, contamination fear group membership, anxiety, and depression were controlled for, disgust sensitivity was found to be the only significant predictor of BAT anxiety and avoidance. Results of this study implicated disgust sensitivity as a "unique vulnerability factor" for behavioral avoidance based on contamination fears. Disgust sensitivity was also found to be a mediator between threat overestimation and contamination fear. In other words, disgust generated from the overestimation of threat likely leads to contamination fear and behavioral avoidance.

Given the demonstrated disgust-mediated behavioral avoidance found in contamination-based OCD, changes in treatment focus may be warranted. The hypothesis that severe disgust reactions may be an overlooked treatment target in contamination-fearful OCD patients was addressed by McKay (2006). This study examined the effectiveness of exposure to disgust stimuli in reducing disgust reactions for OCD. Two groups, one presenting with primary contamination fears and the second with other primary symptoms, were compared. Traditional ERP for the particular participants' primary symptoms was utilized in combination with exposure to non-anxiety provoking disgust stimuli (e.g., used garbage cans, stick food, dirty water). Results demonstrated non-significant decreases in symptom (obsessions and compulsions) severity ratings for both groups after five sessions of exposure for disgust and anxiety. In addition, the group with other primary symptoms showed greater decreases in disgust after five sessions of exposure than the group with primary contamination fears. These findings are consistent with other research suggesting that habituation to disgust occurs slower than for anxiety. Important treatment implications are apparent. It may be that prolonged intense exposure to disgust evoking stimuli may be necessary to relieve symptoms for psychiatric disorders involving disgust as a mechanism.

Therapy/therapist/patient variables

Although most clinicians try to be highly aware of the nature of the therapeutic relationship and the context of the therapy, there is little mention of this in the CBT literature. In treating the OC spectrum disorders, the setting of the therapeutic sessions is a considerably important factor. In vivo exposure requires ingenuity and flexibility on both the therapist's and patients' part and may be conducted in non-traditional settings, such as in a public place or the patient's home. Adequate psychoeducation regarding the process and assessing patients' beliefs and expectations for treatment are necessary.

In addition, patients with OCD may experience considerable anxiety about the setting of the session because an aspect of the therapeutic environment is anxiety provoking. For example, an OCD patient may be unable to tolerate the "dirty" office, experience difficulty crossing the various thresholds from the car to the therapist's office, and so on. These types of factor may need to be assessed and solutions discussed in the early stages of treatment and adjustments made accordingly.

Pacing of exposure exercises and assigning a reasonable level of therapy homework are also key factors in treating OCD. A typical 45 minute therapy session is often not sufficient time for planning and carrying out an exposure exercise. Patients may leave the session at the height of their anxiety, which may result in patient dropout or increased reluctance to participate in treatment. Longer sessions are required to carry out specific ERP exercises and should be planned as needed.

Therapists working with OCD and the spectrum disorders sometimes find it challenging to find the right balance of respecting the patient's right to say no and pushing their patient to engage in exposure exercises. It is prudent to proceed slowly in the beginning stages of treatment in order to develop a strong therapeutic relationship. Individuals vary in their ability to accurately predict their anxiety level during exposures, so if a patient consistently overestimates how anxious he or she will be during a particular exercise but does well with some encouragement, then it is probably safe to push a bit harder than with a person who has a very low tolerance for anxiety and who does not habituate quickly.

The use of humor and creativity is often overlooked in the behavioral treatment literature, but it is worth some attention since it may lead to increased compliance. Engaging in behavioral treatment can be a daunting experience for patients; they willingly attend session after session with the knowledge that the goal is to create anxiety for symptom relief. Incorporating humor into exposure scripts or adding creativity to homework assignments can help patients to feel more comfortable with the process.

Treatment planning

Based on the initial consultation, treatment professionals will likely have begun to compile a list of the patients' obsessions, rigid or irrational thoughts, compulsions, and avoidant behaviors. Data obtained from various self-report measures can also assist clinicians in gathering data necessary for hierarchy construction and pacing of treatment.

In addition, discussing the chronology and development of the particular disorder, activating events, and others' responses can shed significant light on how the symptoms began, evolved, and have been maintained.

This basic information about trigger events, people, and situations, as well as specific responses to these, can also help the treating clinician to develop the basic foundation of the hierarchy. Obtaining baseline measures of the frequency, intensity, and duration of specific compulsive behaviors, combined with data based on direct behavioral observations and planned BATs tends to flesh out the hierarchy, providing a solid framework for developing exposure with ERP exercises and rational disputations to irrational thoughts.

Adjunct therapies to exposure and response prevention therapy

A major criticism of ERP has been patient attrition. Contributing to patient attrition are family variables of antagonism or accommodation, low levels of emotional support, and high expressed emotion. In addition, the challenges of treating patients with post-traumatic stress disorder symptoms and anxiety, because of their relationship problems, their difficulty managing emotions, their inability to tolerate distress, their shame and guilt, and the presence of dissociation or anger reactions, requires the incorporation of approaches other than ERP. Accordingly, other integrative approaches have been developed.

Cognitive therapy

Cognitive therapy, originally developed by Beck, is often used as an adjunct to ERP. Cognitive restructuring involves an examination of the activating event, the beliefs generated, and the consequences that ensue. Following this process, there is a reframing of the belief system in a manner that challenges the negative thought patterns and allows patients to look at their schemas differently.

The Obsessive Compulsive Cognitions Working Group (1997) identified six main domains of thoughts in OCD which should be targeted for effective CT:

- inflated responsibility
- overimportance of thoughts
- excessive concern about the importance of controlling one's thoughts
- overestimation of threat
- intolerance of uncertainty
- perfectionism.

Cognitive distortions frequently experienced by OCD patients include "should statements," magnification, and perfectionism (Yurica and DiTomasso 2001).

Acceptance and commitment therapy

According to Hayes and Pierson (2005), problems emanate from a set of problems described by the acronym FEAR: fusion with your thoughts, evaluation of your experience, avoidance of your experience, and reason-giving for your behavior. The defense against FEAR is accepting one's reactions and being present, choosing a valued direction, and taking action. The ACT approach derives its origins from clinical behavior analysis and, according to Hayes and Pierson (2005), "uses metaphors, experiential exercises and logical paradox to get around the literal content of language and to produce more contact with the ongoing flow of experience in the moment." Thus, ACT utilizes acceptance and mindfulness strategies, coupled with commitment and behavioral change, to increase psychological flexibility.

Use of ACT can facilitate a patient's willingness to experience anxiety and, as such, may increase the patient's ability to participate in ERP (Eifert and Heffner 2003). Decreasing experiential avoidance improves treatment outcome (Hayes et al. 2006). Dalrymple and Herbert (2007) examined the effectiveness of ACT combined with ERP with 19 patients experiencing social anxiety disorder. The first and second sessions were devoted to the theme of willingness as an alternative to controlling unwanted events, while sessions 3–12 focused upon standard ERP. The patients were able to experience anxiety while engaging in social situations and evidenced significant improvement from pretreatment to follow-up, experiencing increased functioning, a better quality of life, and greater control over emotional reactions and external events.

One recent study found clinically significant reductions in compulsions in four OCD patients after eight sessions of ACT (Twohig et al. 2006). The authors reported positive changes in anxiety, depression, decreased experiential avoidance, believability of obsessions, and a need to respond to obsessions. Use of ACT appears particularly helpful when patients are unable to tolerate the anxiety of ERP and display a high overvalued ideation; ACT may be employed previous to or in conjunction with ERP.

The use of ACT to assist a patient in participating without resistance to ERP makes it a useful adjunctive treatment to ERP.

Dialectical behavior therapy

Dialectical behavior therapy was originally developed by Linehan to treat borderline personality disorder with suicidal ideation (Neacsiu *et al.* 2010). It is rooted in mindfulness and behavior therapy and utilizes behavior analysis and exposure to block resistance and damaging and dysfunctional behaviors. Aside from borderline personality disorders, dialectical behavior therapy has shown promising results for substance abuse (Dimeff *et al.* 2000) and eating disorders (Chen *et al.* 2008).

Cognitive-behavioral family therapy

Both clinicians and researchers have long recognized the influence of family variables in terms of the ultimate effectiveness of ERP treatment (Van Noppen *et al.* 1991; Amir *et al.* 2000; Steketee and Van Noppen 2003).

Van Noppen *et al.* (1991) felt that family members tend to exhibit a continuum of behaviors ranging from accommodation ("accommodating style") to rejection ("antagonistic style"). They also distinguish "split families," families who have one member relating in an accommodating style and another member relating in an antagonistic style. Accommodating families tend to be "permissive, over-involved and intrusive," whereas antagonistic families tend to be "detached, rigid, punitive, and critical." Accommodating increases OCSs, and the stress for the patient that emerges from antagonistic familial styles increases stress for the OCD patient, similarly increasing OCSs.

Amir *et al.* (2000) examined familial responses to OCD and their impact on the severity of symptoms, as well as the relationship between accommodation and rejection and treatment outcome. There was a correlation between family distress, accommodation, and rejection and depression and anxiety in family members. There was also a relationship between accommodation and the severity of symptoms at post-treatment.

Occurrence of OCD affects the whole family system. Families often organize around the symptoms and are puzzled about the most helpful actions to take. Educating family members as to appropriate ways of responding can reduce OCSs, aid ERP efforts, and enhance and reinforce autonomy and self-efficacy.

Conclusions

It appears that after 40 plus years of research in the treatment of OCD, ERP is a very effective modality. Despite its efficacy, there are many factors that may complicate its usage; consequently, utilization of adjunct treatments may be necessary. Treatments such as ACT, dialectical behavior therapy, family therapy, behavioral activation and/or purely CT addressing overvalued ideation, depression, and personality disorders may be essential to enhance the efficacy of ERP.

References

Abel J (1993). Exposure with response prevention and serotonergic antidepressants in the treatment of obsessive compulsive disorder. *Behav Res Ther* **3**: 463–478.

Abramowitz JS (1997). Effectiveness of psychological and pharmacological treatments for obsessive-compulsive disorder: A quantitative review of the controlled treatment literature. *J Consult Clin Psychol* **65**: 44–52.

Abramowitz JS, Franklin ME, Kozak MJ, Street GP, Foa EB (2000). The effects of pretreatment depression on cognitive-behavioral treatment outcome in OCD clinic patients. *Behav Ther* **31**: 517–528.

Abramowitz JS, Foa EB, Franklin ME (2003). Exposure and ritual prevention for obsessive-compulsive disorder: Effectiveness of intensive versus twice-weekly treatment sessions. *J Consult Clin Psychol* **71**: 394–398.

Abramowitz J, Taylor S, McKay D (2005a). Potentials and limitations of cognitive treatments for obsessive-compulsive disorder. *Cogn Behav Ther* **34**: 140–147.

Abramowitz JS, Whiteside SP, Deacon BJ (2005b). The effectiveness of treatment for pediatric obsessive-compulsive disorder: a meta-analysis. *Behav Ther* **36**: 55–63.

Abramowitz JS, Taylor S, McKay D (eds.) (2008). *Clinical Handbook of Obsessive-Compulsive Disorder and Related Problems*. Baltimore, MD: Johns Hopkins University Press.

Amir N, Freshman MS, Foa EB (2000). Family accommodation and rejection in relatives of OCD patients. *J Anxiety Disord* **14**: 209–217.

Antony MM, Downie F, Swinson RP (1998). Diagnostic issues and epidemiology in obsessive-compulsive disorder. In Swinson RP Antony MM, Rachman S, Richter RA (eds.) *Obsessive Compulsive Disorder: Theory, Research and Treatment* (pp. 3–32). New York: Guilford Press.

Azrin NH, Nunn RG (1973). Habit reversal: a method of eliminating nervous habits and tics. *Behav Res Ther* **11**: 619–628.

Bagley A, Abramowitz C, Kosson D (2009). Vocal affect recognition and psychopathy: converging findings across traditional and cluster analytic approaches to assessing the construct. *J Abnorm Psychol* **118**: 388–398.

Baer L, Minichiello WW (1990). Behavior therapy for obsessive compulsive disorder. In Jenike MA, Baer L, Minichiello WE (eds.) *Obsessive Compulsive Disorders: Theory and Management* (pp. 203–232). Chicago, IL: Year Book Medical.

Baum M (1965). An automated apparatus for the avoidance training of rats. *Psychol Rep* **16**: 1205–1211.

Baum M (1969a). Extinction of an avoidance response following a period of response prevention in the avoidance apparatus. *Psychol Rep* **18**: 59–64.

Baum M (1969b). Paradoxical effect of alcohol on the resistance to extinction of an avoidance response in rats. *J Compr Physiol Psychol* **69**: 238–240.

Baum M (1970). Effect of alcohol on the acquisition and resistance to extinction of avoidance responses in rats. *Psychol Rep* **26**: 759–765.

Baxter LR, Schwartz JM, Bergmann KS, *et al.* (1992). Caudate glucose metabolic rate changes with both drug and behavior therapy for obsessive compulsive disorder. *Arch Gen Psychiatry* **49**: 681–689.

Bejerot S, von Knorring L, Ekselius L (2000). Personality traits and smoking in patients with obsessive-compulsive disorder. *Eur Psychiatry* **15**: 395–401.

Bienvenu O, Samuels J, Riddle M, *et al.* (2000). The relationship of obsessive-compulsive disorder to possible spectrum disorders: Results from a family study. *Biol Psychiatry* **48**: 287–293.

Boersma K, den Hengst S, Dekker J, Emmelkamp PMG (1976). Exposure and response prevention in the natural environment: A comparison with obsessive-compulsive patients. *Behav Res Ther* **14**: 19–24.

Bolton D, Luckie M, Steinberg D (1995). Obsessive compulsive disorder treated in adolescence: 14 long term case histories. *Clin Child Psychol Psychiatry* **1**: 409–430.

Boulougouris JC, Bassiakos L (1973). Prolonged flooding in cases with obsessive-compulsive neurosis. *Behav Res Ther* **11**: 227–231.

Brakoulias V, Starcevic V (2008). Symptom subtypes of obsessive compulsive disorder: Are they relevant for treatment? *Aust N Z J Psychiatry* **42**: 651–661.

Calamari JE, Wiegartz PS, Janeck AS (1999). Obsessive compulsive disorder subgroups: a symptom-based clustering approach. *Behav Res Ther* **37**: 113–125.

Catts S, McConaghy N (1975). Ritual prevention in the treatment of obsessive compulsive neurosis. *Aust N Z J Psychiatry* **9**: 37–41.

Cath DC, Spinhoven PH, van der Wetering BJM, *et al.* (2000). The relationship between types and severity of repetitive behaviors in Gilles de la Tourette's syndrome and obsessive-compulsive disorder. *J Clin Psychiatry* **61**: 505–513.

Cath DC, Spinhoven PH, Hoogduin CAL, *et al.* (2001). Repetitive behaviors in Tourette's syndrome and obsessive-compulsive disorder with and without tics: What are the differences? *Psychiatry Res* **101**: 171–185.

Charash M, McKay D (2002). Attention bias for disgust. *J Anxiety Disord* **16**: 529–541.

Chen EY, Matthews L, Allen C, Kuo JR, Linehan MM (2008). Dialectical behavior therapy for clients with binge-eating disorder or bulimia nervosa and borderline personality disorder. *Int J Eating Disord* **41**: 505–512.

Christenson G, Pyle R, Mitchell J (1991). Estimated lifetime prevalence of trichotillomania in college students. *J Clin Psychiatry* **52**: 415–417.

Cisler JM, Reardon JM, Williams NL, Lohr JM (2007). Anxiety sensitivity and disgust sensitivity interact to predict contamination fears. *Pers Individ Dif* **42**: 935–946.

Dalrymple KL, Herbert JD (2007). Acceptance and commitment therapy for generalized social anxiety disorder: A pilot study. *Behav Modif* **31**: 543–568.

Deacon B, Olatunji BO (2007). Specificity of disgust sensitivity in the prediction of behavioral avoidance in contamination fear. *Behav Res Ther* **45**: 2110–2120.

Dimeff L, Rizvi SL, Brown M, Linehan MM (2000). Dialectical behavior therapy for substance abuse: A pilot application to methamphetamine dependent women with borderline personality disorder. *Cogn Behav Pract* **7**: 457–468.

Dollard J, Miller E (1950). *Personality and Psychotherapy: An Analysis in Terms of Learning, Thinking and Culture.* New York: McGraw-Hill.

Emmelkamp PME, Beens H (1991). Cognitive therapy with obsessive compulsive disorder: a comparative evaluation. *Behav Res Ther* **29**: 293–300.

Emmelkamp PME, Visser S, Hoekstra R (1988). Cognitive therapy versus exposure in vivo in the treatment of obsessive compulsives. *Cogn Ther Res* **12**: 103–114.

Eifert G, Heffner M (2003). The effects of acceptance versus control contexts on avoidance of panic-related symptoms. *J Behav Ther Exp Psychiatry* **34**: 293–312.

Eisen J, Phillips K, Baer L, *et al.* (1998). The Brown Assessment of Beliefs Scale: reliability and validity. *Am J Psychiatry* **155**: 102–108.

Fallon BA, Javitch JA, Hollander E, Liebowitz MR (1992). Hypochondriasis and obsessive compulsive disorder: overlaps in diagnosis and treatment. *J Clin Psychiatry* **52**: 457–460.

Foa EB (1979). Failure in treating obsessive-compulsives. *Behav Res Ther* **17**: 169–176.

Foa E, Goldstein A (1978). Continuous exposure and complete response prevention in the treatment of obsessive compulsive neurosis. *Behav Ther* **9**: 821–829.

Foa EB, Kozak J (1996). Psychological treatment for obsessive compulsive disorder. In Mavissakalian MR, Prien RF (eds.) *Long-term Treatments of Anxiety Disorders* (pp. 285–309). Washington DC: American Psychiatric Press.

Foa EB, Grayson JB, Steketee GS, *et al.* (1983). Success and failure in the behavioral treatment of obsessive-compulsives. *J Consult Clin Psychol* **51**: 287–297.

Foa E, Franklin M, Kozak M (1998). Psychosocial treatment for obsessive compulsive disorder: literature review. In Swinson RP Antony MM, Rachman S, Richter RA (eds.) *Obsessive Compulsive Disorder: Theory, Research, and Treatment* (pp. 258–276). New York: Guilford Press.

Foa EB, Huppert JD, Leiberg S, *et al.* (2002). The obsessive compulsive inventory: development and validation of a short version. *Psychol Assess* **14**: 485–496.

Foa EB Liebowitz MR, Kozak J, *et al.* (2005). Randomized placebo-controlled trial of ERP, clomipramine, and their combination in the treatment of OCD *Am J Psychiatry* **162**: 151–161.

Folette VM, Smith AA (2005). Exposure therapy. In Freeman A, Felgoise SH, Nezu CM, Nezu AM, Reinecke MA (eds.) *Encyclopedia of Cognitive Behavior Therapy* (pp.185–187). New York: Springer.

George MS, Trimble MR, Ring HA, Sallee FR, Robertson MM (1993). Obsessions in obsessive-compulsive disorder with and without Gilles de la Tourette's syndrome. *Am J Psychiatry* **150**: 93–97.

Goodman WK, Price LH, Rasmussen SA, *et al.* (1989). The Yale–Brown Obsessive Compulsive Scale: II Validity. *Arch Gen Psychiatry* **46**: 1012–1016.

Hachman A, McLean C (1975). A comparison of flooding and thought stopping in the treatment of obsessional neurosis. *Behav Res Ther* **34**: 47–51.

Hasler G, LaSalle-Ricci VH, Ronquillo JG, *et al.* (2005). Obsessive compulsive disorder symptom dimensions show specific relationships to psychiatric comorbidity. *Psychiatry Res* **135**: 121.

Hayes SC, Pierson H (2005). Acceptance and commitment therapy. In Freeman A, Felgoise SH, Nezu CM, Nezu AM, Reinecke MA (eds.) *Encyclopedia of Cognitive Behavior Therapy* (pp.1–4). New York: Springer.

Hayes SC, Barnes-Holmes D, Roche B (eds.) (2001). *Relational Frame Theory: A Post-Skinnerian Account of Human Language and Cognition.* New York: Kluwer Academic.

Hayes S, Luoma J, Bond F, Masuda A, Lillis J (2006). Acceptance and commitment therapy: model, processes and outcomes. *Behav Res Ther* **44**: 1–25.

Hembree EA, Riggs DS, Kozak MJ, Franklin ME, Foa EB (2003). Long-term efficacy of exposure and ritual prevention therapy and serotonergic medications for obsessive-compulsive disorder. *CNS Spectr* **8**: 363–371.

Hodgson R, Rachman S, Marks I (1972). The treatment of chronic obsessive-compulsive neurosis: Follow-up and further findings. *Behav Res Ther* **10**: 181–189.

Hollander E (1993). Obsessive-compulsive spectrum disorders: an overview. *Psychiatr Ann* **23**: 355–358.

Hollander E, Cohen L (1996). Psychobiology and psychopharmacology of compulsive spectrum disorders. In Oldham JM, Hollander E, Skodol AE (eds.) *Impulsivity and Compulsivity* (pp. 143–166). Washington, DC: American Psychiatric Press.

Hollander E, Wong C (1995). Obsessive compulsive spectrum disorders. *J Clin Psychiatry* **56**: 3–6.

Hollander E, Cohen L, Simeon D (1993). Body dysmorphic disorder. *Psychiatr Ann* **23**: 359–364.

Holzer JC, Goodman WK, McDougle CJ, *et al.* (1994). Obsessive-compulsive disorder with and without a chronic tic disorder: a comparison of symptoms in 70 patients. *Br J Psychiatry* **164**: 469–473.

Hoogduin CAL, Duivenvoorden HJ (1988). A decision model in the treatment of obsessive compulsive neuroses. *Br J Psychiatry* **152**: 515–521.

Huppert JD, Foa EB (2005). Severe OCD. In Freeman A, Felgoise SH, Nezu CM, Nezu AM, Reinecke MA (eds.) *Encyclopedia of Cognitive Behavior Therapy* (pp. 347–349). New York: Springer.

Husted DS, Shapira NA, Goodman WK (2006). The neurocircuitry of obsessive-compulsive disorder and disgust. *Prog Neuropsychopharmacol Biol Psychiatry* **30**: 389–399.

Jaspers K (1913). *General Psychopathology.* Berlin: Springer.

Keijsers GP, Hoogduin CA, Schaap CP (1994). Predictors of treatment outcome in the behavioural treatment of obsessive-compulsive disorder. *Br J Psychiatry* **165**: 781–786.

Kushner MG, Won KS, Donahue C, *et al.* (2007). d-Cycloserine augmented exposure therapy for obsessive compulsive disorder. *Biol Psychiatry* **62**: 835–838.

Kishore R, Samar R, Reddy J, Chandrasekhar CR, Thennarasu K (2004). Clinical characteristics and treatment response in poor and good insight obsessive compulsive disorder. *Eur Psychiatry* **19**: 202–208.

Kirk J (1983). Behavioural treatment of obsessional-compulsive patients in routine clinical practice. *Behav Res Ther* **21**: 57–62.

Kozak M, Foa E (1994). Obsessions, overvalued ideas, and delusions in obsessive-compulsive disorder. *Behav Res Ther* **32**: 343–353.

Lawrence NS, An KS, Mataix-Cols D, *et al.* (2007). Neural responses to facial expressions of disgust but not fear are modulated by washing symptoms in OCD. *Biol Psychiatry* **61**: 1072–1080.

Leckman JF, Grice DE, Boardman J, *et al.* (1997). Symptoms of obsessive compulsive disorder. *Am J Psychiatry* **154**: 911–917.

Lee HJ, Kwon SM (2003). Two different types of obsession: autogenous obsessions and reactive obsessions. *Behav Res Ther* **41**: 11–29.

Lee HJ, Telch MJ (2005). Autogenous/reactive obsessions and their relationship with OCD symptoms and schizotypal personality features. *J Anxiety Disord* **19**: 793–805.

Lee HJ, Kim ZS, Kwon SM (2005a). Thought disorder in patients with obsessive-compulsive disorder. *J Clin Psychol* **61**: 401–413.

Lee H, Kwon S, Kwon J, Telch M (2005b). Testing the autogenous-reactive model of obsessions. *Depress Anxiety* **21**: 118–129.

Lindsay M, Crino R, Andrews G (1997). Controlled trial of exposure and response prevention in obsessive compulsive disorder. *Br J Psychiatry* **171**: 135–139.

Maier N (1949). *Frustration: The Study of Behavior Without a Goal*. New York: McGraw-Hill.

Marks IM, Hodgson R, Rachman S (1975). Treatment of chronic obsessive-compulsive neurosis by in vivo exposure. *Br J Psychiatry* **127**: 349–364.

Marks IM, Stern RS, Mawson D, Cobb J, McDonald R (1980). Clomipramine and exposure for obsessive compulsive rituals. *Br J Psychiatry* **136**: 1–25.

Marks IM, Lelliott PT, Basoglu M, *et al.* (1988). Clomipramine, self-exposure, and therapist-aided exposure for obsessive-compulsive rituals. *Br J Psychiatry* **152**: 522–534.

Masellis M, Rector NA, Richter MA (2003). Quality of life in OCD: differential impact of obsessions, compulsions, and depression comorbidity. *Can J Psychiatry* **48**: 72–77.

Mataix-Cols D, Marks I, Greist J, Kobak K, Baer L (2002). Obsessive-compulsive symptom dimensions as predictors of compliance with and response to

behaviour therapy: Results from a controlled trial. *Psychother Psychosomat* **71**: 255–262.

Mavissakalian M, Turner SM, Michelson L (1985). Future directions in the assessment and treatment of obsessive compulsive disorder. In Mavissakalian M, Turner SM, Michelson L (eds.) *Obsessive-Compulsive Disorder: Psychological and Pharmacological Treatment* (pp. 213–228). New York: Plenum Press.

Mawson D, Marks IM, Romm L (1982). Clomipramine and exposure for chronic obsessive compulsive disorders: two year follow-up and further findings. *Br J Psychiatry* **140**: 11–18.

McKay D (2006). Treating disgust reactions in contamination-based obsessive-compulsive disorder. *J Behav Ther Exp Psychiatry* **37**: 53–59.

McKay D, Neziroglu F (1996). Social skills training in a case of obsessive compulsive disorder with schizotypal personality disorder. *J Behav Ther Exp Psychiatry* **27**: 189–194.

McKay D, Neziroglu F (2009). Methodological issues in the obsessive compulsive spectrum. *Psychiatry Res* **170**: 61–65.

McKay D, Neziroglu F, Yaryura-Tobias JA (1997). Comparison of clinical characteristics in obsessive compulsive disorder and body dysmorphic disorder. *J Anxiety Disord* **11**: 447–454.

Meyer V (1966). Modification of expectations in cases with obsessional rituals. *Behav Res Ther* **4**: 273–280.

Miguel EC, Leckman JF, Rauch S, *et al.* (2005). Obsessive compulsive disorder phenotypes: Implications for genetic studies. *Mol Psychiatry* **10**: 258–275.

Mills HL, Stewart A, Barlow DH, Mills JR (1973). Compulsive rituals treated by response prevention: an experimental analysis. *Arch Gen Psychiatry* **28**: 524–529.

Mowrer H (1947). On the dual nature of learning: A reinterpretation of conditioning and problem solving. *Harvard Educ Rev* **17**: 102–148.

Neacsiu AD, Rizvi SL, Linehan MM (2010). Dialectical behavior therapy skills use as a mediator and outcome of treatment for borderline personality disorder. *Behav Res Ther* **48**: 832–839.

Neziroglu F, Khemlani-Patel S (2005). Overlap of body dysmorphic disorder and hypochondriasis with OCD. In Abramowitz JS, Houts AC (eds.) *Concepts and Controversies in Obsessive-Compulsive Disorder* (pp. 163–175). New York: Springer.

Neziroglu F, Neuman J (1990). Three approaches to the treatment of obsessions. *Int J Cogn Ther* **4**: 371–392.

Neziroglu F, Yaryura-Tobias JA (1993). Exposure, response prevention, and cognitive therapy in the treatment of body dysmorphic disorder. *Behav Ther* **24**, 431–438.

Neziroglu F, Steele J, Yaryura-Tobias JA (1990). Effect of behavior therapy on serotonin level in obsessive compulsive disorder. In Stefanis CN (ed.) *Psychiatry: A World Perspective* (pp. 707–710). New York: Elsevier.

Neziroglu F, McKay D, Yaryura-Tobias JA, Stevens K, Todaro J, (1999). The overvalues ideas scale: development, reliability and validity in obsessive-compulsive disorder. *J Res Behav Ther* **37**: 881–902.

Neziroglu F, McKay D, Yaryura-Tobias J (2000). Overlapping and distinctive features of hypochondriasis and obsessive-compulsive disorder. *J Anxiety Disord* **14**: 603–614.

Neziroglu F, Stevens K, McKay D, Yaryura-Tobias JA, (2001) Predictive validity of the overvalued ideas scale: outcome in obsessive-compulsive and body dysmorphic disorders. *J Res Behav Ther* **39**: 745–756.

Neziroglu F, Bubrick J, Yaryura-Tobias JA (2004). *Overcoming Compulsive Hoarding*. Oakland, CA: New Harbinger Press.

Neziroglu F, Henricksen J, Yaryura-Tobias J (2006). Psychotherapy of Obsessive-Compulsive Disorder and Spectrum: Established Facts and Advances 1995–5005. *Psychiatr Clin N Am* **29**: 585–604.

Neziroglu F, Weissman S, Yaryura-Tobias JA, Allen J (2010). Compulsive hoarders: how they are similar to individuals with obsessive compulsive disorder? *J Behav Res Ther* in press.

Obsessive Compulsive Cognitions Working Group (1997). Cognitive assessment of obsessive compulsive disorder. *Behav Res Ther* **35**: 667–681.

Olatunji BO, Sawchuk CN, Lohr JM, de Jong PJ (2004). Disgust domains in the prediction of contamination fear. *Behav Res Ther* **42**: 93–104.

Olatunji BO, Lohr JM, Sawchuk CN, Tolin DF (2007). Multimodal assessment of disgust in contamination-related obsessive-compulsive disorder. *Behav Res Ther* **45**: 263–276.

O'Sullivan G, Noshirvani H, Marks I, *et al.* (1991). Six year follow up after exposure and clomipramine therapy for obsessive compulsive disorder. *J Clin Psychiatry* **52**: 150–155.

Perugi G, Giannotti D, Frare F, *et al.* (1997). Prevalence, phenomenology and co-morbidity of body dysmorphic disorder in a clinical population. *Int J Psychiatr Clin Pract* **1**: 77–82.

Phillips KA, McElroy SL, Keck PE, Pope HG, Hudson JI (1993). Body dysmorphic disorder: 30 cases of imagined ugliness. *Am J Psychiatry* **150**: 302–308.

Phillips M, Marks I, Senior C, *et al.* (2000). A differential neural response in obsessive-compulsive disorder patients with washing compared with checking symptoms to disgust. *Psychol Med* **30**: 1037–1050.

Rabavilas AD, Boulougouris JC, Stefanis D (1976). Duration of flooding session in the treatment of obsessive compulsive patients. *Behav Res Ther* **14**: 349–355.

Rachman S, Hodgson R, Marks IM (1971). The treatment of chronic obsessive-compulsive neurosis. *Behav Res Ther* **9**: 237–247.

Rachman S, Marks I, Hodgson R (1973). The treatment of obsessive-compulsive neurotics by modeling and flooding in vivo. *Behav Res Ther* **11**: 463–471.

Rasmussen SA, Eisen JL (1992). The epidemiology and clinical features of obsessive-compulsive disorder. *J Clin Psychiatry* **53**: 4–10.

Rasmussen SA, Tsuang MT (1986). Clinical characteristics and family history in DSM-III obsessive compulsive disorder. *Am J Psychiatry* **14**: 317–322.

Rauch SL, Jenike MA, Alpert NM, *et al.* (1994). Regional cerebral blood flow measured during symptom provocation in obsessive-compulsive disorder using oxygen 15-labeled carbon dioxide and positron emission tomography. *Arch Gen Psychiatry* **51**: 62–70.

Rauch SL, Baer L, Jenike MA (1996). Treatment resistant obsessive-compulsive disorder: practical strategies for management. In Pollack MH, Otto MW, Rosenbaum JF (eds.) *Challenges in Psychiatric Treatment: Pharmacologic and Psychosocial Perspectives* (pp. 201–218). New York: Guilford Press.

Rector NA, Richter MA, Bagby RM (2005). The impact of personality on symptom expression in obsessive compulsive disorder. *J Nerv Ment Dis* **193**: 231–236.

Salkovskis PM, Warwick HMC (2001). Meaning, misinterpretations and medicine: a cognitive-behavioral approach to understanding health anxiety and hypochondriasis. In Starcevic V, Lipsitt DR (eds.) *Hypochondriasis: Modern Perspectives on an Ancient Malady* (pp. 202–222). London: Oxford University Press.

Samuels J, Nestadt G, Bienvenu OJ, *et al.* (2000). Personality disorders and normal personality dimensions in obsessive compulsive disorder. *Br J Psychiatry* **177**: 457–462.

Saxena S, Maidment KM, Vapnik T, *et al.* (2002). Obsessive compulsive hoarding: symptom severity and response to multi-modal treatment. *J Clin Psychiatry* **63**: 21–27.

Saxena S, Gorbis E, O'Neill J, *et al.* (2009). Rapid effects of brief intensive cognitive behavioral therapy on brain glucose metabolism in obsessive compulsive disorder. *Mol Psychiatry* **14**: 197–205.

Sawchuk CN, Olatunji BO, de Jong PJ (2006). Disgust domains in the prediction of contamination fear: A comparison of Dutch and US samples. *Anxiety Stress Coping* **19**: 397–407.

119

Schienle A, Schafer A, Stark R, Walter B, Vaitl D (2005a). Neural responses of OCD patients towards disorder-relevant, generally disgust-inducing and fear-inducing pictures. *Int J Psychophysiol* **57**: 69–77.

Schienle A, Schafer A, Stark R, Walter B, Vaitl D (2005b). Relationship between disgust sensitivity, trait anxiety and brain activity during disgust induction. *Neuropsychobiology* **51**: 86–92.

Schwartz JM, Stoessel PW, Baxter LR, Martin KM, Phelps M (1996). Systematic changes in cerebral glucose metabolic rate after successful behavior modification treatment of obsessive compulsive disorder. *Arch Gen Psychiatry* **53**: 109–113.

Seishin SZ (2008). A review of the research focusing on the heterogeneity of obsessive compulsive disorder and its potential subtypes. *Psychiatr Neurol Jap* **110**: 161–174.

Shapira NA, Liu Y, He AG, *et al.* (2003). Brain activation by disgust-inducing pictures in obsessive-compulsive disorder. *Biol Psychiatry* **54**: 751–756.

Simpson HB, Liebowitz M, Foa EB, *et al.* (2004). Post-treatment effects of exposure therapy and clomipramine in obsessive compulsive disorder. *Depress Anxiety* **19**: 225–233.

Simpson HB, Zuckoff A, Page JR, Franklin ME, Foa EB (2008a). Adding motivational interviewing to exposure and ritual prevention for obsessive compulsive disorder. *Cogn Behav Ther* **37**: 38–49.

Simpson HB, Foa EB Liebowitz MR, *et al.* (2008b). A randomized, controlled trial of cognitive behavioral therapy for augmenting pharmacotherapy in obsessive compulsive disorder. *Am J Psychiatry* **165**: 621–630.

Solyom L, Sookman D (1977). A comparison of clomipramine hydrochloride (Anafranil) and behaviour therapy in the treatment of obsessive neurosis. *J Int Med Res* **5**: 49–61.

Sprengelmeyer R, Rausch M, Eysel UT, Przuntek H (1998). Neural structures associated with recognition of facial expressions of basic emotions. *Proc Biological Science* **265**: 1927–1931.

Stanley M, Cohen L (1999). Trichotillomania and obsessive-compulsive disorder. In Stein DJ, Christenson GA, Hollander E (eds.) *Trichotillomania* (pp. 225–261). Washington, DC: American Psychiatric Press.

Stanley M, Turner S, Borden J (1990). Schizotypal features in obsessive-compulsive disorder. *Compr Psychiatry* **31**: 511–518.

Starcevic V (2001). Clinical features and diagnosis of hypochondriasis. In Starcevic V, Lipsitt DR (eds.) *Hypochondriasis: Modern Perspectives on an Ancient Malady* (pp. 21–60). London: Oxford University Press.

Steingard R, Dillon-Stout D (1992). Tourette's syndrome and obsessive compulsive disorder: clinical aspects. *Psychiatr Clin N Am* **15**: 849–960.

Steketee G, Frost R (2003). Compulsive hoarding: current status of the research. *Clin Psychol Rev* **23**: 905–927.

Steketee G, Frost R (2007). *Treatments that Work: Compulsive Hoarding and Acquiring. Therapist Guide and Workbook*. New York: Oxford University Press.

Steketee G, Van Noppen B (2003). Family approaches to treatment for obsessive compulsive disorder. *Rev ABPAPAL* **25**: 43–50.

Steketee G, Henninger N, Pollard C (2000). Predicting treatment outcomes for obsessive-compulsive disorder: effects of comorbidity. In Goodman WK, Rudorfer MV, Maser JD (eds.) *Obsessive-Compulsive Disorder: Contemporary Issues in Treatment* (pp. 257–274). Mahwah, NJ: Lawrence Erlbaum.

Storch EA, Merlo LJ, Bengston M, *et al.* (2007). d-Cycloserine does not enhance exposure and response prevention therapy in obsessive compulsive disorder. *Int Clin Psychopharmacol* **22**: 312.

Tolin DF, Woods CM, Abramowitz JS (2006). Disgust sensitivity and obsessive-compulsive symptoms in a non-clinical sample. *J Behav Ther Exp Psychiatry* **37**: 30–40.

Twohig MP, Hayes SC, Masuda A (2006). Increasing willingness to experience obsessions: acceptance and commitment therapy as a treatment for obsessive compulsive disorder. *Behav Ther* **37**: 3–13.

Tsao SD, McKay D (2004). Behavioral avoidance tests and disgust in contamination fears: distinctions from trait anxiety. *Behav Res Ther* **42**: 207–216.

Van Noppen B, Rasmussen S, Eisen J, McCartney L (1991). A multifamily group approach as an adjunct to treatment of obsessive-compulsive disorder. In Pato MT, Zohar J, (eds.) *Current Treatments of Obsessive-Compulsive Disorder* (pp. 115–134). Washington, DC: American Psychiatric Press.

Van Oppen P, de Haan E, Van Balkom AJLM, Spinhoven P (1995). Cognitive therapy and exposure in vivo in the treatment of obsessive compulsive disorder. *Behav Res Ther* **33**: 379–390.

Van Oppen P, van Balkom A, de Haan E, van Dyck R (2005). Cognitive therapy and exposure in vivo alone. *J Clin Psychiatry* **66**: 1415–1422.

Verdellen CWJ, Keijsers GPJ, Cath DC, Hoogduin CAL (2004). Exposure with response prevention versus habit reversal in Tourette's syndrome: A controlled study. *Behav Res Ther* **42**: 501–511.

Warwick H, Salkovskis P (1990). Hypochondriasis. *Behav Res Ther* **28**: 105–117.

Wernicke C (1906). *Grundrisse der Psychiatrie* (p. 416). [*Fundamentals of Psychiatry.*] Leipzig: Thieme.

Welner A, Reich T, Robbins E, Fishman E, Van Doren T (1976). Obsessive-compulsive neurosis: record, followup, and family studies. I. Inpatient record study. *Compr Psychiatry* **17**: 527–539.

Wetterneck CT, Woods DW (2006). An evaluation of the effectiveness of exposure and response prevention on repetitive behaviors associated with Tourette's syndrome. *J Appl Behav Anal* **39**: 441–444.

Whittal ML, Thordarson DS, McLean PD (2005). Treatment of obsessive-compulsive disorder: cognitive behavior therapy vs. exposure and response prevention. *Behav Res Ther* **43**: 1559–1576.

Wilhelm S, Deckersbach T, Coffey BJ, *et al.* (2003). Habit reversal versus supportive psychotherapy for Tourrette's disorder: A randomized controlled trial. *Am J Psychiatry* **160**: 1175–1177.

Wolpe J (1958). *Psychotherapy by Reciprocal Inhibition.* Stanford, CA: Stanford University Press.

Yaryura-Tobias JA, Neziroglu F (1997). *Obsessive Compulsive Spectrum Disorders: Pathogenesis, Diagnosis and Treatment.* Washington, DC: American Psychiatric Press.

Yurica CL, DiTomasso R (2001). *Inventory of cognitive distortions: development and validation of a psychometric test for the measurement of cognitive distortions.* Ph.D Thesis, Philadelphia College of Osteopathic Medicine.

Compulsive hoarding

Christina M. Gilliam and David F. Tolin

Introduction

Compulsive hoarding is a chronic and debilitating condition that represents a significant public health concern. Hoarding has been associated with high rates of occupational impairment, increased health and safety risks, and family and social burden. With an estimated prevalence of 5% (Samuels *et al.* 2008), compulsive hoarding may be as much as twice as common as obsessive-compulsive disorder (OCD). Despite the high prevalence and the significant detrimental impact of compulsive hoarding, our understanding of this condition is limited, lagging well behind that of OCD and other common psychiatric disorders. The aim of this chapter is to provide an overview of the available literature on compulsive hoarding. After a detailed description of the currently proposed definition of compulsive hoarding, we will review the course and associated features of hoarding. Diagnostic classification of compulsive hoarding will be discussed, followed by presentation of the literature on the social and economic burden of compulsive hoarding. Finally, we will review current models and research on the efficacy of various treatments for compulsive hoarding.

Definition

Compulsive hoarding is not a diagnostic category in the current version of the *Diagnostic and Statistical Manual of Mental Disorders* (DSM; American Psychiatric Association 2000) and, therefore, lacks formal diagnostic criteria. Frost and colleagues (Frost and Gross 1993; Frost and Hartl 1996) identified four key elements to conceptualize compulsive hoarding:

Excessive acquiring. Excessive acquiring is not limited to compulsive buying but includes collection of free things and, on rare occasions, stealing. Many hoarding individuals report spending an inordinate amount of time searching for and acquiring objects, with behaviors that have included excessive spending or rummaging through trash bins (Frost *et al.* 1998). Approximately 85% of individuals with self-reported hoarding symptoms report excessive acquisition; family informants report that nearly 95% exhibit excessive acquisition (Frost *et al.* 2007). High levels of compulsive shopping are often reported (Frost *et al.* 1998), suggesting that acquisition may lead to financial distress in addition to clutter.

Failure to discard possessions. Individuals with compulsive hoarding display strong reluctance to discard objects, including those that others would perceive as "trash" or "junk." Although the reasons for saving or failing to discard objects (e.g., sentimental value, beliefs that the object may be useful or needed in the future, beliefs about wastefulness) are similar to those of non-hoarding individuals (Frost and Gross 1993), these beliefs are applied to a greater number of possessions. Attempts to discard items cause substantial emotional distress and, therefore, are avoided.

Clutter that precludes activities for which living spaces were designed. Excessive clutter is the most visible feature of compulsive hoarding. Acquisition and failure to discard are not typically considered pathological unless they result in significant clutter that interferes with the individual's ability to utilize their home. Common interference from clutter includes inability to sleep in beds, sit in chairs, or eat at

Clinical Obsessive-Compulsive Disorders in Adults and Children, ed. Robert Hudak and Darin D. Dougherty.
Published by Cambridge University Press. Copyright © Cambridge University Press 2011.

tables. In severe cases, the clutter prohibits movement through the house or access to certain parts of the home. Clutter in compulsive hoarding is also unique in its degree of disorganization. For example, clutter on top of a dining room table may include kitchen supplies, tools, and clothing. Important documents may be mixed together with junk mail. Difficulty finding objects when needed is a common complaint and often interferes with the ability to pay bills or file tax returns in a timely fashion (Tolin *et al.* 2008a).

Significant distress or impairment in functioning caused by the hoarding. Clutter's interference with basic functions such as cooking, cleaning, moving through the house, and even sleeping can make hoarding a dangerous problem, putting people at risk for fire, falling, poor sanitation, and health risks (Steketee *et al.* 2001a). The clutter and associated safety hazards may at times lead to threats of eviction, or removal of children or the elderly from the home by government agencies (Tolin *et al.* 2008a). Embarrassed by their clutter, many hoarding individuals avoid inviting friends, family, or repair workers to their homes, leading to social isolation, family conflict, and poor housing conditions (Rasmussen *et al.* 2007). Clutter and time spent on acquiring often cause conflict with family members, particularly those that live in the same home (Tolin *et al.* 2008b). Excessive acquisition through compulsive buying may also lead to significant financial distress.

Course and features of compulsive hoarding

Prevalence

Until recently, hoarding was believed to be a relatively rare phenomenon. This estimate was mostly a result of conceptualization of compulsive hoarding as a subtype of OCD and, therefore, making up only a small sample of those with OCD (i.e., less than 1% of total population). This estimate has been challenged by evidence that hoarding often occurs outside of OCD. When researchers sample participants who identify hoarding (rather than OCD) as their primary concern, the rate of hoarding without OCD may be over 80% (Frost

et al. 2006). An epidemiological survey of personality disorders, in which a hoarding-related question was included, reported that approximately 5% responded affirmatively to the question (Samuels *et al.* 2008). Although this result from an epidemiological survey to assess hoarding is clearly a significant contribution to our understanding of hoarding prevalence, hoarding was assessed as part of a diagnostic interview for obsessive-compulsive personality disorder. Future studies to assess the prevalence of hoarding with the use of hoarding-specific assessment instruments are needed to confirm the prevalence rate of hoarding.

Onset and course

Compulsive hoarding appears to be a chronic problem that generally begins in childhood or early adolescence (Samuels *et al.* 2002; Seedat and Stein 2002; Grisham *et al.* 2006; Tolin *et al.* 2010). In studies of individuals with primary compulsive hoarding, 60% of participants reported an onset of hoarding symptoms by age 12, and 80% by age 18 (Grisham *et al.* 2006; Tolin *et al.* 2010), Participants who reported an early onset of hoarding described a gradual, steady progression of their hoarding symptoms, with difficulty discarding typically emerging earlier than acquiring. Once present, hoarding appears to follow a chronic course, with only a minority reporting remission of symptoms (Grisham *et al.* 2006; Pinto *et al.* 2007) and most describing a worsening of symptoms across the lifespan (Grisham *et al.* 2006; Samuels *et al.* 2008).

Demographic features

Age, income, and marital status have consistently been found to be associated with hoarding (Tolin *et al.* 2008a; Samuels *et al.* unpublished data). Hoarding appears to be more prevalent among middle-age and older adults; this may be because of the progressive nature of hoarding, with symptoms worsening as one ages (Grisham *et al.* 2006; Samuels *et al.* 2008). Income is inversely associated with hoarding even after controlling for related socioeconomic factors, such as age, gender, living arrangement, and employment (Wheaton *et al.* 2008; Samuels *et al.* 2008). In one study, 38% of participants with hoarding symptoms reported an income below the national poverty level (Tolin *et al.* 2008a). The presence and severity of hoarding has also been associated with lower rates of marriage (Frost and Gross 1993; Steketee et al. 2000; Samuels et al. 2002; Tolin et al. 2008a), which may be a consequence of hoarding or comorbid disorders or may reflect the protective function served by the presence of a cohabitating partner.

Gender ratios in compulsive hoarding studies appear to be quite diverse, depending on the source of the sample (seeking treatment for hoarding or OCD, or a community sample). In general, women represent a large percentage of those who seek treatment for compulsive hoarding (72–100%; Saxena et al. 2002, 2007; Tolin et al. 2007), although a few studies have found more male than female treatment seekers (29–52%; Steketee et al. 2000; Abramowitz et al. 2003). In non-treatment studies that recruited OCD participants with and without hoarding, equal distribution (Labad et al. 2008; Wheaton et al. 2008) or greater prevalence of men (Samuels et al. 2002) were found among hoarding OCD participants. Similarly, in the general population, twice as many men as women reported hoarding symptoms (Samuels et al. 2008).

Unfortunately, most published treatment studies of compulsive hoarding do not report information on ethnicity/race. When reported in studies of treatment seeking or self-identified individuals with compulsive hoarding, the majority (80–90%) of participants are Caucasian (Tolin et al. 2007, 2008a). An epidemiological survey of hoarding, however, found that race/ethnicity was not related to hoarding, with comparable rates of hoarding among Whites (3.2%) and non-Whites (4.4%; Samuels et al. 2008).

Psychiatric and medical comorbidities

Compulsive hoarding has been associated with high rates of psychiatric and medical conditions. As many as 92% of individuals with compulsive hoarding have other axis I or axis II psychiatric conditions (Frost et al. 2006). Hoarding behaviors have been documented in schizophrenia (Luchins et al. 1992), organic mental disorders (Greenberg et al. 1990), eating disorders (Frankenburg 1984), brain injuries (Eslinger and Damasio 1985), and dementia (Finkel et al. 1997; Hwang et al. 1998). Hoarding individuals are more likely to be overweight or obese (78%), or to suffer from a chronic and severe medical illness (64%) (Tolin et al. 2008a) than are individuals in the general US population (Kessler et al. 1994).

Compulsive hoarding is associated with high rates of personality disorders and maladaptive personality traits. Although hoarding is one of the criteria for obsessive-compulsive personality disorder (American Psychiatric Association 2000), only 15–22% of OCD patients with hoarding were found to have this disorder (Winsberg et al. 1999; Samuels et al. 2007a). Instead, hoarding appears to be associated with high rates of personality disorders/features in general in both clinical and community samples, such as dependent, avoidant, paranoid, and schizotypal (Mataix-Cols et al. 2000; Samuels et al. 2002, 2007; Seedat and Stein 2002; Lochner et al. 2005).

In clinical samples, hoarding often co-occurs with various anxiety, mood, and substance use disorders. Compared with OCD patients without hoarding, those OCD patients with hoarding have higher rates of social phobia, generalized anxiety disorder, and depression, as well as bipolar and substance use disorders (Samuels et al. 2002, 2007a; Fontenelle et al. 2004; Lochner et al. 2005). In a primary hoarding sample, major depressive disorder (58%), social phobia (29%), and generalized anxiety disorder (28%) were more prevalent than was OCD (17%; Frost et al. 2006). Significant hoarding symptoms were also found among patients seeking treatment for anxiety disorders, especially those diagnosed with generalized anxiety disorder (27%), major depressive disorder (38%), and social phobia (14%; Meunier et al. 2006). In the only epidemiological survey of compulsive hoarding, however, Samuels and colleagues (unpublished data) did not find increased rates of axis I disorders associated with hoarding, other than lifetime alcohol dependence (52% vs. 20%).

The drastic differences in rates of axis I comorbidity with hoarding among clinical and community samples may reflect sampling differences, such as gender. When rates of axis I comorbidity were examined among OCD patients with and without hoarding, female participants accounted for much of the difference in rates of comorbidity between these two groups (Wheaton et al. 2008). Specifically, female hoarding participants had significantly higher rates of various axis I disorders, such as bipolar disorder I, substance abuse, panic disorder, and binge-eating disorder than did non-hoarding OCD female participants. Among male participants, only social phobia was found to be more prevalent among hoarding participants in comparison to OCD participants. Other features, such as avoidant personality symptoms and parental psychopathology, were more strongly associated with hoarding among women in a community sample (Samuels *et al.* 2008).

Diagnostic classification for compulsive hoarding

The diagnostic classification of compulsive hoarding has yet to be clearly established. Currently, hoarding's only mention in DSM-IV (American Psychiatric Association 2000) is as one of the eight diagnostic criteria for obsessive-compulsive personality disorder. Traditionally, however, hoarding has been conceptualized as a subtype or dimension of OCD. Some researchers, however, have also noted similarities between hoarding and impulse control disorders and attention-deficit hyperactivity disorder (ADHD). This section discusses the degree of overlap among these diagnostic categories.

Compulsive hoarding and OCD

Compulsive hoarding has traditionally been conceptualized as a subtype of OCD, with some evidence supporting this classification (Frost and Gross 1993; Frost *et al.* 1996, 1998). Hoarding symptoms and OCD symptoms are correlated with one another in both clinical and non-clinical samples (Frost and Gross 1993; Frost *et al.* 1996, 2004). Patients in OCD specialty clinics frequently describe hoarding symptoms (18–33%; Frost *et al.* 1996; Rasmussen and Eisen 1989; Sobin *et al.* 2000; Samuels *et al.* 2002), with 11% identifying hoarding as their primary symptom (Saxena *et al.* 2002). The doubting, checking, and reassurance seeking when attempting to discard objects observed in hoarding have been compared with similar obsessions and compulsions among those with OCD (Rasmussen and Eisen 1992).

In contrast to this, accumulating data suggest that hoarding might not be best conceptualized as a subtype of OCD. The prevalence of hoarding is estimated to be twice that of OCD (Samuels *et al.* 2008), which argues against the conceptualization of compulsive hoarding as a *subtype* of OCD. As many as 83% of primary hoarding patients deny symptoms of OCD (Frost *et al.* 2006), and patients with other anxiety disorders (particularly generalized anxiety disorder) are more likely to endorse hoarding symptoms than are those with OCD (Meunier *et al.* 2006). Although hoarding symptoms correlate with OCD symptoms, they may correlate even more strongly

with other symptoms such as depression (Wu and Watson 2005). Hoarding has consistently emerged as a discrete symptom factor from other OCD symptoms (e.g., checking, washing) in factor analytic studies of OCD symptoms (reviewed by Bloch *et al.* 2008) utilizing the Yale–Brown Obsessive Compulsive Scale (Y-BOCS; Goodman *et al.* 1989). Whereas classic OCD symptoms (e.g., checking, contamination) correlated highly with each other, hoarding demonstrated weaker, more moderate relationships with these symptoms (Wu and Watson 2005; Abramowitz *et al.* 2008).

Grisham and colleagues (2005) have proposed that hoarding with OCD and hoarding without OCD ("pure hoarding") may represent distinct syndromes with different mechanisms and clinical presentation. In their study of hoarding patients with and without OCD, "pure hoarding" patients reported significantly less negative affect and more positive affect than did those with hoarding *and* OCD or OCD alone (Grisham *et al.* 2005). Similar results were found in two other studies; OCD symptoms, but not hoarding symptoms, correlated significantly with negative affectivity after controlling for general distress (Wu and Watson 2005), and those with hoarding reported significantly lower depressive symptoms than did other OCD symptom subgroups (Calamari *et al.* 2004). It has been proposed that the high general psychopathology and greater disability associated with hoarding might largely be occurring in hoarding patients who also have OCD, whereas the lack of insight and recognition reported in the literature might be attributable to "pure hoarding" patients who are experiencing minimal distress (Grisham *et al.* 2005).

Compulsive hoarding and impulse control disorders

Excessive acquiring, one of the four proposed elements of hoarding, shares some similarities with impulse control disorders. Those with compulsive hoarding often report both positive and negative feelings that contribute to excessive acquiring. Positive feelings following the act of acquiring appear similar to those in impulse control disorders following the completion of the impulsive act (e.g., hair pulling, gambling). Excessive acquisition through compulsive buying is common in hoarding (Frost and Gross 1993; Frost *et al.* 1998), and hoarding symptoms are prevalent among compulsive buyers (Frost *et al.* 2002). High levels of hoarding symptoms have also been found among compulsive gamblers (Frost *et al.* 2001). Compared with OCD patients without any hoarding, those with hoarding have a higher rate of trichotillomania and skin picking (Samuels *et al.* 2002). There is some evidence that acquiring behaviors in compulsive buying may be driven by similar beliefs and attachment to possessions found in compulsive hoarding (e.g., possessions equated with an important memory, exaggerated sense of responsibility for possessions; Kyrios *et al.* 2004).

Compulsive hoarding and attention-deficit hyperactivity disorder

Deficits in attention, one of the information processing deficits that are believed to play a key role in compulsive hoarding (see below), resemble symptoms of ADHD. Hoarding individuals report greater symptoms of attentional problems than do community (Hartl *et al.* 2005) and non-hoarding psychiatric (Grisham *et al.* 2007) controls. Using a standardized self-report measure of ADHD symptoms, 12% of hoarding patients met diagnostic criteria for ADHD (symptoms were counted only if the individual scored 1.5 standard deviations or more above the population mean); the majority of these patients meeting diagnostic criteria for ADHD (11%) met the criteria for the combined type of ADHD (Tolin *et al.* 2010). When the childhood-onset criterion was removed, 21% of hoarding patients met criteria for current ADHD. The ADHD symptoms correlated strongly with severity of hoarding symptoms. Neuropsychological testing revealed that hoarding patients exhibited impaired ability to sustain attention (Grisham *et al.* 2007; Tolin *et al.* 2009); specifically, those with hoarding symptoms displayed greater variability in their reaction time, greater impulsivity, and poorer ability to detect the target stimuli.

Social and economic burden of compulsive hoarding

Compulsive hoarding has been associated with high levels of disability or impairment. These impairments include the inability to engage in activities of daily living (e.g., cleaning, cooking) and safety hazards as a result of clutter, work impairment, and the impact of hoarding on the family and community. In severe cases of hoarding, clutter poses a safety hazard, increasing the risk of falling, fire, poor sanitation,

and medical problems, especially among the elderly (Steketee *et al.* 2001a). For some, these safety hazards lead to threats of eviction, or removal of children or elderly from the home by government agencies (Tolin *et al.* 2008a). Involvement of government agencies, including the public health department, is not uncommon. Approximately 64% of surveyed health officials reported receiving at least one complaint of hoarding during a five-year period, with the majority (88%) of these cases being reported because of unsanitary conditions, and most being reported by neighbors (Frost *et al.* 2000). Data from these health officials indicated high rates of safety hazards with hoarding, such as fire hazard or health hazard. There were three reported cases in which hoarding was judged to be directly contributing to death in a fire. In approximately half of reported cases, clutter went beyond the person's home, suggesting that the impact of hoarding extends beyond the individual and immediate family members (Frost *et al.* 2000). There is likely a significant financial impact of hoarding on the community as well because of the cost of involvement of government agencies.

The impact of compulsive hoarding extends beyond the home to the person's work environment. In a large-scale survey of individuals with self-identified hoarding, as many as 7% of individuals reported being on disability benefit because of hoarding and 6% reported being fired from work because of hoarding (Tolin *et al.* 2008a). Even those who were employed reported impaired work productivity, with more than half reporting difficulty finding items at work and describing their workspace as cluttered. Severity of hoarding predicted the number of psychiatric work impairment days, even after controlling for medical conditions. Overall, the degree of reported work impairment associated with hoarding exceeded that found in most anxiety or depressive disorders and was comparable to that reported by individuals with psychotic disorders (Tolin *et al.* 2008a).

Finally, hoarding appears to negatively affect the hoarding individual's family members, as well as the quality of family relationships. Adult children of self-identified individuals with hoarding reported high childhood distress, such as less happiness, difficulty making friends, reduced social contact in the home, high intrafamilial strain, and embarrassment about the condition of their home (Tolin *et al.* 2008b). Family members reported high levels of patient rejection towards the hoarding individual. Degree of patient rejection attitudes worsened with severity of hoarding, severity of clutter during the family member's childhood, and with the family member's perception of the hoarding individual's level of insight about hoarding (Tolin *et al.* 2008b).

A suggested biopsychosocial model of compulsive hoarding

Originally, childhood material deprivation was believed to play a key role in the onset of compulsive hoarding, with hoarding behaviors serving as a compensatory strategy for the fear of future deprivation. However, empirical evidence has not supported childhood material deprivation as a causal factor in hoarding (Frost and Gross 1993). Instead, current models of compulsive hoarding identify various deficits in cognitive processes, as well as maladaptive beliefs and behavioral patterns as underlying mechanisms of hoarding (Frost and Hartl 1996; Steketee and Frost 2003, 2007; Frost and Tolin, 2008). Anecdotal and empirical evidence, including neuropsychological and neuroimaging studies, support the role of these factors in the onset and maintenance of hoarding. Individuals with hoarding appear to have abnormalities in specific brain regions associated with executive functioning, impulse control, and processing of reward value. Like many psychiatric disorders, familial and environmental vulnerability factors have also been identified in compulsive hoarding.

Familial and environmental vulnerabilities

Traumatic or stressful events may play a role in the onset, course, or expression of hoarding. Individuals with hoarding report a greater frequency of lifetime traumatic events than do OCD patients (Cromer *et al.* 2007) and community controls (Hartl *et al.* 2005). The relationship between hoarding and traumatic events remained significant after controlling for age, age of onset, depression, OCD severity, and comorbid conditions (Cromer *et al.* 2007). Higher rates of physical and sexual abuse and post-traumatic stress disorder have also been found in hoarding individuals compared with community controls (Hartl *et al.* 2005). Harsh physical discipline and other childhood adversities, such as parental psychopathology, have also been associated with hoarding (Samuels *et al.* 2008). These stressful life events may be closely related to the onset of hoarding problems. As many as 55% of hoarding individuals report experiencing a

stressful life event that coincided with the onset of hoarding symptoms (Grisham *et al.* 2006); stressful life events are more likely to be reported around the time of symptom onset than at other times (Tolin *et al.* 2010). Samuels and colleagues (2008) found that home break-ins during childhood were associated with adult hoarding. Those who reported a stressful life event at the time of onset had a later age of onset than those who did not (Grisham *et al.* 2006). These findings suggest that stressful life events may not only be related to the presence of hoarding, but also influence the course of hoarding. Some have hypothesized that hoarding may be a compensatory strategy of strengthening one's sense of safety following a trauma or a chaotic childhood environment (Cromer *et al.* 2007), which is consistent with the perception of possessions as sources of comfort and security reported by those with hoarding (Frost *et al.* 1995).

There is evidence to suggest a strong familial component to hoarding symptoms. For example, 84–85% of hoarders described a first-degree relative as a "packrat," compared with 37–54% of OCD patients without hoarding symptoms (Frost and Gross 1993; Winsberg *et al.* 1999). The OCD patients with hoarding have more first-degree relatives with hoarding (12%) or some hoarding symptoms (49%) than do OCD patients without hoarding (3% and 33%, respectively). High correlations of hoarding symptoms have been found among siblings with OCD (Hasler *et al.* 2007). In particular, indecisiveness may be an important aspect of the "hoarding phenotype;" indecisiveness is more common in OCD patients with hoarding (59%) than without (41%) and is strongly associated with hoarding in a relative (Samuels *et al.* 2007a).

Familial vulnerability to hoarding is likely both environmental and genetic. Anecdotally, many hoarding patients report being taught or observing in their parent, from early in life, beliefs and behaviors associated with hoarding (e.g., condemning of "wasteful behavior," observing excessive acquiring in a parent). Several studies also support a genetic factor in hoarding (Lochner *et al.* 2005; Zhang *et al.* 2002; Samuels *et al.* 2007b). Chromosome 14 has been found to have a suggestive link with hoarding among families with OCD (Samuels *et al.* 2007b). Lochner and colleagues (2005) found a higher prevalence of the *L/L* genotype of the catechol-*O*-methyltransferase Val158Met polymorphism among OCD hoarding participants of Afrikaner descent.

Maladaptive cognitive process

Attention

Individuals who hoard report problems sustaining attention to a greater extent than do community samples (Hartl *et al.* 2005) and non-hoarding psychiatric controls (Meunier *et al.* 2006; Grisham *et al.* 2007). These self-reports are corroborated by results of standardized tests of attentional capacity, in which hoarding is associated with diminished non-verbal attention, greater variability in reaction time, greater impulsivity, and poorer ability to detect target stimuli (Grisham *et al.* 2007; Tolin *et al.* 2009).

Anecdotal evidence also suggests that individuals with compulsive hoarding exhibit an apparent attentional bias in which excessive attention is allotted to details that are often unimportant, particularly in relation to possessions (Frost and Tolin 2008). This attentional bias increases the perceived importance of these non-essential details, heightening the importance or uniqueness of a possession, thereby increasing saving behaviors.

Memory

Many hoarding individuals describe poor memory and indicate that they keep certain possessions because of fears that they will forget relevant information or lose an important memory if they discard an object. They state that they prefer to leave objects out in the open (e.g., piling important papers on the table) rather than putting them away (e.g., a file cabinet) because of fear that they will forget where they placed the item or that they possess that item. Standardized tests of memory functioning have revealed that hoarding individuals show impaired delayed recall (both verbal and visual) and use less-effective visual recall strategies than do healthy control participants (Hartl *et al.* 2004). When asked to decide whether or not to discard possessions during functional magnetic resonance imaging (fMRI), hoarding patients displayed greater activity in left parahippocampal gyrus, a region associated with effortful memory search and retrieval (Gur *et al.* 1997; Maguire and Mummery 1999; Yonelinas *et al.* 2001), and suppression of left superior frontal gyrus, a region associated with working memory (du Boisgueheneuc *et al.* 2006), than did healthy control participants (Tolin *et al.* 2008c).

Ironically, despite these apparent memory deficits, individuals with hoarding frequently report overtaxing their existing memory capacity by relying on a memory-based approach to finding objects rather than a category-based approach (Frost and Tolin 2008). In other words, individuals with compulsive hoarding attempt to organize and find items based on visual spatial recall (remembering where an item was last seen) instead of categorical recall (remembering where a certain category of item is usually placed).

Executive function

Difficulty discarding possessions is hypothesized to result, in part, from problems in decision making and categorization. Self-reported indecisiveness has been associated with hoarding in college and community samples (Frost and Gross 1993; Frost and Shows 1993; Steketee *et al.* 2003a). Compared with participants with OCD, hoarding participants reported greater indecisiveness on a self-report measure, and were rated by study clinicians as more indecisive (Samuels *et al.* 2002). Research using the Iowa Gambling Task (Bechara *et al.* 1997), which requires participants to sacrifice immediate rewards in order to maximize long-term gain, shows that OCD patients with hoarding symptoms perform more poorly than do OCD patients without hoarding symptoms (Lawrence *et al.* 2006). This result was not replicated in a separate study of primary hoarding patients, however (Grisham *et al.* 2007). Hoarding participants take significantly longer than do healthy controls to decide whether or not to discard personal possessions (Tolin *et al.* 2008c), although no difference was seen in time to discard items that were not personal possessions.

The ability to categorize possessions, a key skill in maintaining organization, also appears to be compromised in hoarding. When asked to sort their personal possessions, hoarding individuals took longer, and created more categories (with a smaller number of items per category), than did healthy controls or participants with OCD (Wincze *et al.* 2007). This difference was not evident when sorting non-personal household items, although another study of subclinical "packrats" using a similar methodology did show diminished categorization ability for non-owned items (Luchian *et al.* 2007).

Executive functions such as these are commonly associated with frontal cortical regions (Bechara *et al.* 1994; Rolls 2004) and anterior cingulate cortex (Devinsky *et al.* 1995). Case studies have reported the onset of hoarding symptoms in adulthood following insult to these regions, such as frontotemporal dementia (Nakaaki *et al.* 2007) and strokes in mesial frontal areas including the right polar sector and the anterior cingulate cortex (Anderson *et al.* 2005). Resting positron emission tomography studies suggest that hoarding patients show lower glucose metabolism in anterior cingulate cortex as well as posterior cingulate cortex (a region involved in the modulation of frontal cortical regions as well as the anterior cingulate cortex) than do control participants (Saxena *et al.* 2004). When asked to imagine hoarding-related activities during fMRI, OCD patients with primary hoarding symptoms exhibited greater activation in ventromedial prefrontal cortex than did OCD patients without hoarding and healthy controls (An *et al.* 2008). During an actual decision-making task in which participants decided whether to discard possessions during fMRI, hoarding patients showed excessive activity in lateral orbitofrontal cortex compared with healthy controls; furthermore, among hoarding patients, refusal to discard personal possessions was associated with increased hemodynamic response, compared with that seen for control items, in middle frontal gyrus extending into the rostral anterior cingulate cortex (Tolin *et al.* 2008c).

Maladaptive cognitive content

Beliefs about possessions

Maladaptive or exaggerated beliefs about possessions appear to play an important role in compulsive hoarding (Steketee *et al.* 2003b). Many individuals with compulsive hoarding describe a heightened sense of responsibility for possessions (Frost *et al.* 1995; Steketee *et al.* 2003b). Responsibility beliefs include an exaggerated sense of the need to be prepared (by having the appropriate possessions), the safekeeping of possessions, and the utility of objects and avoidance of waste. For many, simply imagining a use for a possession implies that it must be saved for that purpose, even if its use is unlikely. The possibility of being "unprepared," by not having an object needed in a certain situation appears highly aversive to those with hoarding. Other patients have described anthropomorphic beliefs, in which they are excessively concerned about making sure that the possession "goes to a good home" and is unharmed. Individuals with compulsive hoarding may also exhibit an exaggerated need to maintain control over their possessions, which is often demonstrated by an aversion to others

touching, moving, and even sharing their possessions (Frost *et al.* 1995). Perfectionistic beliefs may also inhibit discarding (Frost and Shows 1993; Tolin *et al.* 2008d) by rendering individuals fearful of making decisions because of concerns about making a mistake (e.g., discarding the wrong item). The anterior cingulate cortex abnormalities described above may play a role in perfectionistic beliefs or behaviors, given that region's involvement in error monitoring and the sense of decisions being "wrong" (Carter *et al.* 1998; Kiehl *et al.* 2000; Maltby *et al.* 2005).

Emotional attachment to possessions

Emotional attachments include an overappreciation for the esthetics or sentimental value of objects. In some cases, patients have reported feeling a greater sense of attachment to objects than to other people (Frost *et al.* 1995; Steketee *et al.* 2003b). Comments that objects represent a beloved person, memory, or a part of their identity are frequently reported. For example, possessions are relied upon to define identity or character (e.g., collection of newspaper to define oneself as knowledgeable). Discarding possessions, therefore, is often equated with losing a loved one, an important time in the person's life, or part of the person's own identity. Like many other features of hoarding, misdirected emotional attachment has been associated with abnormalities of the anterior cingulate cortex (Devinsky *et al.* 1995),

Maladaptive behavioral patterns

Behavioral avoidance

Unlike OCD, which is characterized by repetitive, compulsive behaviors, compulsive hoarding is largely characterized by what the person does *not* do (e.g., sort, organize, discard). Even in clinical trials in which sorting is assigned as homework, hoarding patients show an extreme inability or unwillingness to follow through with such tasks (Tolin *et al.* 2007). At a cognitive level, sorting and discarding is inconsistent with the individual's deeply held beliefs about responsibility, emotional attachment, need for control, and so on. At a neural level, such conflict may relate to the finding of excessive activity in lateral orbitofrontal cortex when making decisions about whether to discard possessions (Tolin *et al.* 2008c); this area of the brain has been associated with processing relative reward value, particularly values that are experienced as punishing (Kringelbach and Rolls 2004; Kringelbach 2005). Therefore, sorting and discarding become highly aversive and emotionally laden tasks, which are subsequently avoided. The apparent deficits in attention, memory, and executive function described above likely add to the aversive experience by rendering the process particularly time consuming and cumbersome.

Behavioral disinhibition

Excessive acquisition is thought to be a core feature of compulsive hoarding (Frost and Gross 1993; Frost et al. 1998). Excessive buying is significantly correlated with severity of other hoarding symptoms (Frost et al. 1998, 2002; Coles et al. 2003; Mueller et al. 2007). Other acquired items may be obtained for free (e.g., free brochures, giveaways, and discarded items) (Frost et al. 1998, 2002) or (in some cases) stolen. A recent large survey of 878 self-identified hoarding participants and 665 family informants revealed that, among hoarding participants who met criteria for clinically significant clutter, difficulty discarding, and distress or impairment, approximately 85% reported excessive acquisition. Reports by family informants whose loved one met criteria for clinically significant hoarding indicated that nearly 95% exhibited excessive acquisition (Frost et al. 2007). Excessive acquisition was associated with greater hoarding severity, earlier onset, and related functional impairment. To the extent that excessive acquisition can be considered a form of behavioral disinhibition, this finding would comport well with studies showing impaired functioning in frontal regions of the brain associated with impulse control and anticipation of behavioral consequences (e.g., Bechara et al. 1994; Rolls 2004). Hoarding patients often identify acquiring as one of their most enjoyable activities, elaborating that acquiring elicits various positive emotions ("exciting") and cognitions ("I feel thrifty and smart"). In these instances, acquisition behaviors appear impulsive in that they are positively reinforced appetitive behaviors. Other hoarding patients describe acquisition behaviors that appear compulsive (negatively reinforced strategies for regulating unpleasant emotion). Some, for example, report fear or discomfort when attempting to refrain from acquiring; others report fears that not acquiring will lead to a "missed opportunity" and subsequent feelings of regret; still others report that acquiring serves to modulate negative emotions such as depression (Steketee and Frost 2007).

Poor problem recognition and motivation

Many individuals who hoard can be characterized as possessing limited motivation to change, possibly because of poor insight into the severity of their condition. Although OCD patients display a range of insight into the irrational nature of their obsessions and compulsions, most exhibit at least some insight (Foa et al. 1995). By contrast, clinical observation suggests that individuals with compulsive hoarding problems often display a striking lack of awareness of the severity of their behavior, sometimes denying the problem and often resisting intervention attempts and defensively rationalizing their acquiring and saving (Greenberg 1987; Steketee et al. 2001a; Steketee and Frost 2003). Research reports indicate that many hoarders do not consider their behavior unreasonable (e.g., Frost and Gross 1993; Frost et al. 1996, 2000; Matsunaga et al. 2002; De Berardis et al. 2005; Samuels et al. 2007a; Storch et al. 2007), and that recognition of a problem with hoarding typically does not occur until at least a decade after onset (Grisham et al. 2006). In a large survey ($n = 584$), family members described their hoarding relative as having fair to poor insight, on average. More than half were described as having "poor insight" or "lacks insight/delusional." Ratings of insight were inversely correlated with the hoarding individual's reported level of distress about the problem. Poor insight may be related to impaired functioning in orbitofrontal cortex and prefrontal regions of the brain: these areas are commonly associated with self-awareness and self-regulation, and lesions in these regions have been linked to anosognosia or the failure to recognize deficits (Stuss and Benson 1986; Vogel et al. 2005; Salmon et al. 2006).

The degree to which a problem is recognized likely plays a substantial role in willingness to change behavior. Among residents reported to health departments because of unsanitary housing conditions from hoarding, less than one third were willing to cooperate with health officials to improve their home condition (Frost et al. 2000). Even among those who seek treatment without pressure from government agencies, low motivation has been frequently identified as a barrier to successful treatment (Shafran and Tallis 1996; Hartl and Frost 1999; Christensen and Greist 2001). Low motivation can interfere with successful treatment by leading to early dropout (Mataix-Cols et al. 2002; Tolin et al. 2007), inconsistent attendance (Tolin et al. 2007), and poor compliance with treatment, particularly homework adherence (Hartl and Frost 1999; Steketee *et al.* 2000; Christensen and Greist 2001; Tolin *et al.* 2007). Diminished motivation would also be consistent with the observed abnormalities in the anterior cingulate cortex (Devinsky *et al.* 1995).

Treatment of compulsive hoarding

In general, compulsive hoarding has been associated with a poor treatment response to both pharmacological and behavioral treatment, at least in comparison to the same treatment applied to OCD. Some have hypothesized that poor response to serotonin reuptake inhibitors (SRIs) may result from certain neurobiological abnormalities found in hoarding, such as lower anterior cingulate cortex activity (Saxena *et al.* 2004). Limited motivation also appears to play a role in poor response to behavioral treatments.

Behavioral treatment

Exposure and response prevention (ERP), considered the gold standard for non-pharmacological treatment of OCD, consists of repetitive exposures of discarding as many items as possible, as quickly as possible, while refraining from the rituals of perfectionistic inspection of these objects (Foa and Kozak 1997). Although ERP has been demonstrated to be highly effective for non-hoarding OCD, ERP for compulsive hoarding has produced less-favorable results, with hoarding symptoms predicting premature termination, poor treatment compliance, and poor treatment response (Mataix-Cols *et al.* 2002; Abramowitz *et al.* 2003). In one study of ERP for both hoarding and non-hoarding OCD, fewer participants with hoarding symptoms (39%) met criteria for clinically significant change (Jacobson and Truax 1991) than did OCD patients without hoarding symptoms (59%; Abramowitz *et al.* 2003). In another study, only 25% of hoarding patients demonstrated a 40% or more reduction on the Y-BOCS compared with 48% of non-hoarding OCD patients (Mataix-Cols *et al.* 2002).

Pharmacological treatment

Pharmacological trials of OCD have had mixed results, with, overall, compulsive hoarding appearing to show diminished response to SRIs (Black *et al.* 1998; Mataix-Cols *et al.* 1999; Stein *et al.* 2007). Mataix-Cols and colleagues (1999) examined predictors of

treatment response to various SRIs (clomipramine, fluvoxamine, fluoxetine, sertraline, and paroxetine) among 150 OCD patients. Among those who received an SRI, hoarding was identified as the only predictor of poor treatment response, even after controlling for pretreatment symptom severity. Similar results were obtained in another large-scale, multistudy placebo-controlled trial of escitalopram for OCD (Stein *et al.* 2007).

Not all pharmacotherapy trials, however, find hoarding to be a poor prognostic indicator. In some trials of an SRI for OCD, non-responders were more likely to have sexual obsessions, washing compulsions, miscellaneous compulsions (Shetti *et al.* 2005) or somatic obsessions (Erzegovesi *et al.* 2001), although there was a trend towards non-response with hoarding obsessions (Erzegovesi *et al.* 2001). In one pharmacological study, hoarding and non-hoarding OCD patients fared equally well in response to paroxetine (Saxena *et al.* 2007), although neither group showed a particularly favorable response. Both hoarding and non-hoarding OCD patients in this study demonstrated lower rates of treatment response and reduction in symptoms, as measured by the Y-BOCS, compared with a previous trial of OCD treatment with paroxetine (Black *et al.* 1998).

Cognitive-behavioral treatment

Specific cognitive-behavioral therapy (CBT) for compulsive hoarding has been developed based on the model described above (Frost and Hartl 1996; Steketee and Frost 2003, 2007; Frost and Tolin 2008). This approach utilizes various strategies to address the beliefs about and attachment to possessions, maladaptive cognitive processes, motivational concerns, and behavioral avoidance and disinhibition believed to maintain hoarding symptoms. Preliminary research on CBT for compulsive hoarding appears promising compared with traditional ERP. Case studies (Hartl and Frost 1999; Cermele *et al.* 2001) and uncontrolled clinical trials (Steketee *et al.* 2001b; Saxena *et al.* 2002) reported significant improvement in the core features of hoarding (clutter, difficulty discarding, acquisition). Tolin *et al.* (2007) reported an open trial of CBT for compulsive hoarding, in which 14 patients (10 treatment completers) received 26 individual sessions of CBT, including frequent home visits, over a period of 7–12 months. Significant decreases from before to after treatment were noted on the Saving

Inventory-Revised (SI-R; Frost *et al.* 2004) and Clutter Image Rating (CIR; Frost *et al.* 2008) but not the Severity Rating of the Clinician's Global Impressions (CGI; Guy 1976). The improvement in CGI ratings indicated that 50% of treatment completers were rated "much improved" or "very much improved" at the end of treatment. Homework completion was strongly related to symptom improvement: at post-treatment, four of five patients (80%) rated at or above the median on homework completion were rated as "much improved" or "very much improved" on the CGI, whereas only one patient (20%) rated below the median on homework completion received this rating.

Greater improvements were obtained in a subsequent small randomized controlled trial of CBT versus wait-list control (Steketee *et al.* 2010). This trial placed greater emphasis on motivational interviewing strategies with the aim of improving treatment compliance. The remainder of the treatment protocol was comparable to that used in the open trial. At the end of treatment (26 sessions), 80% of participants rated themselves as "much improved" on a self-rated CGI; 69% received this rating from their clinicians; 60% of participants met criteria for a clinically significant change (Jacobson and Truax 1991) on the SI-R (Frost *et al.* 2004), which is much higher than the rate for clinically significant change with ERP for hoarding, estimated to be 31% (Abramowitz *et al.* 2003). Therefore, CBT for compulsive hoarding appears promising, although future research with larger scale randomized controlled trials are needed to establish the efficacy of this treatment, as well as continued refinement of the treatment protocol.

Directions for future research

We are still in the early stages of understanding compulsive hoarding; indeed, even the basic definition of hoarding is very much a work in progress. In this respect, research on compulsive hoarding has lagged well behind that of OCD. To the extent that hoarding is considered a subtype of OCD (and therefore much of the extant research on the nature and treatment of OCD would be reasonably expected to apply to hoarding), this imbalance is not particularly worrisome. However, to the extent that compulsive hoarding represents a distinct clinical syndrome or disorder (and, as described above, many recent studies suggest this may be the case), our ability to intervene is greatly hampered by the sparse knowledge base. If we assume

that the preliminary estimate of 5% prevalence is accurate, compulsive hoarding may represent a major service gap. Additional research using empirically validated measures of hoarding severity is needed in order to clarify the prevalence of compulsive hoarding in the population.

On a related note, little is known about the racial, ethnic, and gender distributions of compulsive hoarding. As noted above, the one population survey found that the hoarding item was endorsed more frequently by men; however, studies of OCD patients have frequently shown no gender difference in the distribution of hoarding symptoms, and studies of treatment-seeking hoarding patients have included a much higher proportion of women than men. Clearly, more epidemiological research is needed to understand the demographic correlates of hoarding, particularly since hoarding in men versus women may have different clinical profiles, such as different rates of comorbidity and level of psychopathology.

It remains unclear whether compulsive hoarding is best considered a distinct disorder, a clinical syndrome, or multiple disorders. As noted previously, over 90% of individuals with compulsive hoarding appear to meet diagnostic criteria for at least one axis I or axis II psychiatric disorder. One wonders, therefore, to what extent hoarding should be considered a complication of other disorders. For example, it is not known whether the decision-making impairments in compulsive hoarding can be attributed to the attentional difficulties and impulsivity associated with ADHD, the perfectionistic tendencies associated with OCD and obsessive-compulsive personality disorder, or the fatigue and concentration difficulties associated with depression. Furthermore, even if compulsive hoarding "cuts across" these different conditions, it is not known whether subtle but important differences in hoarding behavior (e.g., age of onset, course, specific behavioral impairments) exist across the different subgroups. Advanced taxometric analyses would likely help to clarify these issues.

Several recent studies have yielded promising results regarding the neural correlates of compulsive hoarding. As noted above, these studies seem to converge on abnormalities in frontocortical regions. However, hoarding has been assessed differently across sites (because of the lack of formal diagnostic criteria as well as the absence, until fairly recently, of valid assessment tools), and it is not clear whether all samples were truly drawn from the same population.

In addition, clear and specific links have yet to be drawn between abnormalities in neural function and the overt manifestations of compulsive hoarding such as cognitive processing deficits, maladaptive beliefs, discarding- and acquiring-related behaviors, and comorbidity.

Unlike OCD, for which specific pharmacological and psychological interventions have reliably proven effective, our ability to treat compulsive hoarding requires substantial refining. Only one study to date, an open trial, has prospectively and quantitatively measured response to standardized pharmacotherapy in compulsive hoarders (Saxena *et al.* 2007); in that study, only 28% of compulsive hoarding patients were considered treatment responders on the Y-BOCS and CGI. Although hoarding and OCD patients did not differ in their response to paroxetine, a 28% response rate is disappointing. To the extent that compulsive hoarding overlaps with other disorders, it might be useful to consider venturing beyond SRIs (a treatment selection guided largely by the classification of hoarding as a subtype of OCD) into medications that have proven helpful for these comorbid conditions. For example, psychostimulant or other cognitive-enhancing medications might be employed to combat the attentional difficulties seen in these patients, or mood-stablizing anticonvulsants might be used to decrease behavioral disinhibition.

The CBT approach appears to fare somewhat better, with 50% (Tolin *et al.* 2007) and 69% (Steketee *et al.* 2010) considered treatment responders on the CGI, and 60% considered responders on the SI-R (Steketee *et al.* 2010). While promising, it is noted that true remission was rare, and most patients remained at least somewhat impaired at the end of treatment. Further development of CBT protocols is needed, and it is likely that the major challenge for CBT development will be to combat the substantial problems of motivation and treatment compliance seen across studies. In addition, large-scale randomized controlled trials are needed in order to compare the efficacy of CBT, pharmacotherapy, and their combination.

References

Abramowitz JS, Franklin ME, Schwartz SA, Furr JM (2003). Symptom presentation and outcome of cognitive-behavioral therapy for obsessive-compulsive disorder. *J Consult Clin Psychol* **71**: 1049–1057.

Abramowitz JS, Wheaton MG, Storch EA (2008). The status of hoarding as a symptom of obsessive-compulsive disorder. *Behav Res Ther* **46**: 1026–1033.

American Psychiatric Association (2000). *Diagnostic and Statistical Manual of Mental Disorders*, 4th edn revised. Washington, DC: American Psychiatric Press.

An SK, Mataix-Cols D, Lawrence NS, *et al.* (2008). To discard or not to discard: the neural basis of hoarding symptoms in obsessive-compulsive disorder. *Mol Psychiatry* **14**: 318–331.

Anderson SW, Damasio H, Damasio AR (2005). A neural basis for collecting behaviour in humans. *Brain* **128**: 201–212.

Bechara A, Damasio AR, Damasio H, Anderson SW (1994). Insensitivity to future consequences following damage to human prefrontal cortex. *Cognition* **50**: 7–15.

Bechara A, Damasio H, Tranel D, Damasio AR (1997). Deciding advantageously before knowing the advantageous strategy. *Science* **275**: 1293–1295.

Black DW, Monahan P, Gable J, *et al.* (1998). Hoarding and treatment response in 38 nondepressed subjects with obsessive-compulsive disorder. *J Clin Psychiatry* **59**: 420–425.

Bloch MH, Landeros-Weisenberger A, Rosario MC, Pittenger C, Leckman JF (2008). Meta-analysis of the symptom structure of obsessive-compulsive disorder. *Am J Psychiatry* **165**: 1532–1542.

Calamari JE, Wiegartz PS, Riemann BC, *et al.* (2004). Obsessive-compulsive disorder subtypes: an attempted replication and extension of a symptom-based taxonomy. *Behav Res Ther* **42**: 647–670.

Carter CS, Braver TS, Barch DM, *et al.* (1998). Anterior cingulate cortex, error detection, and the online monitoring of performance. *Science* **280**: 747–749.

Cermele JA, Melendez-Pallitto L, Pandina GJ (2001). Intervention in compulsive hoarding. A case study. *Behav Modif* **25**: 214–232.

Christensen DD, Greist JH (2001). The challenge of obsessive-compulsive disorder hoarding. *Primary Psychiatry* **8**: 79–86.

Coles ME, Frost RO, Heimberg RG, Steketee G (2003). Hoarding behaviors in a large college sample. *Behav Res Ther* **41**: 179–194.

Cromer KR, Schmidt NB, Murphy DL (2007). Do traumatic events influence the clinical expression of compulsive hoarding? *Behav Res Ther* **45**: 2581–2592.

De Berardis D, Campanella D, Gambi F, *et al.* (2005). Insight and alexithymia in adult outpatients with obsessive-compulsive disorder. *Eur Arch Psychiatry Clin Neurosci* **255**: 350–358.

Devinsky O, Morrell MJ, Vogt BA (1995). Contributions of anterior cingulate cortex to behaviour. *Brain* **118**: 279–306.

du Boisgueheneuc F, Levy R, Volle E, *et al.* (2006). Functions of the left superior frontal gyrus in humans: a lesion study. *Brain* **129**: 3315–3328.

Erzegovesi S, Cavallini MC, Cavedini P, *et al.* (2001). Clinical predictors of drug response in obsessive-compulsive disorder. *J Clin Psychopharmacol* **21**: 488–492.

Eslinger PJ, Damasio AR (1985). Severe disturbance of higher cognition after bilateral frontal lobe ablation: Patient EVR. *Neurology* **35**: 1731–1741.

Finkel S, Costa E, Silva J, *et al.* (1997). Behavioral and psychological signs and symptoms of dementia: A consensus statement on current knowledge and implications for research and treatment. *Int J Geriatr Psychiatry* **12**: 1060–1061.

Foa EB, Kozak MJ (1997). *Mastery of Obsessive-Compulsive Disorder: A Cognitive-Behavioral Approach (Therapist Guide).* New York: Oxford University Press.

Foa EB, Kozak MJ, Goodman WK, *et al.* (1995). DSM-IV field trial: obsessive-compulsive disorder. *Am J Psychiatry* **152**: 90–96.

Fontenelle LF, Mendlowicz MV, Soares ID, Viersiani M (2004). Patients with obsessive-compulsive disorder and hoarding symptoms: a distinct clinical subtype? *Compr Psychiatry* **45**: 375–383.

Frankenburg FR (1984). Hoarding in anorexia nervosa. *Br J Med Psychol* **57**: 57–60.

Frost RO, Gross R (1993). The hoarding of possessions. *Behav Res Ther* **31**: 367–382.

Frost RO, Hartl TL (1996). A cognitive-behavioral model of compulsive hoarding. *Behav Res Ther* **34**: 341–350.

Frost RO, Shows DL (1993). The nature and measurement of compulsive indecisiveness. *Behav Res Ther* **31**: 683–692.

Frost RO, Tolin DF (2008). Compulsive hoarding. In Abramowitz JS, Taylor S, McKay D (eds.) *Clinical Handbook of Obsessive-Compulsive Disorder and Related Problems.* (pp. 76–94). Baltimore, MD: Johns Hopkins University Press.

Frost RO, Hartl T, Christian R, Williams N (1995). The value of possessions in compulsive hoarding: patterns of use and attachment. *Behav Res Ther* **33**: 897–902.

Frost RO, Krause MS, Steketee G (1996). Hoarding and obsessive-compulsive symptoms. *Behav Modif* **20**: 116–132.

Frost RO, Kim HJ, Morris C, *et al.* (1998). Hoarding, compulsive buying and reasons for saving. *Behav Res Ther* **36**: 657–664.

Frost RO, Steketee G, Williams L (2000). Hoarding: a community health problem. *Health Social Care Community* **8**: 229–234.

Frost RO, Meagher BM, Riskind JH (2001). Obsessive-compulsive features in pathological lottery and scratch ticket gamblers. *J Gambling Studies* **17**: 5–19.

Frost RO, Steketee G, Williams L (2002). Compulsive buying, compulsive hoarding, and obsessive-compulsive disorder. *Behav Ther* **33**: 201–214.

Frost RO, Steketee G, Grisham J (2004). Measurement of compulsive hoarding: Saving Inventory-Revised. *Behav Res Ther* **42**: 1163–1182.

Frost RO, Steketee G, Tolin DF, Brown TA (2006). Comorbidity and diagnostic issues in compulsive hoarding. In *Proceeding of the Annual Meeting of the Anxiety Disorders Association of America*, Miami, March.

Frost RO, Steketee G, Tolin DF, Renaud S (2008). Development and validation of the Clutter Image Rating. *J Psychopathol Behav Assess* **32**: 401–417.

Frost RO, Tolin DF, Steketee G, Fitch KE, Selbo-Bruns A (2009). Excessive acquisition in hoarding. *J Anxiety Disord* **23**: 632–639.

Goodman WK, Price LH, Rasmussen SA, *et al.* (1989). The Yale–Brown Obsessive Compulsive Scale. II. Validity. *Arch Gen Psychiatry* **46**: 1012–1016.

Greenberg D (1987). Compulsive hoarding. *Am J Psychother* **41**: 409–416.

Greenberg D, Witztum E, Levy A (1990). Hoarding as a psychiatric symptom. *J Clin Psychiatry* **51**: 417–421.

Grisham JR, Brown TA, Liverant GI, Campbell-Sills L (2005). The distinctiveness of compulsive hoarding from obsessive-compulsive disorder. *J Anxiety Disord* **19**: 767–779.

Grisham JR, Frost RO, Steketee G, Kim HJ, Hood S (2006). Age of onset of compulsive hoarding. *J Anxiety Disord* **20**: 675–686.

Grisham JR, Brown TA, Savage CR, Steketee G, Barlow DH (2007). Neuropsychological impairment associated with compulsive hoarding. *Behav Res Ther* **45**: 1471–1483.

Gur RC, Ragland JD, Mozley LH, *et al.* (1997). Lateralized changes in regional cerebral blood flow during performance of verbal and facial recognition tasks: correlations with performance and "effort." *Brain Cogn* **33**: 388–414.

Guy W (1976). *Assessment Manual for Psychopharmacology.* Washington, DC: US Government Printing Office.

Hartl TL, Frost RO (1999). Cognitive-behavioral treatment of compulsive hoarding: a multiple baseline experimental case study. *Behav Res Ther* **37**: 451–461.

Hartl TL, Frost RO, Allen GJ, *et al.* (2004). Actual and perceived memory deficits in individuals with compulsive hoarding. *Depress Anxiety* **20**: 59–69.

Hartl TL, Duffany SR, Allen GJ, Steketee G, Frost RO (2005). Relationships among compulsive hoarding, trauma, and attention-deficit/hyperactivity disorder. *Behav Res Ther* **43**: 269–276.

Hasler G, Pinto A, Greenberg BD, *et al.* (2007). Familiality of factor analysis-derived YBOCS dimensions in OCD-affected sibling pairs from the OCD Collaborative Genetics Study. *Biol Psychiatry* **61**: 617–625.

Hwang JP, Tsai SJ, Yang CH, Liu KM, Lirng JF (1998). Hoarding behavior in dementia. A preliminary report. *Am J Geriatr Psychiatry* **6**: 285–289.

Jacobson NS, Truax P (1991). Clinical significance: a statistical approach to defining meaningful change in psychotherapy research. *J Consult Clin Psychol* **59**: 12–19.

Kessler RC, McGonagle KA, Zhao S, *et al.* (1994). Lifetime and 12-month prevalence of DSM-III-R psychiatric disorders in the United States. Results from the National Comorbidity Survey. *Arch Gen Psychiatry* **51**: 8–19.

Kiehl KA, Liddle PF, Hopfinger JB (2000). Error processing and the rostral anterior cingulate: an event-related fMRI study. *Psychophysiology* **37**: 216–223.

Kringelbach ML (2005). The human orbitofrontal cortex: linking reward to hedonic experience. *Nat Rev Neurosci* **6**: 691–702.

Kringelbach ML, Rolls ET (2004). The functional neuroanatomy of the human orbitofrontal cortex: evidence from neuroimaging and neuropsychology. *Prog Neurobiol* **72**: 341–372.

Kyrios M, Frost RO, Steketee G (2004). Cognitions in compulsive buying and acquisition. *Cogn Ther Res* **28**: 241–258.

Labad J, Menchon JM, Alonso P, *et al.* (2008). Gender differences in obsessive-compulsive symptom dimensions. *Depress Anxiety* **25**: 832–838.

Lawrence NS, Wooderson S, Mataix-Cols D, *et al.* (2006). Decision making and set shifting impairments are associated with distinct symptom dimensions in obsessive-compulsive disorder. *Neuropsychology* **20**: 409–419.

Lochner C, Kinnear CJ, Hemmings SM, *et al.* (2005). Hoarding in obsessive-compulsive disorder: clinical and genetic correlates. *J Clin Psychiatry* **66**: 1155–1160.

Luchian SA, McNally RJ, Hooley JM (2007). Cognitive aspects of nonclinical obsessive-compulsive hoarding. *Behav Res Ther* **45**: 1657–1662.

Luchins DJ, Goldman MB, Lieb M, Hanrahan P (1992). Repetitive behaviors in chronically institutionalized schizophrenic patients. *Schizophr Res* **8**: 119–123.

Maguire EA, Mummery CJ (1999). Differential modulation of a common memory retrieval network revealed by positron emission tomography. *Hippocampus* **9**: 54–61.

Maltby N, Tolin DF, Worhunsky P, O'Keefe TM, Kiehl KA (2005). Dysfunctional action monitoring hyperactivates frontal–striatal circuits in obsessive-compulsive disorder: an event-related fMRI study. *Neuroimage* **24**: 495–503.

Mataix-Cols D, Rauch SL, Manzo PA, Jenike MA, Baer L (1999). Use of factor-analyzed symptom dimensions to predict outcome with serotonin reuptake inhibitors and placebo in the treatment of obsessive-compulsive disorder. *Am J Psychiatry* **156**: 1409–1416.

Mataix-Cols D, Baer L, Rauch SL, Jenike MA (2000). Relation of factor-analyzed symptom dimensions of obsessive-compulsive disorder to personality disorders. *Acta Psychiatr Scand* **102**: 199–202.

Mataix-Cols D, Marks IM, Greist JH, Kobak KA, Baer L (2002). Obsessive-compulsive symptom dimensions as predictors of compliance with and response to behaviour therapy: results from a controlled trial. *Psychother Psychosomat* **71**: 255–262.

Matsunaga H, Kiriike N, Matsui T, *et al.* (2002). Obsessive-compulsive disorder with poor insight. *Compr Psychiatry* **43**: 150–157.

Meunier SA, Tolin DF, Frost RO, Steketee G, Brady RE (2006). Prevalence of hoarding symptoms across the anxiety disorders. In *Proceeding of the the Annual Meeting of the Anxiety Disorders Association of America*, Miami, March.

Mueller A, Mueller U, Albert P, *et al.* (2007). Hoarding in a compulsive buying sample. *Behav Res Ther* **45**: 2754–2763.

Nakaaki S, Murata Y, Sato J, *et al.* (2007). Impairment of decision-making cognition in a case of frontotemporal lobar degeneration (FTLD) presenting with pathologic gambling and hoarding as the initial symptoms. *Cogn Behav Neurol* **20**: 121–125.

Pinto A, Eisen JL, Mancebo M, *et al.* (2007). A 2-year follow-up study of the course of obsessive-compulsive disorder. In *Proceeding of the the Association of Behavioral and Cognitive Therapies*, Philadelphia, November.

Rasmussen J, Steketee G, Frost RO, Tolin DF (2007). Prevalence and associated characteristics of squalor in an internet sample of compulsive hoarders. In *Proceeding of the the Annual Meeting of the Association of Behavioral and Cognitive Therapies*, Philadelphia, November.

Rasmussen SA, Eisen JL (1989). Clinical features and phenomenology of obsessive compulsive disorder. *Psychiatr Ann* **19**: 67–73.

Rasmussen SA, Eisen JL (1992). The epidemiology and clinical features of obsessive compulsive disorder. *Psychiatr Clin N Am* **15**: 743–758.

Rolls ET (2004). The functions of the orbitofrontal cortex. *Brain Cogn* **55**: 11–29.

Salmon E, Perani D, Herholz K, *et al.* (2006). Neural correlates of anosognosia for cognitive impairment in Alzheimer's disease. *Hum Brain Mapp* **27**: 588–597.

Samuels JF, Bienvenu OJ, Riddle MA, *et al.* (2002). Hoarding in obsessive compulsive disorder: results from a case–control study. *Behav Res Ther* **40**: 517–528.

Samuels JF, Bienvenu OJ, Pinto A, *et al.* (2007a). Hoarding in obsessive-compulsive disorder: results from the OCD Collaborative Genetics Study. *Behav Res Ther* **45**: 673–686.

Samuels JF, Shugart YY, Grados MA, *et al.* (2007b). Significant linkage to compulsive hoarding on chromosome 14 in families with obsessive-compulsive disorder: Results from the OCD Collaborative Genetics Study. *Am J Psychiatry* **164**: 493–499.

Samuels JF, Bienvenu OJ, Grados MA, *et al.* (2008). Prevalence and correlates of hoarding behavior in a community-based sample. *Behav Res Ther* **46**: 836–844.

Saxena S, Maidment KM, Vapnik T, *et al.* (2002). Obsessive-compulsive hoarding: symptom severity and response to multimodal treatment. *J Clin Psychiatry* **63**: 21–27.

Saxena S, Brody AL, Maidment KM, *et al.* (2004). Cerebral glucose metabolism in obsessive-compulsive hoarding. *Am J Psychiatry* **161**: 1038–1048.

Saxena S, Brody AL, Maidment KM, Baxter LR, Jr. (2007). Paroxetine treatment of compulsive hoarding. *J Psychiatr Res* **41**: 481–487.

Seedat S, Stein DJ (2002). Hoarding in obsessive-compulsive disorder and related disorders: a preliminary report of 15 cases. *Psychiatry Clin Neurosci* **56**: 17–23.

Shafran R, Tallis F (1996). Obsessive-compulsive hoarding: A cognitive-behavioral approach. *Behav Cogn Psychother* **24**: 209–221.

Shetti CN, Reddy YC, Kandavel T, *et al.* (2005). Clinical predictors of drug nonresponse in obsessive-compulsive disorder. *J Clin Psychiatry* **66**: 1517–1523.

Sobin C, Blundell ML, Weiller F, *et al.* (2000). Evidence of a schizotypy subtype in OCD. *J Psychiatr Res* **34**: 15–24.

Stein DJ, Andersen EW, Overo KF (2007). Response of symptom dimensions in obsessive-compulsive disorder to treatment with citalopram or placebo. *Rev Bras Psiquiatr* **29**: 303–307.

Steketee G, Frost RO (2003). Compulsive hoarding: current status of the research. *Clin Psychol Rev* **23**: 905–927.

Steketee G, Frost RO (2007). *Compulsive Hoarding and Acquiring: Therapist Guide.* New York: Oxford University Press.

Steketee G, Frost RO, Wincze J, Greene K, Douglass H (2000). Group and individual treatment of compulsive hoarding: a pilot study. *Behav Cogn Psychother* **28**: 259–268.

Steketee G, Frost RO, Kim HJ (2001a). Hoarding by elderly people. *Health Social Work* **26**: 176–184.

Steketee G, Chambless DL, Tran GQ (2001b). Effects of axis I and II comorbidity on behavior therapy outcome for obsessive-compulsive disorder and agoraphobia. *Compr Psychiatry* **42**: 76–86.

Steketee G, Frost RO, Kyrios M (2003a). Cognitive aspects of compulsive hoarding. *Cogn Ther Res* **27**: 463–479.

Steketee G, Frost RO, Kyrios M (2003b). Beliefs about possessions among compulsive hoarders. *Cogn Ther Res* **27**: 467–479.

Steketee G, Frost RO, Tolin DF, Rasmussen J, Brown TA (2010). Waitlist-controlled trial of cognitive behavior therapy for hoarding disorder. *Depress Anxiety* **27**: 476–484.

Storch EA, Lack CW, Merlo LJ, *et al.* (2007). Clinical features of children and adolescents with obsessive-compulsive disorder and hoarding symptoms. *Compr Psychiatry* **48**: 313–318.

Stuss DT, Benson DF (1986). *The Frontal Lobes.* New York: Raven Press.

Tolin DF, Frost RO, Steketee G (2007). An open trial of cognitive-behavioral therapy for compulsive hoarding. *Behav Res Ther* **45**: 1461–1470.

Tolin DF, Frost RO, Steketee G, Gray KD, Fitch KE (2008a). The economic and social burden of compulsive hoarding. *Psychiatry Res* **160**: 200–211.

Tolin DF, Frost RO, Steketee G, Fitch KE (2008b). Family burden of compulsive hoarding: results of an internet survey. *Behav Res Ther* **46**: 334–344.

Tolin DF, Kiehl KA, Worhunsky P, Book GA, Maltby N (2008c). An exploratory study of the neural mechanisms of decision making in compulsive hoarding. *Psychol Med* **38**: 1–12.

Tolin DF, Brady RE, Hannan SE (2008d). Obsessional beliefs and symptoms of obsessive-compulsive disorder in a clinical sample. *J Psychopathol Behav Assess* **30**: 31–42.

Tolin DF, Kurtz M, Meunier SA, Carlson S (2009). Neuropsychological impairment in compulsive hoarding. In *Proceeding of the Annual Meeting of the Association of Behavioral and Cognitive Therapies*, New York.

Tolin DF, Meunier SA, Frost RO, Steketee G (2010). Course of compulsive hoarding and its relationship to life events. *Depress Anxiety*, **27**: 829–838.

Vogel A, Hasselbalch SG, Gade A, Ziebell M, Waldemar G (2005). Cognitive and functional neuroimaging correlate for anosognosia in mild cognitive impairment and Alzheimer's disease. *Int J Geriatr Psychiatry* **20**: 238–246.

Wheaton M, Timpano KR, Lasalle-Ricci VH, Murphy D (2008). Characterizing the hoarding phenotype in individuals with OCD: associations with comorbidity, severity and gender. *J Anxiety Disord* **22**: 243–252.

Wincze JP, Steketee G, Frost RO (2007). Categorization in compulsive hoarding. *Behav Res Ther* **45**: 63–72.

Winsberg ME, Cassic KS, Koran LM (1999). Hoarding in obsessive-compulsive disorder: a report of 20 cases. *J Clin Psychiatry* **60**: 591–597.

Wu KD, Watson D (2005). Hoarding and its relation to obsessive-compulsive disorder. *Behav Res Ther* **43**: 897–921.

Yonelinas AP, Hopfinger JB, Buonocore MH, Kroll NE, Baynes K (2001). Hippocampal, parahippocampal and occipital-temporal contributions to associative and item recognition memory: an fMRI study. *Neuroreport* **12**: 359–363.

Zhang H, Leckman JF, Pauls DL, *et al.* (2002). Genomewide scan of hoarding in sib pairs in which both sibs have Gilles de la Tourette syndrome. *Am J Hum Genet* **70**: 896–904.

Chapter 1

Cognitive-behavioral therapy for children and adolescents with obsessive-compulsive disorder

Aureen P. Wagner

Introduction

Childhood obsessive-compulsive disorder (OCD) is a prevalent, distressing, and impairing illness that extends through adolescence and into adulthood. The lifetime prevalence rate of OCD in youth is estimated to be between 2 and 3% (Rapoport *et al.* 2000), which is more common than expected. Childhood OCD resembles adult-onset OCD in the symptom picture and in its waxing and waning course. Like adults, children report obsessions pertaining to fears of germs or contamination, followed by fears of harm to self or others, as well as excessive focus on moral or religious themes. Not all obsessions are anxiety provoking, however. Some children and adults describe vague feelings of discomfort that something is not "just right" until there is a sense of symmetry, closure, or completion. Common rituals experienced by children include washing, repeating, checking, touching, counting, and ordering (Swedo *et al.* 1989). The mean age of onset for childhood OCD may range from 6 to 11 years, as indicated by clinic (Hanna 1995) and community-based (Rapoport *et al.* 2000) studies. Children who have an onset of OCD before the age of 7 years are more likely to be male and to have a family history of OCD than those with OCD of a later onset, suggesting that genetics may play a role in early-onset OCD (Swedo *et al.* 1989).

If left untreated or inadequately treated, OCD may severely disrupt normal development, causing impairment in school performance and in social and family relationships, and extending into adulthood (Adams *et al.* 1994; Piacentini and Bergman 2000). Approximately 80% of adults with OCD report initial symptom onset prior to 18 years of age (Riddle 1998), underscoring the need for early interventions to help youth to overcome OCD symptoms before they become chronic and debilitating. Follow-up studies indicate that, just as for adults, OCD is a chronic disorder for youngsters, with 43–68% still meeting criteria for OCD 2 to 14 years after initial diagnosis (Leonard *et al.* 1993; Bolton *et al.* 1995). However, these sobering statistics may reflect, at least in part, improper diagnosis and treatment at the time of these studies. With recent advances in treatment, the long-term outcome for children with OCD who receive treatment may be much more favorable.

Cognitive-behavioral therapy for childhood OCD

The empirical literature provides strong evidence for the efficacy of exposure-based cognitive-behavioral therapy (CBT) for the treatment of OCD in children and adolescents. Exposure and response prevention (ERP) involves purposeful confrontation of objects or situations that trigger obsessions while simultaneously refraining from the rituals that relieve the anxiety generated by obsessions. The latter technique was developed for adults and was initially considered neither possible nor desirable for children and adolescents. Since the mid-1990s, ERP has emerged as a viable and effective treatment for OCD in children and adolescents, with durable response rates ranging from 60% to 100%, mean symptom reduction rates of 50% to 67%, and maintenance of treatment gains for up to 18 months (March *et al.* 1994; Piacentini *et al.* 1994; Franklin *et al.* 1998; Barrett *et al.* 2004; Pediatric OCD Treatment Study Team 2004). According to Huppert and Franklin (2005), children may even be more likely to recover from OCD than adults because they are generally more malleable in changing their

Clinical Obsessive-Compulsive Disorders in Adults and Children, ed. Robert Hudak and Darin D. Dougherty.
Published by Cambridge University Press. Copyright © Cambridge University Press 2011.

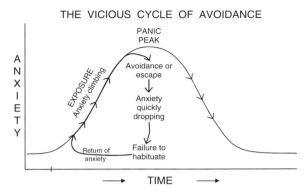

THE VICIOUS CYCLE OF AVOIDANCE

Fig. 10.1 The vicious cycle of avoidance. (From Wagner (2002, 2007). Copyright 2002 by Aureen P. Wagner, Ph.D. Reprinted with permission.)

thinking and behavior, and perhaps less entrenched in their OCD-driven habits. In addition, a supportive family and incentives for participation may provide more impetus for youngsters' success in CBT.

Cognitive-behavioral conceptualization

From a behavioral perspective, OCD is maintained and exacerbated over time via negative reinforcement because compulsions, avoidance, and escape alleviate distress in the moment. As depicted in Fig. 10.1, negative reinforcement occurs when a behavior (avoidance or escape from the fear) is rewarded by the evasion of a negative consequence (the discomfort generated by the obsessions). For instance, when eight-year-old Casey touches crayons, his anxiety about being poisoned begins to rise. He has a strong urge to clean up and rushes to wash his hands. He experiences relief and learns that washing his hands or simply avoiding contact with crayons provides quick reprieve from the distress of obsessions. Casey's neutralizing behaviors are reinforced and strengthened with each successful escape. Paradoxically, neutralizing and avoidance perpetuate OCD rather than alleviate it because they prevent the person from learning that the obsessions are unrealistic and harmless, and abate on their own.

According to cognitive models of OCD, obsessions elicit negative appraisals that evoke distress and fuel neutralizing behaviors such as rituals and

avoidance. The maintenance of OCD in adults implicates beliefs pertaining to inflated personal responsibility; overimportance of thoughts; excessive concern about the need to control one's thoughts; overestimation of threat, guilt or shame about one's thoughts; intolerance of uncertainty; and perfectionism (Foa and Kozak 1985; Obsessive Compulsive Cognitions Working Group 1997). The role of cognitive appraisals in childhood OCD is less clear, as investigations in this area are constrained by children's limited cognitive development.

The most commonly proposed mechanism for the effectiveness of ERP is that the process of autonomic habituation leads to the dissipation of anxiety when exposure is sustained and frequent. Additionally, ERP allows the realization that obsessive fears do not materialize even in the absence of rituals. Although exposure is considered the mainstay of treatment for OCD, cognitive strategies are closely integrated into exposure treatment when patients are assisted in changing inaccurate beliefs about feared situations (e.g., learning that feared consequences did not occur or that the patient's fear did not remain forever). Cognitive strategies can be a very helpful addition to ERP in enhancing the patient's readiness for treatment, thereby priming and preparing the child for ERP. They may also increase treatment acceptance and adherence, sustaining the motivation, persistence, and effort required for exposure.

Experts recommend CBT alone or in combination with selective serotonin reuptake inhibitors as the first-line treatment for OCD in youngsters (March *et al.* 1997a; Pediatric OCD Treatment Study Team 2004). However, it is estimated that many, if not most, children and adolescents with OCD do not receive CBT. One reason for this unfortunate situation is that many clinicians are not trained in CBT for OCD or in negotiating the unique developmental challenges that arise in the treatment of youngsters. In addition, making the leap from science to everyday clinical practice can be challenging because treatment protocols that are developed in research settings are not always easily adapted to the realities and constraints of community practice. An appreciation of the developmental challenges in working with youngsters is the stepping stone for disseminating evidence-based CBT to clinical practice settings where it is most needed.

Developmental challenges

A wide range of developmental differences between children and adults arising from age, maturity, and conceptual and language development may complicate the application of CBT with children. Recognition of these differences sets the groundwork for implementing developmentally tailored treatment.

First, OCD in children may be difficult to detect and diagnose for a variety of reasons. Children may not be able to recognize, label, or articulate their obsessions or fear triggers. A typical response of "I just have to do it," or "I don't know" may mislead caregivers into believing the child's behaviors are willful. Primary presenting complaints of irritability, agitation, aggression, withdrawal, or decline in school functioning may mask OCD and may be mistaken for oppositional behavior, poor motivation, laziness, or non-compliance. Children may keep their OCD a secret and parents may be unaware of the presence or severity of symptoms (Rapoport *et al.* 2000). Sensitive but direct interviewing by the clinician may be necessary to uncover obsessions and rituals that may underlie initial complaints. True OCD must also be differentiated from normal developmental rituals and fears that are commonplace in childhood.

Diagnosis is also confounded by the fact that OCD in children is a highly comorbid condition. Up to 80% of youngsters meet criteria for an additional disorder under *Diagnostic and Statistical Manual of Mental Disorders,* 4th edition (DSM-IV; American Psychiatric Association 1994) criteria (Pediatric OCD Treatment Study Team 2004) and up to 50% display multiple comorbidities, most commonly other anxiety disorders (26–75%), depressive disorders (25–62%), behavioral disorders (18–33%), and tic disorders (20–30%) (Zohar 1999; Rapoport *et al.* 2000). Depression is more common among adolescents with OCD than in children and may be reactive because it often occurs after the onset of OCD. Comorbidity complicates the course of illness in OCD as well as the treatment outcome (Albano *et al.* 1999).

In addition, children and adolescents vary tremendously in the level of future orientation, ability to delay gratification, self-reliance, maturity and internal motivation they bring to CBT. Because children rarely seek treatment for themselves and are usually referred by adult caregivers, they may be more motivated to get help avoiding their fears rather than overcoming them. Young children are generally present oriented and, therefore, less likely to appreciate the prospect of future improvement. Consequently, they may be reluctant to tolerate the potential anxiety of ERP to achieve future gain. Compliance with ERP homework exercises can be particularly challenging because most children normally dislike and avoid homework. As a result, children may require substantial structure, supervision, and assistance from the therapist and parents to participate effectively in CBT.

Children's misconceptions about the nature of OCD and fears of being "crazy" may affect their motivation for treatment. They are less likely than adults to realize that their symptoms are senseless and excessive. Although older children may have good insight, shame may lead them to minimize their symptoms. Children are more likely to passively succumb to obsessions and rituals, and they may fear treatment because ERP can be counterintuitive and daunting at first glance. The child's lack of ability to introspect or give specific examples of symptoms or triggers may limit the therapist's ability to design effective treatment.

Finally, children live in the context of a family, and parents are an integral part of their lives. Piacentini and Bergman (2000) noted that family members of children with OCD participate in rituals and provide reassurance more frequently than do family members of adults. The child may exert coercive control over the household with angry outbursts if family members fail to comply (Bolton *et al.* 1983). Parents, therefore, often feel coerced into participating in rituals or accommodating OCD behaviors in order to appease the child and avoid conflict. Families of children with OCD may exhibit increased levels of expressed emotion, parent–child conflict, and parental OCD (Waters and Barrett 2000).

Protocols for CBT in children have included developmental adaptations such as psychoeducation, age-appropriate language, cognitive strategies for dealing with anxiety, use of gradual exposure, and rewards in treatment (March *et al.* 1994; Piacentini *et al.* 1994). Carefully assessing developmental issues, devising appropriate adaptations, and building a child and family's "treatment readiness" prior to the initiation of treatment may be vital to successful outcomes.

Active parent involvement in the child's treatment may also increase efficacy and long-term gains from treatment (Waters *et al.* 2001; Piacentini *et al.* 1994). Failure to recognize and address developmental issues may result in rushing into treatment precipitously in response to the sense of urgency elicited by the child's symptoms. Children, parents, and even clinicians may abandon treatment prematurely when the initial rise in anxiety elicited by ERP seems intolerable to the youngster.

The implementation of a developmentally sensitive CBT protocol for childhood OCD that is flexible and feasible for clinicians in primarily clinical settings is described below.

Child-friendly cognitive-behavoiral theray for children and adolescents

The Worry Hill CBT treatment protocol for OCD is designed to be appealing and user-friendly for the child, parent, and therapist. A detailed description of the protocol is available in Wagner (2003, 2007). The four sequential phases in the protocol are described below and illustrated with a case example at the end of this chapter. Each phase is focused on completing specific goals or building on skills that have been mastered in the previous phase. The number of sessions in each phase is flexible to allow customization to the child and family's unique needs. The average treatment extends over 10 to 20 sessions (the 50-minute clinical hour), depending on the severity and complexity of the case. Straightforward OCD may be treated in as few as six sessions.

Phase I Biopsychosocial assessment and treatment plan

Phase I lays the essential foundation for successful treatment and may extend over one to three sessions. A biopsychosocial assessment focuses on a complete and sensitive understanding of the child's OCD symptoms in the context of the child's overall health, strengths and limitations, family, and social and school functioning. Initial diagnosis is followed by OCD symptom analysis and a treatment plan.

Initial evaluation and diagnosis

The first step in the evaluation is to establish a diagnosis of OCD, assess baseline severity and impairment, and identify potentially difficult areas for

treatment. The assessment should target current and past fears, rituals and triggers, events surrounding the onset of symptoms, frequency and context of symptoms, degree of distress and impairment, comorbid conditions, medical and developmental history, family history, social relationships, and functioning at home and school (Pinto and Francis 1993). Structured diagnostic interviews for children provide more reliable diagnosis; however, time and resource constraints may make them infeasible in clinical settings.

Clinical interview of parent(s)

In addition to describing the child's symptoms, parents are valuable in providing a chronology of events, developmental history, comorbid symptoms, family history, and functioning, of which children might not be aware.

Clinical interview of the child

Although the child may not be the best historian, it is important for the clinician to gauge the child's insight and experience of symptoms, level of distress, and motivation for treatment. Interview of the child is geared towards obtaining answers to many questions. Does the child perform rituals to relieve anxiety or prevent bad outcomes? How is each fear connected with each ritual? What would happen if he or she did not do a ritual? How does the child know when enough has been done? What makes the child feel better and what makes the thoughts dissipate? Does the child believe he or she can overcome these fears? Is the child hopeful and optimistic or does he or she feel defeated and dispirited? The clinician must be empathic and resourceful in order to engage children of various ages and levels of maturity, elicit trust, and query thoughts and rituals with the level of detail necessary for effective treatment.

Self-report and parent ratings

In addition to the clinical interview, several other measures with established psychometric properties yield clinically useful before and after treatment data and can be efficient and time saving in the clinical setting. They can be administered, scored, and reviewed prior to the first appointment, thereby allowing the clinician to target areas for closer assessment during the initial visits. The Child Behavior Checklist (Achenbach and Edelbrock 1991) is a parent-report measure that allows assessment of a broad range of symptoms that point to both OCD and comorbid conditions. The Leyton Obsessional Inventory-Child Version (Berg *et al.* 1988) is a self-report measure of obsessive thoughts suitable for children aged 10–18. Twenty Yes/No items cover areas such as dirt–contamination, numbers–luck, school-related thoughts, and general obsessive thoughts. For each thought endorsed as present, the youngster rates the degree to which the thought interferes with functioning on a scale of 0 (none) to 3 (a lot). The child's overall anxiety can be assessed on the Multidimensional Anxiety Scale for Children (March *et al.* 1997b). The Child OCD Impact Scale (Piacentini *et al.* 2001), completed by parent and child, provides information on the impact of OCD on the child's school, social and family/home functioning.

Clinician ratings

Several single-item clinician rating scales, which take about a minute each to complete, are highly practical in clinical settings. The National Institutes of Mental Health Global Obsessive–Compulsive Scale (NIMH-GOCS) rates OCD severity and impairment. A score of 7 indicates clinically meaningful OCD symptoms, and scores of 13 to 15 indicate very severe symptoms. The NIMH Clinical Global Impressions (CGI) scale provides an overall judgment of impairment from 1 (not at all ill) to 7 (extremely ill). The CGI Improvement (CGI-I) scale allows ratings of improvement during and after treatment on a scale of 1 (very much improved) to 7 (very much worse).

Symptom analysis

A close examination of specific obsessions, compulsions, triggers, the nature and frequency of parental participation and assistance with rituals helps the clinician to design targeted and effective exposures. The Children's Yale–Brown Obsessive-Compulsive Scale (CY-BOCS; Scahill *et al.* 1997) is often the starting point for this information. The CY-BOCS assesses obsessions and compulsions in terms of time consumed, interference, distress, resistance, and control. Scores of 0–9 are considered subclinical, 10–18 mild, 18–29 moderate, and 30 or above indicative of severe OCD.

Biopsychosocial treatment plan

The therapist must use the information derived from the assessment to develop a treatment plan that is designed to improve the well-being of the child, not just the obsessions and compulsions. The child may need treatment to help to rebuild social skills and to improve self-esteem, family relationships, and academic functioning. The OCD symptoms should generally be treated first, unless other issues interfere with the treatment. For example, severe depression or family conflict may need to be treated before a child can engage in CBT.

Feedback and education

The nature, course, prognosis, and contributing factors involved in OCD should be discussed with the child and parents. Blame and shame from misunderstanding OCD as a character weakness or the result of poor parenting should be eliminated. The child and parents should be offered all viable treatment options including CBT, medication, or a combination of both, and given assistance in making the optimal choices for the child. The therapist should discuss the pros and cons of each option, be explicit about what each treatment involves, the focus and commitment required of parents and child, the possible duration of treatment, and when results may be expected. Families who opt for medication should be referred to a child psychiatrist.

Phase II Building treatment readiness

Phase II is focused on planned and active preparation for treatment. The literature suggests that motivation and compliance are essential to treatment success. However, guidelines for optimizing the child's motivation are far less clear. Children may be quite reluctant to confront their fears because they are more cognizant of their immediate distress than they are of the long-term benefit of overcoming anxiety.

Cultivating treatment readiness is in itself an integral part of the treatment. Devoting one to three sessions cultivating treatment readiness in the child and parent is a worthwhile investment that enhances participation, compliance, and the ease of implementation of ERP. The four steps in building treatment readiness are described below.

Stabilization of the child and family crisis

In the typical clinical setting, families seeking help for a child's OCD frequently present in a state of crisis. There is a sense of urgency and high expectancy for immediate relief when children are unable to function and parents may be at their wits' end. It is easy to unwittingly launch into ERP prematurely in response to the urgency of the situation. A child who is

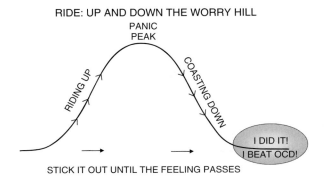

RIDE: UP AND DOWN THE WORRY HILL

PANIC PEAK

RIDING UP

COASTING DOWN

I DID IT!
I BEAT OCD!

STICK IT OUT UNTIL THE FEELING PASSES

Fig. 10.2 The Worry Hill. (From Wagner (2002, 2007). Copyright 2002 by Aureen P. Wagner, Ph.D. Reprinted with permission.)

Rename the thought. *"That's OCD talking, not me."*
Insist that YOU are in charge! *"I'm in charge. I choose not to believe OCD."*
Defy OCD. *"I will ride up the Worry Hill and stick it out until I can coast down."*
Enjoy your success, reward yourself. *"I did it! I beat OCD. I can do it again."*

overwhelmed and struggling to function may not have the wherewithal to consider CBT and ERP may backfire if the child becomes frightened while confronting fear triggers.

Stabilization begins with providing accurate information about OCD, dispelling myths and misconceptions, acknowledging the impact of OCD on the child and family, removing blame and shame, reducing conflict, and building alliances in the family. The therapist describes OCD as a neurobehavioral illness that results from a glitch in the brain that sets off a "false alarm" when there is no real danger. Stabilization also involves providing the child with respite from the dual challenges of OCD and everyday living through flexible expectations and temporary accommodations at home and at school. In severe situations, the child may need medication to reduce the severity of symptoms prior to engaging in CBT.

Parents who are highly distressed also need support, stress management, and conflict-resolution techniques to regain equilibrium before they can support their child during ERP. A "no blame, no shame" approach helps to reduce hostility, guilt, and polarization in the family.

Effective communication

Perhaps the most critical part of treatment readiness is helping children and families understand how rituals and avoidance strengthen OCD, as well as key CBT concepts of exposure, habituation, and anticipatory anxiety. Obsessive-compulsive disorder is overcome by confronting fears (exposure) and learning that they are false alarms, experiencing habituation (getting used to the anxiety, much like getting used to the cold water in the swimming pool), and understanding that confronting fears seems harder before it is done than when it is actually being done (anticipatory anxiety).

Understanding and accepting the vital concepts of exposure, habituation, and anticipatory anxiety, and the ability to tolerate anxiety during ERP, may be crucial to motivation and compliance. A child's success in treatment might hinge on this understanding; yet, these are not intuitive concepts. When children do not understand CBT, they are unnecessarily intimidated and consequently unmotivated. The metaphor of the Worry Hill (Wagner 2002, 2004) was developed to communicate key CBT concepts effectively in child-friendly language. It places significant emphasis on the child's comprehension, acceptance, and temporal experience of anticipatory anxiety, exposure, and habituation as the tools that make ERP easier for the child.

The Worry Hill depicts the relationship between exposure and habituation. The bell-shaped curve of the Worry Hill (Fig. 10.2) illustrates the rise in anxiety when exposure to a feared situation takes place. Anxiety increases steadily as exposure continues and may reach a peak. If, on the one hand, the child persists with exposure, autonomic habituation sets in and anxiety automatically begins to decline. On the other hand, if the child succumbs to rituals or avoids the fear trigger, habituation is interrupted and obsessions are inadvertently strengthened by negative reinforcement (escape from an aversive situation). The Worry Hill is explained to children as follows: "Learning how to stop OCD is like riding your bicycle up and down a hill. At first, facing your fears and stopping your rituals feels like riding up a big Worry Hill, because it's tough and you have to work very hard. If you keep going and don't give up, you get to the top of the Worry Hill. Once you get to the top, it's easy to coast down the hill. But you can only coast down the hill if you first get to the top."

Most parents and children are not aware that habituation of anxiety is an automatic physiologic process and takes place naturally if anxiety is endured for a reasonable length of time. This lack of awareness and inability to tolerate increasing anxiety may lead them to readily succumb to rituals to escape the anxiety. When a child understands the metaphor of the Worry Hill, it is often an "aha!" experience. Parents and children who are educated about the Worry Hill prior to beginning treatment appear to be less anxious and more motivated to engage in treatment.

Effective persuasion

Persuasion involves helping children see the necessity for change, the possibility for change, and the power to change. Children are more readily persuaded once they have an accurate understanding of OCD and CBT. The child must be helped to see the benefits of overcoming OCD; this convinces the child of the necessity for change. Providing information about CBT outcomes helps children to learn that OCD can be successfully overcome, and that many others have done it. They are able to see the possibility for change. Finally, the child must know that he or she has the power to change. The child must understand that he or she can take charge and take control of OCD instead of letting it take control. The therapist's genuineness, credibility, and empathy build the rapport and trust that persuade the child to consider taking the risks of treatment.

Collaboration between parent, child and therapist

Collaboration, not coercion, sets the tone for the treatment and makes the child a vital partner in recovery. The child, parent, and therapist have different but complementary roles to play in the child's treatment.

Proactively defining each of these roles before treatment begins can preempt the conflict and frustration that can ensue from misunderstanding. It also corrects the misattribution of power to the therapist.

The therapist's role is to guide the child's treatment, the child's role is to RIDE (rename, insist, defy, enjoy, as described below) the bicycle up and down the Worry Hill, and the parent's role is to RALLY for the child (recognize OCD episodes; ally with your child; lead your child to the RIDE; let go so your child can RIDE on his own; yes, you did it! Reward and praise). The metaphor of the Worry Hill is extended to help children and parents clearly to understand their respective roles in treatment. The child's role is described as follows: "No one else can ride a bicycle for you. You have to do it for yourself. In the same way, only you can face your fears and make them go away. No one else can do it for you." The parents' role is conveyed as follows: "You can help your child get ready for the ride by selecting the right bicycle and gear and holding on to the seat if he's unsteady. Eventually, you must let go and let your child ride for himself. Your child cannot ride on his own until you let go of the seat."

With the therapist's guidance, the child must be involved in setting goals and deciding the pace of treatment, as is suitable to the child's age and maturity. The child is more likely to be invested in his or her recovery when the child can perceive that he or she has control over it. It is a good rule of thumb to wait to begin ERP until the child voluntarily expresses willingness to proceed. Children generally agree to participate in treatment when they are well informed and given the choice. When a child declines to participate despite proper preparation, it may be a good indicator that the child is truly not ready for CBT and, therefore, unlikely to benefit from it. Additional preparation may be necessary or other options such as medication may need to be considered. For some children, CBT may have to be deferred temporarily and attempted later when they are older, more mature, or more willing.

Phase III The RIDE up and down the Worry Hill

Phase III may extend between sessions 4 and 15 and consists of separate sessions with the child plus joint sessions with the child and parents. During this phase, the child actively engages in ERP.

Symptom monitoring

Symptom monitoring provides targets for exposure as well as data for ongoing evaluation of treatment response. The child and parents list all OCD symptoms and record their frequency on easy-to-use monitoring sheets known as the "OCD Diary." Parents may assist younger children or record for them.

"Fear temperature"

Fear temperature ratings are analogous to the "subjective units of distress" used in the treatment of adults, and allow children to rank exposure targets from least to most difficult. Children rate their fear temperature on a Fear Thermometer, a graduated scale from 1 ("no anxiety") to 10 ("out of control") that teaches them to differentiate, quantify, and communicate levels of anxiety to the therapist and parents.

Gradual exposure

Gradual exposure involves progressing in small sequential steps from the least-feared to the most-feared situations. It is recommended that exposure with children should be gradual, as children may not be able to participate in ERP if they become overwhelmed by anxiety. Gradual exposure is described to the child as "riding up little hills before tackling the big one." The relatively easy success experienced during gradual exposure provides positive reinforcement and boosts the child's self-confidence and willingness to attempt subsequent exposures. The child's fear temperature ratings are used to construct a gradual exposure hierarchy that proceeds from least difficult to most difficult triggers.

Exposure and response prevention

The four-step RIDE acronym encompasses the steps that the child or adolescent must take to successfully tackle the Worry Hill. The RIDE was designed to simplify ERP for children and adolescents, enhance preparedness for treatment, and foster endurance of anxiety until habituation takes place. It includes both cognitive and behavioral techniques such as externalizing, distancing, and taking control of OCD thoughts; exposure; and self-reinforcement. The acronym helps to break down ERP into concrete, finite steps that structure and clarify the ERP process.

The first two steps, "rename and insist" are aimed at preparing the child's belief system in anticipation of exposure. They include perspective taking, reframing, and distancing from OCD and empowerment to take back control.

Step 1: rename the thought

The first step involves recognizing OCD thoughts as unrealistic and external to the child's rational self. Young children may find it helpful to personify OCD as the "Worry Monster" or "Mr. Right" whereas adolescents usually prefer to refer to OCD by its name. This technique of externalizing OCD has been used by March and Mulle (1994) with children.

Step 2: insist that *you* are in charge!

The second step fosters a shift in attitude from passive acquiescence to active assertion. It helps the child to recognize and utilize the power of choice. Instead of readily succumbing to OCD, the youngster can choose to take active control over his or her thoughts and actions. Statements such as, "I am in charge, not OCD" and "I'm going to choose not to believe the tricks that OCD plays on my mind," help the child to build the self-confidence and endurance needed to embark on exposure.

Step 3: defy OCD, do the OPPOSITE of what it wants

The third step of the RIDE signals the beginning of ERP, which requires a change in behavior. This is the most critical step, as this is the core exposure strategy. The therapist first instructs the child in the steps of the RIDE, then models the procedure and asks the child to follow suit. For instance, the therapist shows the child how to touch the "contaminated" door handle and then asks the child to do the same. Modeling allows the child to see that the therapist is willing to assume the same risks that are asked of the child.

Step 4: enjoy your success, reward yourself

The final step allows the child to review success and to take due credit for his or her efforts and courage. Children can learn to give themselves positive feedback and internalize success with self-talk, such as, "I did it! I can do it again. Now I deserve to be good to myself."

Guiding through the RIDE steps

Coaching or instruction in each of the four RIDE steps is followed by therapist modeling, behavioral rehearsal, frequent practice, and reinforcement until the child masters the steps. In addition to the auditory mnemonic aid of the RIDE acronym, the Worry Hill Memory Card (Fig. 10.2) provides a visual mnemonic aid to the child.

Rewards

Rewards bridge the gap of delayed gain from treatment and provide children with the immediate incentive to participate and maintain motivation. Not all youngsters need rewards, as some may be inherently motivated to overcome OCD. The child must be rewarded for *effort* rather than success because effort reflects the desired behavior. Praise and attention are preferable to material rewards, although young children often need tangible rewards.

The parents' role: RALLY

Working closely with parents and families may enhance the chances of success in treatment. Specific parental behaviors that support and reinforce the child's RIDE are discussed in each session. The RALLY steps are tailored and put into action as per the specific circumstances for each child and family, including the child's age, maturity, specific symptoms, degree of parental involvement in symptoms, and the nature of the parent–child relationship. Targets for working with parents include helping them to take care of themselves in order to take better care of their children; reducing parental assistance and participation in the child's symptoms; and increasing positive family interactions, communication, problem-solving and child management skills. Proactive discussion of realistic expectations about the duration and course of treatment, as well as the time frame and nature of improvement, removes misconceptions and ensuing disillusionment with treatment.

Frequent practice

Frequent and diligent practice of ERP is crucial for mastery of anxiety. Weekly graphs of progress and fear temperature ratings give the child and family tangible evidence of progress. The therapist assigns daily "practice" in writing after each session in order to reduce the chances that assignments are forgotten or misunderstood. (The word "homework" is best avoided because children often have negative conditioned associations with it.) Incomplete assignments are usually a sign that there is some obstacle to the child's participation. Sometimes, the child is willing and enthusiastic in the therapists' office but becomes afraid when returning home. Parents may not be able to provide the supervision or structure that allows the child to focus on completing ERP exercises. Exercises may not be working as expected because the child terminates ERP prematurely before habituation has taken place, or replaces overt rituals with silent mental rituals.

Success in CBT may be limited until barriers to full participation are removed. Maintaining daily phone contact with patients during the early stages of the RIDE can preempt many of these problems. Parents and children are asked to leave a message every day, letting the therapist know how the practice is proceeding. This not only increases accountability but also allows the therapist to intervene quickly if things are not proceeding as expected.

Phase IV After the RIDE

Phase IV signals the end of treatment and should begin when the child has mastered the RIDE, parents RALLY effectively, and the child's OCD symptoms have decreased at least moderately.

Preparation for slips and relapses

Parents and children need to be prepared for the reality that OCD "slips" or relapses can happen either unexpectedly or at times of stress and transition. When prepared, they are more likely to have an organized and productive response, and less likely to become demoralized. Relapse-recovery training involves having realistic expectations, recognizing the early signs of relapses, keeping things in perspective, and intervening immediately. The metaphor of falling off a bicycle is used to suggest that when a slip occurs, OCD should be confronted head on by doing ERP exercises even more vigorously. "When you fall off your bicycle, you pick yourself up. If you made no attempt to get up, you wouldn't get anywhere. If you want to move on, you get up, dust yourself off, survey the damage, attend to it, and get right back on that bicycle." It is important that the child and parents not fall into the trap of avoiding the feared situation.

During this phase, there is a shift in focus to building self-reliance in the child. The child initially gets substantial guidance and support during ERP from therapist and parents. However, once the child has experienced success and knows the process, the therapist and parent must gradually phase out their assistance in order to foster the child's self-reliance in managing OCD. The more self-reliance the child develops, the better equipped he or she is for future recurrences of OCD. The child is encouraged to begin to design his or her own exposures during this phase of treatment. Parents are encouraged to redirect the child who seeks help in coping to first ask, "What do *you* think you need to do with that OCD thought?" rather than providing suggestions reflexively.

Treatment completion and booster sessions

There must be significant recognition of the child's efforts and success when treatment is completed. Treatment outcome is assessed via CY-BOCS post-treatment scores, CGI-I ratings, changes in "fear temperature," and parent and child ratings of percentage improvement. Periodic booster sessions after treatment enhance the maintenance of treatment gains. Booster sessions should be scheduled prior to completion of treatment to reduce the rate of attrition.

Case example

Daniel, a 12-year-old seventh grader was referred by his pediatrician for treatment of obsessions that his muscles would atrophy through electronic and magnetic waves. He was an accomplished athlete on his school team and was, therefore, very concerned about losing his athletic prowess. Daniel had not received any prior treatment for his fears.

Phase I Biopsychosocial assessment and treatment plan (three sessions)

Biopsychosocial assessment consisted of interview of Daniel and his parents, telephone interview with his school counselor, review of medical records, and administration of self-report measures and rating scales.

Six months prior to referral, Daniel had experienced a significant escalation of worries that his muscles would be damaged by electrical and magnetic waves emanating from various items such as TV remote control devices, game controllers, cell phones,

batteries, magnets, antennas, and even UPC codes on grocery packaging. Daniel avoided being in the proximity of these items. What initially seemed like a little extra caution soon became a preoccupation. Daniel could not be in the same room when the TV was on, could not hold any electronic or magnetic device, and seemed to panic if family members inadvertently pointed any remote control devices in his direction. He became afraid of electricity, light switches, plug outlets, and electrical cords. Daniel did not like being near his parents' car keys, and sat as far as possible away from them in the car. He was terrified of static electricity in his clothing, fearing that it would attract magnetic and electrical waves. Daniel became very nervous about perceived unfamiliar smells, dust that could permeate his lungs, and food that he thought was slightly exposed or that had "foreign" objects on it such as a small black speck. He would not touch food packages that had UPC codes on them and would only eat if the food was separated from its packaging. He did not like going to stores and avoided being near UPC scanners.

Daniel repeatedly sought reassurance, asking his parents if they thought his muscles might atrophy. In addition, he would verify, up to 50 times a day, that his muscles were still working by running in the yard for 20 minutes; flexing, shaking, and pointing his limbs; and kicking a soccer ball. Regardless of snow or rain, Daniel insisted on going outside to engage in his checking rituals. If unable to check, Daniel would panic and become enraged.

Daniel lived with both parents and three teenage siblings. His family was supportive and understanding. They had tried to reason with him and to explain that there was nothing to fear and gave him reassurance to assuage his distress. Family members were vigilant not to inadvertently point the TV remote or cell phone in Daniel's direction. With regard to family history, Daniel's deceased maternal grandmother was reported to have experienced severe OCD for most of her adult life.

At school, Daniel visited the counselor's office daily and asked to call his mother. He asked his mother for reassurance over the phone and often requested that she pick him up from school so that he could return home and verify that his muscles were still working. Daniel reportedly had outbursts of anger if she did not comply with his demands. Daniels grades had deteriorated from B/C to C/D over the previous six months.

He reported that he could not concentrate on his work at school. He had frequent nighttime awakenings and was unable to complete school work or homework. Socially, Daniel was reported to be well liked at school, although with no close friends.

As a toddler and young child, Daniel was reported to get upset if his hands were sticky or dirty, and to insist on washing them. His socks had to feel "just right" and he would not wear shirts unless the tags were cut off them. He would not eat if anyone was near his food for fear that they would sneeze or cough on it, and sat away from everyone when eating.

Daniel's symptoms met criteria for a DSM-IV diagnosis of OCD. His score on the CY-BOCS was 25, suggesting notable distress and functional impairment. Daniel's symptoms merited a score of 8 on the NIMH-GOCS and 4 on the CGI. Daniel acknowledged that he did not like being afraid and expressed motivation to overcome his fears.

Phase II Building treatment readiness (two sessions)

The diagnosis of OCD was described to Daniel and his parents, along with information about its course, risk factors, prognosis, and treatment options. Daniel and his family were relieved of blame and shame for the OCD, and the focus was on fostering hope and optimism about recovery. The metaphor of the Worry Hill was presented, and the roles of therapist, child, and parent were discussed at the outset. The importance of willingness to change and compliance with treatment were emphasized. Daniel clearly understood the Worry Hill and the RIDE and was able to explain it to his parents. Daniel's parents were enthusiastic in their commitment to RALLY for him.

Phase III The RIDE up and down the Worry Hill (eight sessions)

Daniel and his parents completed the daily diary to monitor the nature, context, and frequency of obsessions and rituals. Daniel was able to differentiate between realistic and obsessive worries, to label the latter as "false alarms," and to rate his fear temperature on the feeling thermometer. Daniel and the therapist worked together to construct an exposure hierarchy with the following items (fear temperatures for each item are in parentheses): Therapist to hold a cell phone a few feet away from him (3), hold a cell phone (4), point a cell phone at his face (5), plug in toaster (5), unplug toaster (5), hold a box with a UPC code (6), touch the cell phone to his face (7), eat at a table with the cell phone on it (7), hold and point TV remote control at himself (8), click remote control device on his body (8), hold car keys and click the pad while pointing to body (9), unlock car doors using car keys (9), touch electrical cord ends on unplugged toaster (10), rub clothing on body to generate static electricity (10), and finally, rub static-filled hands on face (10). Daniel knew that, while he engaged in exposures, he would need to refrain from urges to check his muscles or to ask for reassurance.

After coaching in the RIDE steps, Daniel was ready to begin ERP. He engaged in gradual exposure to the first item on the hierarchy by allowing the therapist to hold a cell phone about 10 feet away from him. He recognized that his obsessive thoughts were not realistic and distanced himself from them by saying, "That's just a false alarm." The therapist then pointed the cell phone at herself and then suggested he try letting her point it at him for the count of one.

Daniel used the Worry Hill Memory Card as a reminder of the RIDE steps. The therapist used the feeling thermometer to rate changes in his anxiety every 30–60 seconds initially and every two to five minutes subsequently from beginning to end of each exposure. Daniel talked himself through ERP by saying, "I'm going to ride up the Worry Hill now. It's going to be tough going up the hill, but if I stick it out, I'll get to the top of the hill. Once I'm at the top, it will be easy to coast down the hill. I won't quit until the bad feeling passes. I won't give in to the rituals."

As Daniel engaged in ERP to feared triggers, his anxiety escalated and peaked and then automatically began to decline, because habituation set in. Daniel rode to the top of the Worry Hill and then enjoyed the coast down the other side. He was surprised that exposure wasn't as upsetting as he had expected and that he tolerated the anxiety. As expected, his anxiety followed the curve of the Worry Hill, dropping from 8 to 2. The time was then gradually increased until Daniel could point the cell phone at himself for 5 to 10 minutes. Habituation occurred within 2 to 10 minutes. Daniel received frequent praise and was encouraged to take credit for his effort and success. He was pleased with himself and his parents were pleasantly surprised at his willingness to take the risk. Daniel's fears decreased with repeated exposures, and his anxiety habituated faster with practice.

Daniel then progressed through each task on the hierarchy, using the same process for ERP and habituation. He practiced each ERP exercise daily at home and recorded it in his OCD diary. His parents gave him reminders and encouraged him, but Daniel managed the practices himself. Daniel generally habituated to the initial anxiety within five minutes.

Daniel's parents learned how to RALLY for him by reinforcing the message of the Worry Hill and the steps of the RIDE, providing support during exposure exercises and gradually withdrawing participation in his rituals. Strategies to help Daniel to express frustration appropriately and contain angry outbursts were presented. Daniel's parents learned stress-management strategies for themselves. Reassurance seeking was gradually weaned by preparing Daniel ahead of time for a change in parental response, redirecting Daniel to consider if his fear was realistic or an OCD false alarm, and to answer the questions himself. His parents gradually decreased the number of reassurances down to once. These steps were role-played during the therapy session before the parents implemented them at home.

Phase IV After the RIDE (four sessions)

At the end of six sessions of ERP, Daniel and his parents reported 80% improvement in his symptoms and overall functioning. His CY-BOCS score was 4, NIMH-GOCS score was 2 and CGI-I score was 1. Daniel was no longer checking his muscles nor was he asking for reassurance. Daniel's parents reported feeling more confident about helping him to manage his OCD. His counselor at school reported a decline in visits to her office. Daniel stopped calling his mother from school.

Booster sessions scheduled at periodic intervals (e.g., 4, 8, 14, and 22 weeks and every 12 weeks thereafter for two years) were focused on review of progress, identification of areas of difficulty, and recapitulation of strategies.

Daniel experienced a minor relapse four months after treatment was completed, when the approach of the summer school recess triggered memories of the onset of his OCD the previous year. Daniel's mother also reported that his OCD symptoms were less evident when he was busy, and he did not like having "down time" on his hands. Relapse recovery steps were reviewed and implemented, and Daniel successfully overcame the resurgence of fears within a week. As Daniel's symptoms improved again, he became lax with his daily practices and the OCD became worse again. Daniel was then able to understand the connection between daily practice and improvement in his symptoms. Daniel also learned to estimate the probability that his fears would come true, given the evidence that they had not come true in a year, and that they had not come true for his family members either, even though they did not engage in avoidance and protective rituals.

At 18 months post-treatment, Daniel's score on the CY-BOCS was 3, in the normal range. Other than occasional rituals that did not cause distress or interference, Daniel was reported to be doing very well at home and at school.

Conclusions

Knowledge about childhood OCD and its treatment has progressed tremendously since the mid 1990s, thanks to significant research and clinical attention to the disorder. The use of CBT, which was once considered neither feasible nor suitable for children, is now recommended by experts as the treatment of choice for OCD in youngsters. Clinicians are now better able to provide youngsters with symptom relief as well as the skills to manage OCD in the long term and to lead productive lives.

However, there are many obstacles to be overcome before this recommendation translates to real benefit for children and families who struggle to cope with OCD. Parents, pediatricians, teachers, and school professionals, who function as gatekeepers for timely recognition and referral of children, often do not have the knowledge or tools to detect OCD until it is severe. Moreover, most children who are diagnosed still do not receive CBT because there is a dearth of clinicians with the requisite skills. The application of CBT with children calls for expertise in treating children, familiarity with developmental and family issues, a sound therapeutic relationship with the child and the family, and facility in adapting and customizing standard treatment protocols.

The Worry Hill represents a universal, cross-cultural metaphor because children as young as four, adolescents, and even adults across most cultures can relate to the idea of riding a bicycle up a hill. Parents, siblings, and teachers find the metaphor equally helpful in understanding how CBT works. The easy acronym, logical steps, and visual features of the Worry Hill and RIDE are simple to grasp, remember, and recall, even in the midst of anxiety, reducing chances of premature termination of exposure and habituation. The metaphor is comprehensive and readily lends itself to a description of most elements of treatment and recovery. In addition, the Worry Hill protocol clearly and proactively delineates the roles of therapist, child, and parent in the treatment and places strong emphasis on "treatment readiness" as a precursor to beginning ERP.

We know that CBT works. Efforts to help youngsters with OCD must emphasize wider dissemination of accurate information about OCD and CBT to parents, school personnel, and healthcare professionals, and in-depth training opportunities for clinicians.

References

Achenbach T, Edelbrock C (1991). *Manual for the Child Behavior Checklist and Revised Child Behavior Profile.* Burlington, VT: University of Vermont.

Adams GB, Waas GA, March JS, Smith MC (1994). Obsessive compulsive disorder in children and adolescents: the role of the school psychologist in identification, assessment, and treatment. *Sch Psychol Q* **9**: 274–294.

Albano A, March J, Piacentini J (1999). Cognitive behavioral treatment of obsessive-compulsive disorder. In Ammerman R, Hersen M, Last C (eds.) *Handbook of Prescriptive Treatments for Children and Adolescents* (pp. 193–215). Boston, MA: Allyn & Bacon.

American Psychiatric Association (1994). *Diagnostic and Statistical Manual of Mental Disorders*, 4th edn. Washington, DC: American Psychiatric Press.

Barrett P, Healy-Farrell L, March J (2004). Cognitive-behavioral family treatment of childhood obsessive-compulsive disorder: a controlled trial. *J Am Acad Child Adolesc Psychiatry* **43**: 46–62.

Berg CZ, Whitaker A, Davies M, Flament MF, Rapoport JL (1988). The survey form of the Leyton Obsessional Inventory-Child Version: norms from an epidemiological study. *J Am Acad Child Adolesc Psychiatry* **27**: 759–763.

Bolton D, Collins S, Steinberg D (1983). Treatment of obsessive-compulsive disorder in adolescence: a report of fifteen cases. *Br J Psychiatry* **142**: 456–464.

Bolton D, Luckie M, Steinberg D (1995). Long-term course of obsessive-compulsive disorder treated in adolescence. *J Am Acad Child Adolesc Psychiatry* **34**: 1441–1450.

Foa E, Kozak M (1985). Treatment of anxiety disorders: implications for psychopathology. In Tuma AH, Maser J (eds.) *Anxiety and the Anxiety Disorders* (pp. 421–461). Hillsdale, NJ: Erlbaum.

Franklin M, Kozak M, Cashman L, *et al.* (1998). Cognitive-behavioral treatment of pediatric obsessive-compulsive disorder: an open clinical trial. *J Am Acad Child Adolesc Psychiatry* **37**: 412–419.

Hanna G (1995). Demographic and clinical features of obsessive-compulsive disorder in children and adolescents. *J Am Acad Child Adolesc Psychiatry* **34**: 19–27.

Huppert JD, Franklin ME (2005). Cognitive-behavioral therapy for obsessive-compulsive disorder: an update. *Curr Psychiatr Rep* **7**: 268–273.

Leonard HL, Swedo S, Lenane M, *et al.* (1993). A two- to seven-year follow-up study of 54 obsessive compulsive children and adolescents. *Arch Gen Psychiatry* **50**: 429–439.

March J, Mulle K, Herbel B (1994). Behavioral psychotherapy for children and adolescents with obsessive-compulsive disorder: an open trial of a new protocol-driven package. *J Am Acad Child Adolesc Psychiatry* **33**: 333–341.

March J, Frances A, Kahn D, Carpenter D (1997a). Expert consensus guidelines: treatment of obsessive-compulsive disorder. *J Clin Psychiatry* **58**: 1–72.

March J, Parker J, Sullivan K, Stallings P, Conners K (1997b). The Multidimensional Anxiety Scale for Children (MASC). *J Am Acad Child Adolesc Psychiatry* **36**: 554–565.

Obsessive Compulsive Cognitions Working Group (1997). Cognitive assessment of obsessive-compulsive disorder. *Behav Res Ther* **35**: 667–681.

Pediatric OCD Treatment Study Team (2004). Cognitive-behavioral therapy, sertraline, and their combination for children and adolescents with obsessive-compulsive disorder: the Pediatric Obsessive-Compulsive Disorder Treatment Study Randomized Controlled Trial. *JAMA* **292**: 1969–1976.

Piacentini J, Bergman RL (2000). Obsessive-compulsive disorder in children. *Psychiatr Clin N Am* **23**: 519–533.

Piacentini J, Gitow A, Jaffer M, Graae F, Whitaker A (1994). Outpatient behavioral treatment of child and adolescent obsessive-compulsive disorder. *J Anxiety Disord* **8**: 277–289.

Piacentini J, Jaffer M, Bergman RL, McCracken J, Keller M (2001). Measuring impairment in childhood OCD: Psychometric properties of the COIS. *Sci Proc Am Acad Child Adolesc Psychiatry* **48**: 146.

Pinto A, Francis G (1993). Obsessive-compulsive disorder in children. In Hersen M, Ammerman RT (eds.) *Handbook of Behavioral Therapy with Children and*

Adults: A Longitudinal Perspective (pp. 155–165). New York: Allyn & Bacon.

Rapoport J, Inoff-Germain G, Weissman M, *et al.* (2000). Childhood obsessive-compulsive disorder in the NIMH MECA study. Parent vs. child identification of cases. *J Anxiety Disord* **14**: 535–548.

Riddle M (1998). Obsessive-compulsive disorder in children and adolescents. *Br J Psychiatry* **173**: 91–96.

Scahill L, Riddle M, McSwiggin-Hardin M, *et al.* (1997). Children's Yale–Brown Obsessive Compulsive Scale: reliability and validity. *J Am Acad Child Adolesc Psychiatry* **36**: 844–852.

Swedo S, Rapoport JL, Leonard H, Lenane M, Cheslow D (1989). Obsessive-compulsive disorder in children and adolescents: clinical phenomenology of 70 consecutive cases. *Arch Gen Psychiatry* **46**: 335–341.

Wagner AP (2002). *What to do When Your Child has Obsessive-Compulsive Disorder: Strategies and Solutions.* Rochester, NY: Lighthouse Press.

Wagner AP (2003). Cognitive-behavioral therapy for children and adolescents with obsessive-compulsive disorder. *Brief Treat Crisis Interv* **3**: 291–306.

Wagner AP (2004). *Up and Down the Worry Hill: A Children's Book about Obsessive-Compulsive Disorder and its Treatment*, 2nd edn. Rochester, NY: Lighthouse Press.

Wagner AP (2007). *Treatment of OCD in Children and Adolescents: A Professional's Kit*, 2nd edn. Rochester, NY: Lighthouse Press.

Waters T, Barrett P (2000). The role of the family in childhood obsessive-compulsive disorder. *Clin Child Fam Psychol Rev*: 173–184.

Waters T, Barrett P, March JS (2001). Cognitive-behavioral family treatment of childhood obsessive-compulsive disorder. *Am J Psychother* **55**: 372–387.

Zohar A (1999). The epidemiology of obsessive compulsive disorder in children and adolescents. *Psychiatr Clin N Am* **8**: 445–460.

Community support and societal influences

Elaine Davis

Introduction

Mental disorders around the globe are associated with poverty, marginalization, and social disadvantage (Lancet Global Mental Health Group 2007). Improving the quality of life for people dealing with mental health issues cannot be accomplished solely within the professional mental health community. While professional treatment opportunities for people struggling with mental health issues are critical interventions to enhance the well-being of this population, engagement of a range of individuals throughout society from various backgrounds is crucial to overcoming stigma and working towards high quality of life.

Community volunteers, consisting of people struggling with mental health disorders as well as their family members, friends, employers, religious communities, and social networks have the potential to provide valuable resources to promote the well-being of individuals affected by mental health issues as well as the well-being of society as a whole. These enlightened people can provide a variety of supplemental support within both the social and economic spheres to complement formal mental healthcare. It is clear that developing strategies to improve the outcome of mental health intervention outside of the professional healthcare sector is necessary. Support can be offered on a variety of levels.

Individuals with obsessive-compulsive disorder (OCD) often have difficulty making friends because of the fear of others discovering their symptoms (Gallup Organization 1993) and can feel misunderstood by family, friends, and even their physicians (Black and Blum 1992). In addition to these emotional considerations, there is a substantial health cost; the social and economic costs associated with OCD were estimated at approximately $8.4 billion in 1990

(DuPont 1995). Clearly, the well-being of these individuals is closely tied to the community in which they live and interact. Support is critical for their mental, physical, emotional, and financial well-being. Without knowledge of the societal influences on their disorder and empowerment to overcome these challenges, individuals with OCD are unlikely to perform at their full potential. This is a loss not only to the individual and their family but also to the population as a whole.

This chapter outlines some of the major community and societal influences on the mental health community as a whole and the OCD community in particular. It is by no means inclusive. While the chapter begins with subjects that are tangible resources for this sector, it then considers areas of society that are not directly targeted to people with mental illness.

Support groups

Support groups are probably the most tangible means of community involvement in the OCD population. Support groups have long offered companionship and information for people coping with diseases or disabilities. Encouraging the individual to share their fears, struggles, and accomplishments in a safe environment among others who truly understand the obstacles being faced complements the treatment process. Tips on dealing with all aspects of life are shared by people who have put them to the test. Individuals become empowered to help themselves and can extend their own experience to help others when they feel a part of something larger. Quite often, people with OCD feel extremely isolated because of the secretive nature of their disorders, and they believe that they have never met another person suffering with their condition. Support groups address this isolation. They may also impact on individuals'

Clinical Obsessive-Compulsive Disorders in Adults and Children, ed. Robert Hudak and Darin D. Dougherty.
Published by Cambridge University Press. Copyright © Cambridge University Press 2011.

underlying illness representations. An illness representation is a person's understanding of, usually, their own illness, which has in many cases been shown to have a major impact on self management (Cameron and Leventhal 2003).

Whether the group is designed to accommodate people with general anxiety disorders, OCD or a specific target population within the OCD spectrum, support groups offer an invaluable service. Support groups have been organized to address a wide variety of specific topics, for example body dismorphic disorder, trichotillomania, body-focused repetitive behaviors, and hoarding. Groups may also form to target a defined population, such as children, teens, college/graduate students, males, females, homosexuals, professionals, athletes, and so on. Groups are also available for parents, spouses, siblings, offspring and other support people. Even these groups may be segregated by the age of the relative or friend who has OCD, for example parents of young children versus parents of adult children, or by the specific area of concern for their loved one, for example children of hoarders. These divisions into more specialized topics can facilitate in the cohesiveness of the groups as they share more traits in common. These groups may be available in a face to face setting but many people are also turning to online support groups

There are several different formats for support groups for people suffering from OCD. Some groups are professionally assisted and therapeutic in nature. These highly structured support groups often serve as a bridge between the therapist's office and the more traditional support group setting. Other support groups are less structured and serve as an informative, supportive, informal empathetic environment for people coping with OCD. They are often led and organized by people who suffer from OCD. While the less-formal mutual support group is still very prevalent, other more highly defined and goal-oriented support groups organized by lay people are emerging to help to augment OCD therapy. Obsessive Compulsive Anonymous (OCA) and Clutterers Anonymous (CLA) groups follow a 12- step program. The GOAL groups ("Giving Obsessive-Compulsives Another Lifestyle") help individuals to target specific aspects of their illness with defined tasks to complete between meetings.

For many, support groups are therapeutic. However, with the exception of professionally assisted support groups, these sessions are not intended to be a substitute for professional therapy. Seeking the help of a qualified mental healthcare professional for individuals suffering from OCD should be a major step in managing this disorder. Support groups are designed to augment and extend this more formal therapeutic environment. Support groups do, however, often provide a motivation for individuals to seek treatment.

Determining the right type of support group for a particular individual will involve many factors. A few universally helpful aspects are groups that are caring, compassionate, active, vibrant, and offer a true sense of community (Grohol 2004). Groups where support and opinions are offered in a respectful, considerate manner have been shown to be of a greater benefit to the members. Disagreements should be handled in a courteous manner and little time should be afforded to "pity parties." Groups that have a steady, active community and group leaders or moderators who take an active role in helping the community are generally more successful. New members should be welcomed and informed of the guidelines for membership. Groups that retain membership for long periods tend to foster a tight community in which the members learn about and care for the other members. No group is likely to meet all of an individual's needs nor will any one group display every beneficial aspect. Remember that younger groups may not have had the chance to develop a sense of community or may not seem to be as active as others. If the potential is evident, it may be worth continuing attendance. More established groups may at first seem daunting to new members until they begin to form relationships within the group.

The goals of the individual may also influence the type of group they seek. The following sections are designed to offer a brief synopsis of several types of support groups offered in the OCD community.

Professionally assisted support groups

Professionally operated support groups are facilitated by professionals who do not share the problem of the members. These group leaders may include social workers, psychologists, or members of the clergy. The facilitator controls discussions and provides other managerial service. This kind of group is generally organized as a group therapy setting to extend the individual treatment sessions. The therapist directs the group discussions and activities. Members often pay a fee per session, which may or may not be underwritten by insurers. Such professionally operated groups are often found in institutional settings, including hospitals, drug-treatment centers, therapist offices, and correctional facilities. Often, this type of support group may run for a specified period of time.

Therapist-led groups, like others, provide a safe and supportive environment for people to actively address their symptoms with others who are also working to overcome similar issues. Facilitation by a trained mental health professional keeps the group on track and provides access to evidence-based treatment strategies. Individuals who are addressing specific symptoms that have been particularly problematic often thrive in these sessions. The group environment encourages members to attempt more productive coping strategies. Often these strategies are difficult for an individual to tackle on their own but the support of others who know just how difficult it is to face these particular challenges can help to reduce the anxiety to a level where it no longer serves as a barrier. The encouragement of the other group members along with the guidance of the therapist leader allows the individual to achieve a greater therapeutic benefit.

Peer-led support groups

Peer-led or mutual support groups are defined as groups of people sharing a similar problem who meet regularly to provide emotional support. As they apply to OCD, these groups are typically facilitated by an individual or individuals suffering from OCD, although many are assisted, most often in the founding years, by professionals donating their time. Usually, the facilitators are individuals who have largely learned to manage their OCD symptoms. In these meetings, participants may discuss specific topics, such as medication, symptoms, cognitive-behavior therapy, relevant websites, and so on. The goal of these support groups is informational, not therapeutic. However, they allow for the sharing of practical knowledge that mental health professionals can overlook. These groups capitalize on the potential benefits of socially supportive interactions. These groups can serve to fill in for the deficiencies in more natural support systems of family and friends, who do not have the experiential knowledge of the disorder.

Guest speakers may be invited to talk about a specific topic of interest to the group. Often these speakers are professional mental healthcare providers, legal experts in the field of disability benefits, or other professionals who deal with issues concerning mental health. Mutual support groups usually are held in informal settings such as a local school, library, or church. There is usually no fee for mutual support groups unless there is a fee for the room or other incidental expenses. A mutual help support group is fully organized and managed by its members, usually volunteers. These groups are also referred to as fellowships, peer support groups, mutual help groups, mutual aid self-help groups, or just self-help groups.

The majority of these groups are loosely organized so as to change as needed given different issues facing the group. They are the mainstay of peer self-help network. These groups allow individuals with OCD to gain a sense of community; often this setting is the first opportunity for these people to truly believe that they are not alone in their struggles.

Twelve step groups

Two types of group, which are more structured member-led groups, are based on the 12-step program originally developed at Alcoholics Anonymous. These groups include OCA and CLA.

There is a network of OCA groups throughout the USA and groups are now emerging worldwide. The OCA describes itself as a fellowship of people who share their experience, strength, and hope with each other so that they may solve their common problem and help others to recover from OCD. The only requirement for membership is a desire to recover from OCD. There are no dues or fees. The OCA is not allied with any sect, denomination, political group, organization or institution; it does not wish to engage in any controversy, neither endorsing nor opposing any causes. The primary purpose is to recover from OCD and to help others facing similar struggles. The members remain anonymous at the public level to allow the sharing of personal stories, knowing that they will remain in the confidence of those who attend the meetings. The philosophy maintains that following this program with the support of the other members of the group present at the meetings can reduce or eliminate the cycle of obsessions and compulsions that are difficult to overcome when faced alone.

Generally the group begins with a formal presentation or reading from the OCA manual given by the group leader. Limited time is allowed to each member to share their story or current struggles within the format of a rotating topic. No pressure is exerted on individuals to share during this part of the session. Discussions are encouraged to focus more on the tools of recovery that can ultimately bring relief from OCD. While sharing feelings of pain and frustration are part of the process, talking directly from the obsession is considered counter-productive. Socializing and networking following the end of the formal meeting time is encouraged to build personal connections to others in the group. This fellowship leads to continued contact between meetings and "sponsorship" of newer members by those who have advanced on their road to recovery and are committed to the principles of the group. Members are encouraged to write about their personal issues, resentments, fears, and so on, rather than acting them out in unhealthy, compulsive ways. Prayer and/or meditation are also encouraged in this recovery program.

The CLA system is similar but focuses more specifically on people dealing with hoarding issues. This fellowship is likewise based on suggestion, interchange of experience, rotation of leadership, and service. As with the OCA, the CLA does not collect dues and is not affiliated with any public or private organization, political movement, ideology, or religious doctrine; it takes no position on outside issues. This organization lists meetings around the world and also supports a phone-in group. Additional information about the specific structures of the groups and contact information is given at the end of this chapter.

The GOAL groups

The GOAL groups somewhat merge the concept of consumer-led and therapist-assisted groups. The original group was started by a psychologist and an OCD sufferer in 1981. This individual saw the advantage of continuing to have sufferers work on exposure and response prevention (ERP) therapy in a group to prevent relapse following discharge from formal therapy. A therapist is present at every GOAL group meeting; however, their function is to provide technical information and they usually do not facilitate the group. The group is most often led by an individual who suffers from OCD.

The GOAL group meetings are divided into three distinct parts: discussion of a previously agreed-upon OCD-related topic, participation in small groups to devise behavioral goals, and informal socializing. Its atmosphere is one of compassion, not commiseration, and its manner is one of inspiration and encouragement, not coercion.

The full group participates in a discussion of some OCD-related topic that is selected by the group leader or is the consensus of the group at a prior meeting. Each member present will be given an opportunity to share feelings and thoughts on this topic or may elect not to speak if he or she so wishes. This part of the session allows for cohesion of the group. It also serves as an introduction for new members to become more familiar with the group prior to initiating the more structured portion of the session.

Following the more formal discussion, the group then breaks down into more symptom- or experience-focused groups. Led by a recovering obsessive–compulsive, each small group will help each of its members formulate a specific and concrete goal to accomplish in the interval before the next support-group meeting. This extension of the individual's ERP therapy should advance the member in the attempt to recover his or her life from obsessive-compulsive behavior. While encouraged to perform these assignments, each individual is allowed the freedom to accept or decline the task.

Socializing at the end of the sessions allows everyone to come back together as a larger group. Camaraderie among the group is facilitated in this manner. Also, after a session of confronting one's anxiety, this time allows for a period of "decompression" from the hard work to be faced. Members have the opportunity to come to know one another on a more personal basis, seeing them as more than their disorder – as a person as a whole. As with the other support groups discussed above, relationships are formed during this portion of the group, often facilitating a means of support between meetings.

These groups occasionally provide a format to allow a presentation from a professional guest speaker. The members then participate in a question-and-answer session. These interludes from the normal structure of the group serve to educate the members on issues of concern to the OCD community. Often these presentations allow the group to devise novel topics of discussion to be used in the first portion of future meetings, which may not have been considered without this influx of information. These sessions tend to move directly to socializing with refreshments without breaking out into small groups. The presenter is encouraged to stay for this informal gathering to allow members who did not feel comfortable asking questions in a group session to interact with the professional.

Online support groups

Since at least the early 1980s, the Internet has provided a venue for support groups. These groups are particularly helpful in offering support to people in remote geographical areas. Groups can be designed to allow individuals to exchange messages in real time or facilitate the exchange between members who may connect to a network at a convenient time in their life to leave messages for others to read at their leisure. Chat rooms, e-mail, usenet, internet bulletin boards, and FaceBook pages have become popular methods of communication for peer-to-peer self-help groups and among facilitated support groups.

Online support groups offer anonymity that is not possible in face to face settings, which may allow for the discussion of difficult or embarrassing issues (Eysenbach 2003). This type of forum also allows members to speak in an environment free from some inhibiting social constraints, allowing people to free themselves to speak more openly. This online disinhibition can result in people being more confident and outgoing but may in certain instances result in more aggressive traits being displayed as well. Care needs to be exerted by the group facilitator to ensure that deliberately provocative or insulting posts, known as flaming, by members of the group towards the more fragile individuals is not allowed to occur or persist.

This forum presents a unique advantage in how people manage the exchange of information. Swapping addresses and discussing helpful websites is facilitated by the easy access to these sites to all the members. There is often no need to attempt to remember a specific piece of information, such as a treatment provider's contact number, provided during a discussion. No pen or paper need be found, the information is at the person's disposal. Likewise, many of these forums provide for an archive of past discussions to allow for members to search for needed information when it becomes relevant to their situation.

While most online support groups offer many of the same advantages of the traditional face to face groups, they may risk isolating individuals who would most benefit from a more rounded social interaction. As often the mere act of leaving the home environment is crucial to the recovery of some individuals, online support groups may allow these people to continue to isolate themselves in what they consider a safe environment. Online groups do offer a form of social interaction and many close relationships are often formed with participation over time; however, the absence of physical contact does limit the extent of the benefits of such relationships.

Advantages and disadvantages of support groups

Evidence for the efficacy of mutual help groups has been extensively reported in the medical literature, although some discrepancies are noted in the outcome measure for improvement. When reviewing studies that employed criteria used by professionals to measure "psychiatric outcomes" such as reduction of symptoms, hospitalizations or need for medication, Pistrang *et al.* (2008) reported that 7 of 12 studies indicated a benefit for members of mutual support groups over individuals who did not participate in such interventions. They further report that in the five studies that did not show a clear benefit for support group members, no negative effects were observed. Other studies that have focused on the type of life changes which are less empirically measured, such as terms of identity, spiritual development, sense of being cared for, or social well-being, are more likely to indicate a benefit for participants (Humphreys 2000; Davidson 2003). While the differences in structure and outcome of mutual support groups, which set them apart from professional interventions, are quite valuable and should not be overlooked, it is difficult to measure the benefits realized in these settings. However, in attempting to more clearly define the parameters for measuring outcome, often the dynamic of the group is inevitably altered, thereby distorting the initial aim of the study.

Both the facilitators and the members of support groups need to guard against their resource being misused by people intent on deceiving others. Some individuals only pretend to suffer from OCD and can often divert the attention of the group off their intended dialogue by relating struggles with their feigned symptoms or try to glean sympathy with additional made-up diagnoses (Feldman 2000). Others may be seeking to find information to be used against members of the group or other individuals with OCD. While most online sites work hard to remain secure, the programs designed to keep information private are constantly under attack. Discovering that a group has been infiltrated can be devastating. Confrontation is probably the most reliable way of ferreting out these nefarious individuals. While both face to face and internet groups are vulnerable to these extremely infrequent problems, online groups currently report more issues with this type of behavior. Perhaps the most important lesson is that all members must carefully balance empathy with circumspection.

Each person should do their best to educate themselves prior to implementing the offered advice of other group members. Individuals must be careful to fully weigh the possible detrimental outcomes of basing their healthcare decisions on information obtained from the group that is not seeded in evidence-based medicine. Even non-treatment-related advice should be carefully implemented to guard against passing along detrimental coping strategies.

Starting a support group

Therapist-led support groups are generally formed by the professional who will lead the group. Occasionally an institution will wish to provide these services and will essentially hire an appropriate mental health provider to facilitate the group. This does not mean that the people who would most benefit from the formation of such a group cannot persuade a therapist to provide their services to such an endeavor. This may involve contacting many OCD therapists to find one or more willing to devote their time to this project.

If the desire is to form a group under the OCA, CLA or GOAL format, guidance can be obtained as to the particulars of running these types of group. Websites are available to provide guidance and the International OCD Foundation has provided materials in the past to anyone wishing to start a GOAL group. The following discussion applies to general suggestions of how to begin the path to bring a support group to life. Most of these suggestions apply to the formation of any self-help group. Some tips may not be relevant for the various specialized groups.

Forming a support group takes motivation, common sense, and determination. While enthusiasm is a powerful tool, it is important to proceed with a well thought out plan for the group. Begin by ensuring that a group does not already exist in the area which fills this need. Contact local mental health advocacy groups. These groups often have listings of active support groups in the area and can offer practical advice for start-up information. They will also be useful in helping to advertise the group once it is running. Often it is helpful to attend other self-help groups as a guest to get a sense of what aspects of the group work well

and may be incorporated into the formation of the new group.

Determine a group of people who share the goal of starting a new group. There will be enough work to go around. This group can help to define the early goals and structure of the group. Often people engage the help of a mental health professional in the initial organization of the group. This can offer a level of expertise and impartiality that can aid the smooth start up of a group, but the role of this therapist should be clearly defined to all involved. While the group's focus may evolve over time, keeping the goals simple at first will facilitate a learning curve for the group leaders. Decide which part of the OCD community the group is hoping to target.

Explore possible venues for the group meetings. Many community buildings have space available for these groups. Schools and libraries are likely sources of a meeting room. Churches are also popular choices but consideration should be given to people who may not be comfortable meeting in a house of worship. Hospitals and clinics are additional sources of meeting space. Access to parking and/or public transportation is helpful. Ensure that all financial requirements are discussed up front including any possible requirement to show proof of insurance. If free accommodation cannot be found, a source of funding needs to be determined. This may require that a fee be charged to attend the group, partnering with an advocacy group, or finding private funding.

Decide how often the group will meet and set an inaugural meeting date, allowing for sufficient time to advertise the group. If there is flexibility in the room availability and with the personal schedules of the planning committee, the initial meeting can be used to determine if the proposed meeting time is optimal. Plan for a more structured meeting for this date but do not try to incorporate too many activities. The bulk of the meeting will most likely be devoted to discussion of the organization of the group. The goal is to make the members feel welcome and invested in the group, and to give a clear sense of purpose. Go in with an open mind, the group dynamic may alter the intended structure of the group but also keep a grasp on the initial goals set forth. Make sure that the work will be kept within reasonable means.

Once the groundwork is laid, it is time to get the word out. Contact as many mental health professionals in the area as possible. Provide them with a simple, uncluttered flyer that introduces the group that they can distribute to their patients who may wish to attend. Hopefully you can encourage them to also pass the flyer on to their colleagues to do the same. The flyers should clearly state the name of the group, the extent of the support offered, meeting location, starting and ending times as well as contact information. Post these notices in areas where you are most likely to target the intended audience. Enlist the help of mental health advocacy groups in your area to help to spread the word. Investigate the possibility of advertising via the Internet through e-mail blasts and notices on appropriate websites. Explore avenues to public service announcements, free advertisements in local papers, and notify appropriate government agencies of your existence. Make sure that contact information is provided and adequately monitored to ensure that people who are timid about joining can speak to someone prior to attending.

Once the group has had its initial meeting there are a few tips to ensure that it thrives. Begin the meetings on time. Welcome everyone and allow members to introduce themselves if desired while keeping in mind that some members may be reluctant to disclose a great deal of personal information at first. Emphasize confidentiality and how it applies to your group. Remind everyone that pictures should not be taken without receiving the permission of everyone prior to snapping the shot. Describe the group's purpose, guidelines, and rules of order especially when welcoming new members. Review the agenda if you have one prepared. It is often good practice to note the ending time making sure that everyone understands that they may leave early if they need to do so. Plan appropriate activities if desired, which may include inviting speakers, engaging in planned discussions, or holding social activities. Attempt to deal with practical matters such as announcements or group business quickly. End the meeting with a few short positive remarks to leave people with a sense of accomplishment and a desire to return.

Establish a set of rules to ensure appropriate behavior and hold everyone accountable to the rules. While you do not want to become punitive, an environment where everyone is striving to improve themselves and offer support to others will only be enhanced by keeping the meetings orderly and fostering trust. Remember a support group is not unconditional. It is based on a person's willingness to change. Consider having "active listening" training sessions to help members to improve their verbal and non-verbal communication skills. Learn to redirect from predominately negative discussions by directing the members to list common and unusual methods to combat OCD. Re-evaluate the group periodically to ensure that the meetings are still serving the members needs.

The rewards of helping implement and sustain a mutual self-help group can far outweigh the duties involved. But keep in mind that one goal of the group is to allow a sense of empowerment to all the members. Ask members if there is anything that could make the group an even more rewarding experience and follow up on suggestions and comments. Engage members of the group by asking for volunteers to help to plan and facilitate meetings on topics of personal importance. Group members need to be convinced that the group is meeting a need for them. Once they "buy in," this will help to ensure the longevity of the group as well as give members an opportunity to use their talents and gifts for the good of the group. Reward members who abide by the rules and actively participate over time by asking them to mentor new group members. Always showcase the good examples. As rewarding as it may be to foster and facilitate a group yourself, watching members grow into this position can be doubly rewarding.

Family to family education program

Family members of mentally ill patients are called upon to provide considerable care regarding the illness, treatment, and the sequelae of their loved one's illness. This expectation has grown through increasing deinstitutionalization, mandates of least restrictive care, and changing commitment laws. Little or no resources are afforded to these individuals by the mental health establishment to face these significant challenges and the privacy mandates enforced by the US Health Insurance Portability and Accountability Act and comparable legislation in other countries often shut out the people who are in fact being asked to shoulder this increasing burden of care.

The family to family education program is a structured, peer-led 12 week self-help class designed to aid the family members of people with serious mental illness. Designed by a psychologist and family member, it seeks to address unmet family needs (Burland 1995). This widely available program is firmly rooted in the community and aims to provide both information and support. The curriculum focuses on both coping with stress and trauma recovery and is based on a belief that families follow a predictable path through three stages of emotional responses: dealing with catastrophic events, learning to cope, and finally moving towards advocacy. Graduates of this program report a sense of increased empowerment and reduced subjective burden (Dixon *et al.* 2004). Participants are provided with an understanding of mental illness, the mental healthcare system, and self-care. The curriculum is also intended to normalize reactions such as shock, disorientation, and grief resulting from the traumatic diagnosis of their loved one.

Tools are introduced over the period of the program to help participants to implement new ideas that aim to improve their life situation. These skills reduce the anxiety, despair, anger, and guilt often displayed by family members as they try to negotiate their new life path. Fear of the next hurdle they will encounter can be reduced as they feel that they possess the ability to face these challenges. Participants learn that their attempts to control this illness and the actions of the affected person are counter-productive for both parties. Change can ensue in how they treat themselves, their ill relative, other members of the family, and the community at large.

Participants also gain an understanding and empathy about living with a mental illness from first-person experiences, allowing them to gain a level of tolerance of the nature of their loved one's illness. Combining this knowledge with the tools offered by this program often improves communication between family members and consumers (Lucksted *et al.* 2008). Sometimes, however, negative emotions are provoked by attendance in this class. Knowledge gained pertaining to the mental health system can lead to doubts about the correct diagnosis and treatment protocols of their loved ones. Frustration about the plight of individuals struggling with mental health and the stigma involved in this diagnosis can be intensified during this curriculum. Increasing the understanding of the nature of their relative's suffering can also lead to a sense of despair over the futility of trying to relieve the pain experienced by these individuals (Lucksted *et al.* 2008).

This course allows people to realize they are not alone in their situation and allows them to share experiences with other people who truly understand the demands placed upon them. These copyrighted classes are currently sponsored by the National Alliance on Mental Illness (NAMI). This group provides the training for the peer leaders and facilitates running the groups in areas across the USA. Class schedules can

be obtained from the website of this organization or by contacting a local NAMI chapter.

It is important to note that the curriculum for this course is broad based when it focuses on explaining mental illnesses. The material devoted to OCD is minimal and some techniques taught may be inappropriate for this disorder. It is recommended that people with a family member diagnosed with OCD attending the class look to other sources for information to understand the nature of this particular diagnosis while reaping the myriad of beneficial general information offered by this course.

Charitable and advocacy organizations

Charitable and advocacy groups offer an organized community effort to support and raise awareness of a variety of specific health issues. These groups range in structure from all volunteer grassroots associations to highly structured, professionally run organizations that employ staff to facilitate their efforts. The majority of these groups are not-for-profit organizations operating within governmental guidelines of the country of origin.

Many consumer-run mental health organizations emerged in the 1970s. These early groups tended either to emphasize personal empowerment and recovery (Weitz 1984) or to focus on advocacy by engaging in political action to protect patients' rights (Chamberlin 1978). Both types were working to promote the well-being of mental health patients, the former often working with mental health professionals to provide informal support while the latter were often created in reaction to the adverse conditions of mental health institutions common at that time. Today, most organizations at least loosely work in concert with today's far more enlightened mental health professional community to complement efforts providing a better quality of life for mental health consumers. Support services range from peer support to drop-in programs. Advocacy groups have now shifted their focus from battling inhumane hospital conditions to helping to secure housing, employment, education, awareness, and access to effective treatment. Regardless of the path chosen by these organizations, all have realized a role in mental health reform by influencing values in the lives of the targeted populations (Nelson *et al.* 2008). The availability of resources to conduct any of the activities often determines the scope of programs offered by these groups. Social influences such as community interest, transient populations, and reluctance of individuals to "go public" also shape the focus of a given group. Despite financial and human resource limitations, these charitable and advocacy groups are, for the most part, quite adept at maximizing their activities to enhance the outcomes for their target audience.

The overall organization of the group often has a great influence on the longevity of the group and the length of individual membership. Paid staff allow for a stable environment as well as enhancing the work output for the group. These groups are poised to serve a larger community, achieve a more widespread dissemination of services and awareness, and serve the needs of individuals who are in a stage of their illness that requires a higher level of guidance to attain the services required to realize a more stable level of mental health. On the one hand, foundations with professional staff are also more likely to weather the periods of upheaval that all these groups tend to experience. On the other hand, groups which encourage the consumers themselves to take active roles in running the organization foster a sense of "ownership" of the group as well as enhancing an environment of empowerment. Individuals taking leadership roles in these groups often realize a positive, psychological well-being as giving help to others is often more strongly associated with this outcome than simply receiving help (Roberts *et al.* 1999). As they feel a greater sense of belonging, these individuals tend to continue involvement in the group long after the initial issues for which they sought help have been resolved.

A variety of not-for-profit profit groups are available to the OCD community. Some of these organizations focus solely on OCD while others address issues of a variety of mental disorders including OCD. A common thread of the OCD-focused groups is to guide individuals in their journey to find a qualified OCD treatment provider and/or support group services. These groups also serve as a resource for general information about OCD, some providing more extensive information than others. Most of these groups were formed by OCD sufferers who were frustrated with the status quo when they began their own journey to recovery. All show an incredible dedication to helping the OCD community and desire to increase understanding of the true nature of this disorder.

The International OCD Foundation

The International OCD Foundation (IOCDF), formerly the Obsessive Compulsive Foundation, is an organization with a mission to raise awareness among policy makers and the general public about OCD, educate the mental health community about the latest treatments and research, connect people suffering from OCD with treatment providers, and advance research opportunities for more effective treatments. The organization began in 1986 as a group of 12 people with OCD and grew from a small grassroots effort to a national foundation with affiliated local groups in multiple US states who serve to promote the mission on a local level. The IOCDF is based in the USA with the majority of its resources currently devoted to promoting its mission within its home country. Membership has expanded beyond the USA and efforts are being made to expand the informational resources to include treatment providers and support services in other countries where current OCD organizations do not exist.

The IOCDF serves as a resource of general information about OCD and related disorders and treatment options via the website as well as through articles, pamphlets, books, and video tapes. Members receive a quarterly newsletter providing information about the latest advances in treatment and research as well as inspirational stories from individuals and their families struggling with OCD. The IOCDF maintains a list of psychiatrists, psychologists, social workers, nurses, and mental health counselors who have indicated an interest in treating OCD and related disorders as well as maintaining lists of support groups and other support services. These databases are available free of charge online and dedicated staff members also dispense this information when people call into the office seeking more personal guidance.

To further its goal to educate the public and professional sectors, the organization sponsors a three day annual conference. This event is attended by individuals with OCD and their families and friends, as well as by mental health treatment providers and academics involved in research into issues involving OCD and related disorders. Early in its tenure, the IOCDF recognized a need to expand the pool of clinicians able to offer effective behavioral therapy to people struggling with OCD and related disorders. The Behavior Therapy Institute was formed to address this issue. Experts in the field of cognitive-behavior therapy and its application specifically to OCD lead a three-day intensive course for practicing mental health professionals. Classes are kept small to maximize student–teacher interaction and follow-up supervision is available via phone consultations with an assigned "advisor."

The IOCDF is also emerging as a major source of funding for promising young researchers dedicated to advancing the knowledge into the causes and treatment of OCD and related disorders. Fostering a sense of international cooperation, the IOCDF initiated a collaboration of established research groups working on identifying genetic components of OCD. This network of centers dedicated to genetic studies has been able to pool genetic samples and data, which has benefited all involved and advanced the field beyond that possible with individual efforts alone.

The OCD Centre Manitoba

The OCD Centre Manitoba is a not-for-profit organization that provides support, education, and information to members, family, friends, and professionals, and promotes psychosocial research into OCD. With a permanent office and two part-time staff, this group is able to provide confidential consultations for people new to a diagnosis of OCD and can help to make referrals both within the provincial medical system as well as to private therapists. A library service is also provided for all members of the centre.

This organization provides support groups, peer counseling, information, and education. They also work to support and promote research as well as coordinating communication between healthcare professionals, community services, and those affected by OCD.

Ontario Obsessive Compulsive Disorder Network

The Ontario Obsessive Compulsive Disorder Network is a not-for-profit organization focusing on self-help groups; it provides a web-based directory of clinical services and community resources, responds to inquiries, and offers support and referrals via email and telephone. Listings are provided for various regions within of the province. This group hopes to expand their efforts in the near future to help to raise the awareness of OCD and the people it touches.

OCD Ireland

OCD Ireland is an organization that began in 2002. The organization was founded by sufferers, family members, and interested mental health professionals who were concerned with the limited resources available in Ireland for people with OCD, body dysmorphic disorder, and trichotillomania, as well as the general lack of awareness about these disorders. OCD Ireland decided that its goal would be to provide support to people who have any of these three disorders as well as to provide assistance for their family members, friends, and caretakers. OCD Ireland makes it clear that their group provides support, not treatment. They encourage all members to seek out and engage in an effective OCD treatment protocol.

The organization provides two main services: free informational talks and support groups. The nine seminars each year are provided by a leading specialist in each area. OCD Ireland offers general support groups for OCD, body dysmorphic disorder, and trichotillomania, as well as a family support group. OCD Ireland advocates attending the mindfulness training seminars listed on their website. Mindfulness, a relaxation technique, can help people with OCD to learn to observe their thoughts without allowing the anxiety to rise or engaging in a ritual.

OCD-UK

OCD-UK is a national charity, independently working with and for people with OCD. The objective of this organization is to make a positive and meaningful difference in the everyday lives of people affected by OCD by providing accessible and effective support services and by campaigning for improved access and quality treatment and care for people with OCD to ensure that every person affected by OCD receives the quality of treatment and care that they deserve. OCD-UK facilitates a safe environment for people affected by OCD to communicate with each other and provide mutual understanding and support.

OCD-UK was founded in November 2003 by two OCD sufferers. Both felt that OCD was still not widely recognized and that a more proactive approach was needed to bring the problems faced by people suffering with OCD into the public spotlight. OCD-UK became an officially registered charity on 14th April 2004.

OCD-UK continues to work both alone and in partnership with other charities and organizations to provide information and practical and emotional support for anyone affected by OCD. This is achieved through a telephone information line, e-mail support service, facilitated support groups, and through fully moderated online discussion forums. Their advocacy service provides independent and confidential advice and practical support to people affected by OCD, which enables people to have a voice in the services that they receive, the decisions that are made about their lives, and to safeguard their rights. OCD-UK actively supports and participates in non-invasive ethically approved research projects that work towards a better understanding of the illness and treatments.

This organization also acts as an independent advocacy body for people affected by OCD. Part of that work involves working closely with individuals to help them to access treatment where the local National Health Service system has failed them. The group has begun to focus on fostering a sense of community for children struggling with OCD by organizing fun, social activities.

Website addresses for each of these groups are listed in the Resources section.

Additional groups offering help

A number of international groups dedicate themselves directly to aiding people struggling with OCD. Details of many of these can be obtained at a website that provides contact information for OCD organizations and support groups in many countries including the USA, UK, Australia, Belgium, Denmark, France, Germany, Holland, Iran, Italy, Norway, Sweden, and South Africa (see Resources at the end of this chapter). The lack of individual mention of these groups within this chapter should not be construed as any negative reflection of these groups. Communication issues prevented a full investigation of the services offered. Other groups undoubtedly exist that were not identified by the Internet searches during the research for this chapter.

Groups have also formed to focus on particular aspects of OCD and related disorders. The Tricotillomania Learning Center (TLC) is dedicated to helping people with body-focused repetitive behaviors such as hair pulling or skin picking. The TLC is committed to information dissemination, education, outreach, alliance building, and support of research into the cause and treatment of these disorders. The Children of Hoarders (COH) group is dedicated to support individuals who grew up in a hoarding environment and/or had or currently has a parent or in-law that hoards. The group shares insights and experiences amongst its members with a goal to providing tips that may be of use for their situation. There are no doctors or therapists facilitating the board; the discussions are all from family members.

Within the USA as well as in other countries, groups are available to address general mental health issues. The Anxiety Disorders Association of America is concerned with OCD and related disorders while also focusing on general anxiety disorder, panic disorder, social anxiety disorder, post-traumatic stress disorder as well as specific phobias. The NAMI works for patient rights and aims to wipe out the stigma of mental illness of all types. Other groups which help to support the mental health community include Mental Health America, the Foundation for Mental Health, Freedom From Fear, Peace of Mind Foundation, Peer Support and Advocacy Network, National Anxiety Foundation as well as many others. Internationally, the list is also extensive and readers are encouraged to seek out these organizations on their own if their country does not have a group specifically focused on OCD. While these groups may not be able to offer specific support for OCD, they can be a source of general support and a sense of community within the mental health community at large.

The school environment

Children spend a significant portion of their time in school. Teachers and other school personnel become a large factor in their lives. While the primary goal of schools is to serve as learning centers, these institutions have become key settings for preventative practices (Malti and Noam 2008). Health problems of all types are often identified first by school personnel, who bring the concern to the attention of the parents. Teachers and school service personnel see these children performing in structured activities, which can indicate a specific problem if the child is struggling to complete these tasks. Evaluating a child's achievement of developmental milestones is a key element in both education and childhood mental health intervention and, therefore, teachers have the specialized knowledge of what children should be capable of achieving at given stages of their lives. Teachers are exposed to many children throughout their career and may be more able to recognize problems they have likely observed in the past. Teachers, however, should avoid being diagnosticians. While they are trained in childhood development, they are not bone fide medical personnel. Pointing out a potential problem for further investigation, however, is well within their scope.

Families provide the core support structure for children, especially those with mental illness (Blair *et al.* 2003). However, social and economic pressures of Western society have placed restraints on the abilities of parents and guardians to provide the depth of support often necessary to deal with children suffering from emotional and mental disorders. Community support systems have likewise become taxed. Schools often are expected to play a greater role in the well-being of these children.

Once a child is diagnosed with a mental illness, a common response of school systems is to refer this child, if disruptive or troubled, into separate classrooms. Most parents, policy makers, and mental health professionals support an "inclusionary model" for the education of the majority of these students. The well-being of the individual child is believed to be greatly enhanced by remaining within the mainstream. Teachers and school administrators, however, often feel the pressure within the classroom as statistically they will need to deal with one to four children with mental illness on top of those with learning disabilities as well as other health issues within a particular class. They must look to the overall benefit of the class as a whole. Rational and workable accommodations need to be established so that both the class and the individual are afforded the best environment to excel academically.

Both Section 504 of the US Rehabilitation Act of 1973 and the Individuals with Disabilities Education Act require that students with mental illness be placed in the least restrictive environment, mandating that reasonable accommodations be made to keep the student in the classroom. Ideally a 504 plan will be developed for a child struggling with OCD. This type of plan is put in place for medical reasons and should be revised as needed. The benefit of having a child classified under Section 504 is that the plan is considered temporary. If at any point the child recovers to the point that accommodations are no longer required for optimal performance, the plan is removed from the school records. If a child's OCD is severe, it may be more beneficial to work under the more structured Individual with Disabilities Education Act. At this

point, the school would write and periodically review an Individual Education Plan (IEP). Federal guidelines are in place to define the format and scheduled reviews of this plan. An IEP follows the child throughout their school career and becomes a permanent part of their school record.

Both the 504 plan and an IEP can promote children's mental health and allow for continuity of expectations and accommodations from the classroom to home. It is beneficial to involve parents in both the writing and the periodic review of the plan. Parents can provide information about behavior outside of school that should aid in a better picture of the overall progress of the child. Parents are often also able to enlist the help of the child's therapist in setting reasonable accommodations for the classroom environment.

A child struggling with OCD will often be able to mask their disorder for some time and only begin to show signs of this disorder at times of high stress. Behavioral changes or patterns can sometimes be seen to indicate that a child may have OCD. Students may begin to show a pattern of tardiness or absenteeism because of their inability to ready themselves in the morning because of cleaning rituals, reassurance seeking, or fear of contact with the other students. Schoolwork many lag behind schedule because of the child's need to ensure perfection on a paper or examination, showing up as constant erasing or revising of work. Children may spend an inordinate time in the bathroom cleaning up, often resulting in rough or chapped hands, or need to spend time ensuring that everything is placed correctly in their desk, locker, or book bag. Certain phrases may be constantly repeated or the child may continually perform tapping or counting patterns. These children may begin to exhibit signs of eating disorders or depression, which can accompany OCD. Despite the numerous warning signs, OCD is extremely underrecognized in adolescents and children (Chs. 7 and 10).

Teachers should work with parents, school psychologists, or, when possible, the outside therapist treating the child. Generally, simple accommodations for students struggling with OCD can achieve enormous gains in both academic and social success. Tests can be arranged to be taken on a computer if a student is spending an inordinate time erasing. Extra time can be afforded on homework assignments, with contracts signed by the student and teacher clearly defining reasonable deadlines for the long-term assignments of older children. Group tasks may also help the student to keep on track and not allow them to bog themselves down with minutia or revisions. Older children can be enrolled in classes to teach them more effective methods of note taking when it appears they are falling behind because of the desire to record every word uttered during a lesson (Purcell 1999).

Responsible older students can be given a universal hall pass and/or a "quieting area" can be set up in the classrooms for younger students to afford them time to pull themselves together when anxiety rises too high for them to sit unobtrusively in the classroom. Affording children a set number of times they can make a trip to the bathroom without receiving prior consent can often relieve the anxiety arising from the thought of having to go wash up as well as the anxiety of needing to call attention to themselves when they need to publicly ask for permission. Methods can be employed to reduce class time spent reassuring a child by either limiting the number of these types of question that can be asked or providing time after the end of class to go over these issues. All these accommodations should be in place prior to the actual need to implement them so as to minimize the attention drawn to the student.

Both the 504 plan and the IEP for a child with OCD should be reviewed as the child's situation changes. Often, obsessions will change in nature, requiring new accommodations and relaxing of ones no longer required for optimal functioning. As the child progresses through their behavioral therapy outside the classroom, they may be asked by their therapist to engage in situations that are new or anxiety provoking. Communication is critical during these times to understand why these changes are occurring and to be ready for negative outcomes when things do not go well. Often children will have a period after treatment begins where schoolwork may become even more of a burden as the child ramps up their ERP "homework." Just as one would relax the standards for a child undergoing a medical intervention, so must the teacher be ready to accommodate the child in this situation. Smooth transitions for these children should not be expected and even situations that were handled with grace on a previous occasion may prove to be challenging at another time.

The demeanor of the teacher towards the specific needs of a child fighting OCD can go a long way towards making the child feel safe in the classroom environment. As much of the anxiety exhibited in OCD stems from the perceived possibility of encountering the feared stimulus, simply knowing that the adult controlling the child's environment understands the challenges faced because of the OCD can often reduce the intensity and frequency of the obsession. Teachers who foster an environment of acceptance and compassion will often translate these attitudes to the child's peers in the classroom. As children with OCD are often ostracized or picked on by their fellow students, the social development of these children can be severely undermined. Strategies for reducing bullying in the social environment often play a large roll in the well-being of children facing OCD.

The teacher also needs to keep in mind the overall progress of the class as a whole. Patience is a key issue when dealing with students suffering from OCD, as frustration can always be looming in these situations. At times, the teacher will need to decide to move the class on without a student who is caught up in the rituals associated with their disorder. This often proves to be more productive than to engage in a futile confrontation of the ritualistic behavior preventing the child's immediate participation. When possible, the student should be allowed to rejoin the class when they find themselves ready to do so. Advance communication can also facilitate a "signal" agreed upon by both teacher and student as to when the child requires intervention to help to break free from the ritualistic cycle, as well as one for when the child feels confident that they can break free on their own. Involving the full class in relaxation techniques can allow the time for a child with OCD to reduce anxiety and frustration without singling out the student. It may even help to relieve mounting tension in the other students as well as the teacher in times of rising stress.

Teachers and school counseling personnel should consult with each other to ensure that a consistent plan is implemented throughout the school day when children are changing classes, as well as at the end of the year/beginning of the following school year as the child changes grades. While assessments will certainly need to be made as the child progresses through the school system, knowledge of what has worked in the past can help to facilitate the process. The school administration needs to be supportive of the teacher's efforts both in these transitions and as the process begins in their own classroom. "In service" training on OCD should be encouraged as, given the incidence of OCD in the pediatric population, dealing with this child's OCD in the classroom is unlikely to be a unique situation.

Parents encountering schools or teachers who fail to understand or recognize the particular struggles of their child can easily become frustrated. It is up to parents to advocate for their child. Educating yourself about your child's difficulties in the classroom, therapy, and the law is important. Sometimes the parent may be able to suggest ways that the child can work around their obstacles on their own. Parents need to be honest with themselves as to the true limitations placed on the child by a teacher and to remember that the teacher has the wider concern of the full class as well as your child. Therapists rarely have the time or desire to step into these situations directly but may be able to give you or your child advice on how to proceed. They are also often willing to review a 504 plan or IEP to make sure that it is touching on the correct issues and have suggestions for other areas which may need attention.

While parents need to advocate for their child, they also need to make sure that the process of working out a desirable situation for their child does not become adversarial. Often enlisting the help of a principal, counselor, school psychologist, or another teacher can help to relieve some of the tension in a parent–teacher discussion. Success may be achieved by attempting to educate a reluctant teacher about the nature of OCD in a non-threatening or diminutive manner. Parents should also keep in mind that school counselors rarely, if ever, receive formal training concerning OCD within the curriculum of their formal degree program, and training for schools psychologists can be equally lacking in this area. Parents should be ready to help to educate individuals serving in these supportive roles as well as teachers as they try to find a solution for their child's education. Discuss the possibility of moving the child to a different classroom that is more accommodating if discussions with individual teachers fail to progress. When an individual teacher or other employee is particularly helpful in working with a child and the parents, writing a letter of praise to this individual and providing a copy to the principal or superintendent can go a long way to foster an environment of mutual respect.

Some parents decide to move their child from a public school system and place them in a parochial or private institution that is more open to addressing the child's needs. When this is possible, it can be the best solution for your child. This may not be an option for all families as the financial burden may be beyond their reach. Home schooling is another avenue that is pursued. Caution should be used when making this choice as increasing the isolation of the child can seriously deter from their overall recovery and serve to increase their shame about their disorder. As these children often already have issues deterring their social development, home schooling can further degrade this area of the child's life.

If despite the parent's best efforts, the situation is not resolved and the child is in danger of falling behind either academically or developmentally, they may need to seek additional help. A variety of governmental and civic rights agencies can help when matters become dire. Most states have an office of dispute resolution or a similarly named agency that is dedicated to resolving these types of issue. Employing these agencies should not be considered until other less-adversarial methods have failed.

It should be noted that many of the same issues which face students in a classroom are shared by adults in the workplace. The laws which protect children in the academic environment also protect these individuals. Some of the practical advice offered in this section may be adapted to a place of employment. Employers are required to make reasonable accommodations but the individual must be capable of producing the work product required of that position. Individuals may be offered alternative positions within the company if their OCD does not allow for them to complete tasks of the original job despite efforts to provide the accommodations. Termination is a legal possibility if no reasonable solution can be found despite a concerted effort in this matter

The media

The media has become an overwhelming force in society. News is available 24 hours a day through the cable news networks, radio, and internet news services as well as via the more traditional printed forms of news. Dramatic television programming and movies are almost universally accessible. Advertisements are ubiquitous throughout everyday living. The impact of the media begins early. By the time most American children enter school, they have spent the equivalent of three school years watching television (Wahl 2003). Given the profound influence of the media on the attitudes and beliefs of our society, these industries are bound to have a direct effect on the mental health community as well as the community at large. Opinions and prejudices about mental illness are often formed long before a person meets someone dealing with these issues.

While not universal, both the entertainment and news media often portray the mentally ill in an overdramatic and distorted fashion. An emphasis is often placed on the dangerousness, unpredictability, and criminality of the mentally ill. These portrayals are generally accompanied by negative reactions of the community to this population, including fear, ridicule, and rejection. The viewing public is also often left with the belief that there is little that can be done to help these people recover or become productive members of society or, conversely, indicate that recovery is simply a matter of "pulling oneself together." Reinforcement of the stigma placed on these very real medical conditions and acceptance of negative attitudes is often a consequence.

Media images have a profound effect on people with mental illness and their families. The impact on their self-image, willingness to seek treatment, and ultimate recovery are often negatively affected. Fear of being "found out" is enforced by intolerance and hostility often displayed by the general community. Individuals become so scared of being labeled as mentally ill that they prefer not to receive either a diagnosis or the treatment available. As a consequence, many people with mental illness limit their social activities, thus increasing their feelings of isolation.

However, many positive steps have been established in recent years. More programming and stories are being offered that do show a glimmer of hope. Reporters are often seen to be doing more background research and attempting to tell a more complete story when it comes to mental illness. Reality shows are covering topics that would not have been conceived several years ago, and while many still do not portray an accurate image of the topic, others are approaching a more desirable level. Entertainment industries often do attempt to consult with knowledgeable agencies who can guide them in their portrayals of characters with a mental illness.

The entertainment media

The entertainment industry rarely portrays characters with OCD as violent or dangerous; however, an emphasis on these characters as eccentric or overly neurotic is quite common. In reality, most people with OCD rarely display their compulsive behaviors in public. In fact, to the outside world most people with OCD display traits that are highly prized: cleanliness, orderly, attentive to detail, and overtly responsible. Most of the compulsive behavior which would be considered "odd" is saved for private moments, as people with OCD are quite adept at hiding or camouflaging these acts. Rarely have films or dramatic television programs shown a person with OCD as someone privately locked in a debilitating cycle of meaningless rituals that they feel compelled to perform despite recognizing their senselessness.

While writers and producers can be somewhat forgiven for exercising "artistic license" in these inaccurate portrayals, it is frustrating to the OCD community that the myths about OCD are perpetuated so effectively. One has to understand that the entertainment industry exists for the purpose of entertainment. While many do attempt to use their media for social change, they can only do so by engaging a wide audience. They have limited time and avenues to introduce the viewer to the characters. It is rarely possible to convey the turmoil occurring within a person's mind on the screen without a more tangible means of communication. Therefore, the audience is shown an actor portraying a physical representation of an auditory delusion in the case of schizophrenia and the character with OCD tends to overperform compulsions, often in what would be inappropriately public situations for an actual person suffering from OCD.

One major fault of this industry in handling issues of OCD in particular and mental health in general is its portrayal of the treatment process. While we have come a long was from *One Flew Over the Cuckoo's Nest* and the *Snake Pit*, which emphasized oppressive and inhumane effects of psychiatric treatment, the mental health field is still often portrayed as unbalanced, malevolent, or ineffectual. Little progress has been made by the entertainment industry to indicate that people with mental illness can and do recover or become productive members of society. Most characters pursuing treatment for OCD are shown in offices participating in talk therapy or running to the psychiatrist's office for a quick fix of pills. Often, the only effects of treatment displayed are negative outcomes. The difficult journey of effective treatment for OCD and the ultimate regaining of one's life is not part of the story line. Both the people suffering from OCD and the general public need to be educated about more realistic outcomes.

Occasionally, OCD has taken center stage in the entertainment industry's products. Unfortunately, many of the characters are portrayed as "unlikable." Jack Nicholson won an Academy Award for his over-the-top portrayal of an author with OCD in *As Good As It Gets*. Despite guidance by an OCD advocacy group, this depiction had little basis in reality. His symptoms became the reason that he was socially inept rather than the underlying fact that the character himself was not a particularly nice guy. The con man portrayed by Nicholas Cage in *Matchstick Men* did have more redeeming qualities despite his chosen life style. This movie also did a better job of showing the compulsive behavior as occurring behind closed doors. Only those closest to him were aware of these activities but, even then, exhibited little compassion or understanding of the underlying pathology. While ultimately portrayed as a victim, at least the film did not base the victimization on the mental illness.

The *Aviator*, starring Leonardo DiCaprio, may be the most accurate on-screen depiction in a feature film of a person struggling with OCD. This balance may have resulted from two main factors. The script was based on the life of Howard Hughes, long believed to have suffered from OCD, and the leading actor understood the illness from his own personal battles with this disorder. While this movie does emphasize the eccentricity of the main character, it is not a far-fetched message. It is commendable that this movie was able to depict the extreme sense of shame that most people with OCD experience concerning their symptoms. In one particular scene, the audience witnesses the extreme distress of the main character when his illness leaves him unable to force himself to hand a towel to a physically handicapped individual in a public restroom.

Another topic that is touched upon in this film is that wealth and power can at times be a hindrance in the treatment of mental illness. With a staff of hundreds and a seemingly endless supply of funds, Howard Hughes was able to go to great lengths to accommodate his disorder. Little effective treatment was available in the lifetime of this person, but his economic situation certainly may have perpetuated his suffering. His ability to fully succumb to his self-perpetuating compulsive behavior probably enhanced his downfall and may have helped to lead to his reclusive suffering.

In the situation comedy *Monk*, the central theme of the show is based on OCD. Adrian Monk, a detective on medical leave from the police department because of his uncontrolled OCD, is played by Tony Shalhoub. His OCD fluctuates between helping to advance his career and serving as a detriment to both his life and work. While serving as one of the best examples of the media conveying the sense of angst that is central to the struggle with OCD, this character's OCD is so over the top and public that the unrealistic characterization of someone with OCD makes this show a favorite target of the OCD community. It can be difficult to watch a humorous take on such a debilitating illness for someone who truly understands the struggle to battle OCD. The popularity of the show can also make raising public awareness of the true nature of OCD difficult.

One should note, however, that while this show may perpetuate many myths about OCD, the show does a wonderful job of showing that people who can look beyond the symptoms to the actual person underneath can find a wonderful individual to celebrate and love. Very few forays into the world of mental illness in the entertainment media can boast a more accurate portrayal of the support systems that are available to people with OCD.

Medical dramas often deal with the issue of OCD as do other dramatic and comedy programs. In medical dramas, often an incidental character playing a doctor is introduced to the show. A common scenario is for this doctor to spend hours in the bathroom following a shift or procedure scrubbing their hands. While at least accurately indicating that the compulsive behavior is not public, frequently they are "caught" by another member of the medical team. These characters soon appear to be forced to leave their position as their OCD makes it impossible to practice medicine despite the fact that our current medical system employs many individuals affected by this disorder. While television does appear to be making many advances in its portrayal of OCD and other mental health concerns, there still is room for improvement.

"Talk shows" are also a main venue for dissemination of information about OCD. While many of the less-respectable formats will often work to highlight the more bizarre behaviors of people with OCD, often during "sweeps" month, in recent years more shows have been taking an interest in presenting a more accurate representation of OCD and the treatment of this disorder. People who were willing to come forward to tell their story in the early years were often led into treacherous interviews that did not present the image they had wished to portray. Editing of these pieces was often done for maximum entertainment value rather than educational and factual content. These early pioneers did, however, help to pave the way for others to come forward. From the lessons learned during these past interviews, recent volunteers were able to arrive better prepared to direct the "spin" of the story to a more realistic and empathetic story.

In literature too, OCD also frequently serves as a central or important theme. The nature of the written word does allow for creative treaties of OCD, which can more accurately describe the nature of this illness as it pertains to the character. Authors are free to spend more time within the character's mind to convey an accurate account of a person's thought process. This can help to create a sense of empathy and compassion in the reader towards a mind experiencing a mental illness. Freed from the restraints of conveying a visual representation of the mental illness and given a much broader landscape for character development, books have greater latitude to handle mental illness in a more thorough manner. More time can also be spent on background research as authors are not as limited by the looming deadlines of film and television.

The news media

More and more often it seems that a journalist's job is to sell the news not merely to tell the news. A good story must capture the public's attention. Violent incidents are highly likely to capture a wider audience. But today's society has a desire to know "why" these events occur. Mental illness has become a favorite facet on which to hang these incidents. Soon after a story of a mass or particularly horrific violence breaks, the news agencies begin to examine the perpetrator's background for any sign of mental illness as well as bringing in commentary from medical reporters to "guess" at the mental health status of those involved.

The occurrence of OCD has recently been creeping into these types of report. It makes sense to the public audience that a person "obsessed with the attention of another individual" can lead to a central role in these brutal real-life dramas. Unfortunately, the use of the word "obsessed" in these reports is most often in lay terms, not in the clinical sense. The jump from the idea of a person who is actually "preoccupied with a love interest" to a reported diagnosis of OCD is becoming far too common in the reporting of these events, even

when that report is made by a member of the medical community. It is unfortunate that the mental health professionals who are the most versed in discussing the true nature of mental illness are reluctant to be interviewed following the reports of these violent acts. Given the poor understanding of OCD in particular, this often leads to very erroneous depictions of the nature of this illness.

In balance, the news media can be and is a powerful source for mental health information. Public interest stories often run that help to dispel the stereotype of those with mental illness as being "violent or out of control." More often too the news media has begun to focus on positive outcomes of mental health treatment. Morning news programs and talk shows have begun to run segments on OCD and the time is taken to invite notable experts in the field to give an accurate portrayal of this disorder. Newspapers and internet reports, which often have greater time and space than the broadcast news to devote to personal accounts of struggles with mental health, have played a significant role in educating the public about the true nature of mental health. It is often a matter once again of capturing the interest of a wider audience that detracts from the impact of these accounts.

Commercial advertising

Effective advertisements create an environment that convinces people that they need a particular item even if prior to viewing or listening to these advertisements, the audience was unaware of the product. Very often these advertisements are specifically aimed at exploiting fear. By increasing the anxiety of the viewer over a particular situation, they can convince the public that this one product is all that stands between them and illness, death, destruction, acceptance, and so on. These messages have proven to be enormously effective in raising the anxiety of the general public, while the message can be elevated to increased heights in the segment of the population that already suffers from anxiety disorders. It also blurs the line at which the level of fear does actually fit into a pathological model as opposed to what would be considered normal. Society at large has now become what has been termed "germophobic" as a result of the increase in antibacterial products on the market. People with OCD have a harder time deciding which of their fears are real and which are inflicted upon them by their illness or commercial message. Medical personnel have a harder time recognizing the more subtle signs of a patient who shows signs of OCD. Patients and treatment providers become frustrated with these exaggerated advertisements.

Despite efforts to educate the public about the misconceptions involved in these messages, their pervasiveness in our daily lives is overwhelming. The trend is also to disguise the emotional issues in reports that appear to be from valid scientific sources. We are constantly bombarded by this media in various forms until is it is difficult to discern what information is based in fact. For the community dealing with issues involving OCD, these advertisements very often serve as triggers for their illness to manifest itself in their lives.

Commercial advertising is a part of our society. People within the OCD community need to be aware of the potential influence it may have on the intensity and pattern of symptoms displayed. Knowledge of this stimulus may help both the OCD sufferer and their therapist to deal with issues before they become cumbersome. People struggling with OCD may be advised to turn off the television, close the magazine, switch radio stations, limit web searches or avoid driving routes filled with billboards. This advice may also apply to news stories pertaining to public health and safety issues, which may also feed obsessions.

Conclusions

The promotion of mental health improves the quality of life of individuals and the mental well-being of the whole population (Rutz 2006). A survey of people with mental illness and their families conducted in Australia indicated that "less stigma" was rated highest in a list of topics which would "make their lives better," further indicating a desire that the community would "understand that they were not lazy or weak" and that recovery is more than "pulling yourself together" (Hocking 2003). Stigma contributes to loneliness and distress as well as a failure to seek or find adequate treatment. It contributes to discrimination in housing, employment, education, politics, and social structure. Mental health and well-being are fundamental for quality of life; they are basic elements of social cohesion, productivity, peace, and stability in the living environments (*Mental Health Action Plan for Europe* and *Mental Health Declaration for Europe*; WHO Regional Office for Europe 2005a, 2005b).

Mental illness stigma is not a problem limited to the general population. Discriminatory beliefs are also inherent in the medical field. Physicians and other healthcare workers are less likely to diagnose psychiatric patients with somatic illnesses (Kuey 2008). This may be a contributing factor to the premature death rate of people with mental illness (Coglan *et al.* 2001) as medical conditions such as cardiovascular disease are ignored or labeled as delusional. The sector of the medical profession that should be the most on guard in regard to this stigmatization is also implicated in this problem. One study found that mental health professionals had a similar rate of negative stereotypes and attitude about restrictions towards people with mental illness as did the corresponding group of lay people included in the study (Nordt *et al.* 2006). Psychiatrists often ignore medical comorbidities in their patients, and the mental illnesses of patients in the care of physicians focusing on medical issues are often overlooked or dismissed. Clearly, more effective education is required for healthcare workers in this area, which should reach those currently in practice as well as those still in their initial training.

Reducing the isolation of people struggling with OCD will take a concerted effort. This community needs to work with other sectors of the mental health population to begin to break down the walls that face all individuals living with mental illness. They also need to work within the OCD population to champion their own cause. Only by increasing the general awareness about the difficulties facing people with OCD can the sense of "strangeness" of these individuals begin to be dissipated. Participating in support groups, classes, and group therapy sessions, as well as joining charitable and advocacy groups, can reduce the feeling of isolation and provide a personal feeling of empowerment. Given the support of these services, it is hoped that these individuals can begin to become beacons of light in educating the unenlightened public. Simply by taking the time to tactfully explain the impact of erroneous or thoughtless statements on an individual basis can help. On a more grandiose scale, working with others in the OCD community to help to shape the message from the media or governments will continue to expand the message. Targeting the younger population in schools or other facilities where this population gathers may help to reduce the perpetuating stigma associated with OCD and other mental disorders. Demystifying these topics in children will not only help to break the cycle of discrimination but may also promote good mental health practices when the early signs of mental illness appear in themselves or their friends.

It is hoped that the topics covered in this chapter will provoke thoughtful insight in the reader so as to identify other areas of our global community that may exert sway over the expression and intensity of an individual's OCD, as well as how this illness is perceived by society. Many of the opinions shared were intended also to foster an understanding that the industries and sectors exerting these influences are not necessarily malevolent, but simply providing a service that is not directly concerned with OCD. Understanding the objective of these industries and agencies may allow for the OCD community to better tolerate these influences as well as to find more productive methods to persuade them to shape their message to better reflect the reality of OCD. It is hoped that with knowledge gained to recognize the commercial and social sectors which may increase the distress caused by OCD, one can learn methods to counteract the negative aspects of these influences on the disease process and gain acceptance for their existence in society.

References

Black DW, Blum NS (1992). Obsessive-compulsive disorder support groups: the Iowa model. *Compr Psychiatry* **33**: 65–71.

Blair M, Stewart-Brown S, Waterston T, Crowther R (2003). *Child Public Health.* New York: Oxford University Press.

Burland J (1995). Journey of hope: a family-to-family self help education program. *Self Help* **6**: 20–22.

Cameron LD, Leventhal H (eds.) (2003).*The Self-regulation of Health and Illness Behavior.* London: Routledge.

Chamberlin J (1978). *On Our Own: Patient-controlled Alternatives to the Mental Health System.* Toronto: McGraw-Hill.

Coglan R, Lawrence D, Jablensky A (2001). *Duty to Care: Physical Illness in People with Mental Illness.* Perth: University of Western Australia.

Davidson L (2003). *Living Outside Mental Illness: Qualitative Studies of Recovery in Schizophrenia.* New York: New York University Press.

Dixon L, Lucksted A, Stewart B, *et al.* (2004). Outcomes of peer-taught 12-week family-to-family education program for severe mental illness. *Acta Psychiatr Scand* **109**: 207–215.

DuPont RL, Rice DP, Shiraki S, Rowland CR (1995). Economic costs of obsessive-compulsive disorder. *Med Interface* **8**: 102–109.

Eysenbach G (2003). The impact of the Internet on cancer outcomes. *CA Cancer J Clin* **53**: 356–371.

Feldman MD (2000). Munchausen by Internet: detecting factitious illness and crisis on the Internet. *South J Med* **93**: 669–672.

Gallup Organization (1993). *A Gallup Study of Obsessive Compulsive Disorder Sufferers.* Princeton, NJ: Gallup Organization.

Grohol JM (2004). *What to Look for in Quality Online Support Groups.* http://psychcentral.com/archives/support_groups.htm (accessed 12 August 2010).

Hocking B (2003). Reducing mental illness stigma and discrimination-everybody's business. *Med J Aust* **178**: S47–S48.

Humphreys K (2000). Community narratives and personal stories in Alcoholics Anonymous. *J Community Psychol* **28**: 495–506.

Kuey L (2008). The impact of stigma on somatic treatment and care for people with comorbid mental and somatic disorders. *Curr Opin Psychiatry* **21**: 403–411.

Lancet Mental Health Group (2007). Scale up services for mental disorders: a call for action. *Lancet* **370**: 1241–1252.

Lucksted A, Stewart B, Forbes CB (2008). Benefits and changes for family to family graduates. *Am J Community Psychol* **42**: 154–166.

Malti T, Noam GG (2008). The hidden crisis in mental health and education: the gap between student's needs and existing supports. *New Direct Youth Dev* **120**: 13–29.

Nelson G, Janzen R, Trainor J, Ochocka J (2008). Putting values into practice: public policy and the future of mental health consumer-run organizations. *Am J Community Psychol* **42**: 192–201.

Nordt C, Rossler W, Lauber C (2006). Attitudes of mental health professionals toward people tihe schizophrenia and major depression. *Schizopr Bull* **32**: 709–714.

Pistrang N, Barker C, Humphreys K (2008). Mutual help groups for mental health problems: a review of effectiveness studies. *Am J Community Psychol* **42**: 110–121.

Purcell J (1999). Children, adolescents and obsessive-compulsive disorder in the classroom. *ERDS Guides* 1–22.

Roberts LJ, Salem D, Rappaport J, *et al.* (1999). Giving and receiving help: interpersonal transactions in mutual self help meetings and psychosocial adjustment of members. *Am J Community Psychol* **27**: 841–868.

Rutz W (2006). Social psychiatry and the public mental health: present situation and future objectives; Time for rethinking and renaissance? *Acta Psychiatr Scand* **113**: 95–100.

Wahl OF (2003). Depictions of mental illnesses in children's media. *J Ment Health* **12**: 249–258.

Weitz D (1984). "On Our Own": a self help model. In Lumsden DP (ed.) *Community Mental Health Action: Primary Prevention Programming in Canada* (pp. 312–320). Ottawa: Canadian Public Health Association.

WHO Regional Office for Europe (2005a). *Mental Health Action Plan for Europe: Facing the Challenges, Building Solutions.* Copenhagen: WHO Regional Office for Europe, http://www.euro.who.int/document/mnh/edoc07.pdf (accessed 11 August 2010).

WHO Regional Office for Europe (2005b). *Mental Health Declaration for Europe, Facing the Challenges, Building Solutions.* Copenhagen: WHO Regional Office for Europe, http://www.euro.who.int/document/mnh/edoc07.pdf (accessed 11 August 2010).

Resources

The following list are some, but not all, resources that may prove useful (accessed 14 August 2010).

Children of Hoarders http://www.childrenofhoarders.com/bindex.php

Clutters Anonymous http://sites.google.com/site/clutterersanonymous

Family to family education program; National Alliance on Mental Illness www.nami.org

International OCD Foundation http://www.ocfoundation.org/

National Alliance of the Mentally Ill (NAMI) www.nami.org

Obsessive Compulsive Anonymous www.obsessivecompulsiveanonymous.org

OCD Centre Manitoba http://www.ocdmanitoba.ca/

OCD Ireland www.ocdireland.org/

OCD Organizations and Support Groups http://www.geonius.com/ocd/organizations.html

OCD-UK http://www.ocduk.org/

Ontario Obsessive Compulsive Disorder Network http://www.ocdontario.org/

Tricotillomania Learning Center http://www.trich.org/

12 The family in the treatment of obsessive-compulsive disorder

Andrea Allen and Stefano Pallanti

Introduction

Familial factors have been implicated in the development, maintenance, and exacerbation of obsessive-compulsive disorder (OCD). At the same time, the presence of someone with OCD in a family often has a severe, negative impact on the family, and the stress that creates is likely to exacerbate the obsessive-compulsive symptoms. These intricate factors have led to research on the inclusion of family members in OCD treatment. Although the body of literature on this is not large, and more research is needed, it has become clear that the involvement of family members in treatment can be very valuable. Their involvement in treatment can ease the stress on the family, help them to avoid inadvertently maintaining or exacerbating the OCD, and enable them to actively support the patient's treatment and recovery.

Family quality of life

The occurrence of OCD clearly impairs the psychological well-being and quality of life of those who suffer from it (Hollander et al. 1996; Stein et al. 1996; Koran 2000), but OCD also has a severe impact on patients' family members. The caregiver burden in OCD is actually similar to that found for severe mental disorders such as schizophrenia (Kalra et al. 2008). Family members are affected in many different ways; day-to-day life can be complicated, stressful, and frustrating, with many psychological ramifications.

On a practical level, many family members become very involved in the patient's OCD by helping in the performance of rituals and modifying household routines (Rachman and Hodgson 1980). Shafran et al. (1995) found that 90% of family members report that the family member's OCD interferes with their own life. Many patients with severe, chronic OCD are dependent on their families for essential day-to-day activities (Steketee 1997). Families often have to make up excuses for the absence of the patient at social gatherings or even to cover up hospitalizations. Families may keep the disorder a secret. Concealment is a frequent issue; many families attempt to conceal the illness from others and often only some family members are informed. Most attempt to prevent the patient's OCD behaviors in public and may avoid joint activities to avoid the embarrassment and annoyance. For some, framing odd behaviors as quirks seems preferable to labeling them OCD. In some instances, the patient demands that the disorder be kept a secret and will not allow the family member to have a confidant to share their burden with.

Research has found that these families with a member with OCD have a lower quality of life in terms of psychological well-being, physical well-being, and social relationships; family members of patients with OCD tend to report a high level of personal distress, depression, marital discord, and disruption to their own social and personal lives (Cooper 1996; Amir et al. 2000; Renshaw et al. 2000; Barrett et al. 2001). Family members grieve the loss of the relationship they had hoped for with the patient and what they had hoped for the patient's life. Obviously, having a parent with OCD can be a serious problem for a child or teenager.

Stigma is known to be a serious problem for those suffering from severe metal illness (Phelan and Link 1998; Crisp et al. 2000) and their families (Wahl and Harman 1989; Phelan et al. 1998); it is also an issue for OCD. A study of OCD patient families in Germany (Stengler-Wenzke et al. 2004) found a broad range of stigmatizing experiences.

In one study (Stengler-Wenzke et al. 2006), three of the four domains of the World Health Organization

Clinical Obsessive-Compulsive Disorders in Adults and Children, ed. Robert Hudak and Darin D. Dougherty.
Published by Cambridge University Press. Copyright © Cambridge University Press 2011.

Quality of Life Assessment-Bref (WHOQOL Group 1998) – physical well-being, pyschologicalwell-being, and social relationships – were lower for family members of patients with OCD than in the general population in Germany. These differences were small but statistically significant. The pyschologicalwell-being domain includes negative mood, sadness, anxiety, dissatisfaction with self, enjoyment of one's life, and the meaning of life; relatives of patients with OCD must deal with the chronic illness of their family member and struggle with understanding and accepting their bizarre thoughts and behaviors (Stengler-Wenzke *et al.* 2004, 2006). The physical well-being domain includes somatic symptoms of depression such as sleep, fatigue, and pain, as well as problems in coping with daily life and with physical health. The social relationship domain covers socializing outside of the family and social leisure activities. These three domains all seem to be impaired by the presence of a household member with OCD.

The role of the family in OCD

Family members can become involved in OCD to an extent rarely found in other mental illnesses. The families are often drawn deeply into the illness given that OCD symptoms can become all-encompassing. Patients with OCD can place intense demands on their families to provide reassurance and participate in, or at least facilitate, their behavioral rituals. Thus, individuals with OCD can dominate the family. Family participation can operate both directly (e.g., participation with the rituals, interference with or intrusion into the rituals) and indirectly (e.g., modification in the family's lifestyle around the symptoms).

There also can be conflict among family members about how best to deal with the demands made by the person with OCD (Amir *et al.* 2000; Stengler-Wenzke *et al.* 2004). Van Noppen and colleagues (1997) suggested a continuum from accommodating to antagonizing: that is, from families who assist in the OCD rituals to those that resist and on to those that oppose or even attempt to stop the rituals. Of course, there are also situations where one family member takes an antagonistic stance and another is accommodating. In such cases, family discord can be expected and this can be very severe. Often, individual family members are inconsistent – sometimes being accommodating and other times being critical or hostile. Regardless of whether the family rejects the symptoms or

accommodates to them, they are often inextricably involved in the disorder.

Accommodation

It has long been documented that many families accommodate to patients' OCD symptoms, whether these patients are adults or children (Rachman and Hodgson 1980; Allsopp and Verduyn 1990; Livingston-Van Noppen *et al.* 1990). Studies focusing on accommodation have found that the majority of family members accommodate to the patient's symptoms; this is true for both outpatients (100% for adolescent OCD in Bolton *et al.* 1983; 88% in Calvocoressi *et al.* 1995; 60% in Shafran *et al.* 1995) and inpatients (97% in Stewart *et al.* 2008).

Families of patients with OCD adjust their behavior in many different ways. Family members can offer reassurance, take over household responsibilities from the individual with OCD, participate in the rituals, or adjust their own daily routines to follow some or all of the OCD rules. Calvocoressi (*et al.* 1995) found that half or more of the family members they studied reassure the patients (53%), participate in the behavioral rituals (50%), or assume responsibility for the patient's chores (59%). Specific examples of accommodation include not touching the patient, helping to decontaminate the home, showering upon entering the house, or not being able to cook because the stove is covered with hoarded papers. Family members also may adjust to always being late or generally having trouble getting out of the house because they have to wait for, or help with, the checking of windows and faucets before they can leave (perhaps including unplugging appliances). One might be unable to put down the newspaper, a pen, or any other object without having it quickly thrown out or put away.

Accommodation occurs for different reasons, including to calm and support the individual with OCD and to make life easier for the family in general. For example, family members may believe that it would take longer for their relative to finish their rituals if they did not help them (Calvocoressi *et al.* 1995). The more angry and anxious the patient's reaction is to the family refusing to help, the more likely the family members are to accommodate (Calvocoressi *et al.* 1995). Half the family members reported being verbally or even physically abused by the patient and nearly one third reported that the patient suffered severe or disabling anxiety

Table 12.1 Parental attitudes associated with obsessive-compulsive disorder in children

Attitudes	Studies
High expressed emotion	Leonard *et al.* (1993); Bressi and Guggeri (1996); Waters and Barrett (2000); Renshaw *et al.* (2003)
Low affection	Cavedo and Parker (1994); Hafner (1998); Alonso *et al.* (2004).
Low support	Valleni-Basile *et al.* (1995)
Overprotection, overcontrol	Cavedo and Parker 1994); Hafner (1998); Alonso *et al.* (2004);
Low confidence in child's ability, low reward of independence	Barrett *et al.* (2002)
High anxiety	Kohlmann *et al.* (1988)
Perceived lack of control over external events	Capps *et al.* (1996); Chorpita and Barlow (1998)

(Calvocoressi *et al.* 1995). Accommodating family members try to avoid conflict and have difficulty setting limits on the patients.

Whatever the motivation, accommodation has a negative impact on both the patient and the family, but many families do not realize that accommodation backfires. Accommodation is not good for the patient as it increase the severity of the OCD. In addition, it harms the family. Their intent may be to make things easier for the patient and themselves; however, in reality accommodating increases stress and adversely affects the functioning of the family (Magliano *et al.* 1996; Livingston-Van Noppen *et al.* 1990; Amir *et al.* 2000). The greater the involvement of families with OCD rituals, the greater the distress in the families ($r = 0.72$) and the more rejecting their attitudes toward the patient ($r = 0.67$) (Calvocoressi *et al.* 1995). It is important to keep in mind that accommodation is related to negative feelings toward the family member, because such negative attitudes from family members exacerbate patient symptoms, as will be discussed below

Note that although there is a clear negative impact to accommodation, this does not mean that the family members are causing OCD, but rather they are caught up in maintaining the disorder in some ways (Calvocoressi *et al.* 1995; Waters and Barrett 2000).

Antagonism

Some family members are antagonistic, critical, and hostile towards the patient's symptoms and consistently refuse to support or be involved in the ritualistic behavior; others react this way some of the time. Examples of antagonistic family involvement include

criticism of the patient for performing rituals, treating them as though they could control the behavior but are choosing not to, attempting to stop the patient with OCD from performing rituals, and forced traumatic exposure to the feared stimulus. As with accommodation, family members who react to the patient's OCSs in a hostile or critical way may also unwittingly be increasing the frequency and/or severity of the rituals.

Several family characteristics have been found to be associated with OCD. One prominent one is high expressed emotion. Expressed emotion refers to a family environment characterized by hostility, criticism, and/or emotional over-involvement. There is preliminary evidence from child studies to suggest that high expressed emotion or one of its components is characteristic of families with an OCD child (Hibbs *et al.* 1991; Leonard *et al.* 1993; Bressi and Guggeri 1996; Waters and Barrett 2000; Renshaw *et al.* 2003). Other parental characteristics that are associated with OCD development in children are low affection (Cavedo and Parker 1994; Hafner 1998; Alonso *et al.* 2004), low support (Valleni-Basile *et al.* 1995), overprotection or overcontrol (Cavedo and Parker 1994; Hafner 1998; Alonso *et al.* 2004), low confidence in the child's ability, and low reward of independence (Barrett *et al.* 2002) (Table 12.1). Barrett and colleagues (2002) found that OCD families were less confident in their children's abilities, granted the children less autonomy and were less competent in using flexible problem-solving techniques. Such parental attitudes are hypothesized to create avoidance, caution, and fearfulness in their children, which may contribute to the development of OCD (Henin and Kendall 1997).

Table 12.2 Factors associated with treatment non-response in obsessive-compulsive disorder

	Factor	Study
Individual	Baseline severity of obsessive-compulsive symptoms	Ginsburg *et al.* (2008)
Family environment	Family dysfunction	Ginsburg *et al.* (2008)
	Parental high expressed emotion	Leonard *et al.* (1993)
	Parental hostile criticism	Chambless and Steketee (1999)
	Parental emotional overinvolvement	Chambless and Steketee (1999
	Family accommodation	Amir, Freshman, and Foa (2000)

Moreover, factors such as high parental anxiety (Kohlmann *et al.* 1988) and perceived lack of control over external events (Capps *et al.* 1996; Chorpita and Barlow 1998) are also hypothesized to be relevant to the exacerbation of childhood OCD.

Cognitive style in the family

According to cognitive theorists, information processing may play a central role in the development and maintenance of obsessional problems (Salkovskis 1985, 1998; Rachman, 1993, 1997, 1998). Current psychological models of OCD propose that the way in which people interpret their thoughts is an important maintaining factor (Salkovskis *et al.* 1995; Rachman 1997). Individuals with OCD tend to believe that their intrusive thoughts and urges have meaning, that they are dangerous or immoral, and that they are able to prevent harm occurring either to their self or a vulnerable person (Salkovskis *et al.* 1995). So, they tend to adopt actions in an attempt to prevent feared catastrophes and reduce harm (Salkovskis 1985) and will, therefore, turn to compulsions and neutralizing behaviors. Several authors have identified a cognitive style that may be uniquely involved in the development of OCD, namely inflated responsibility (Salkovskis *et al.* 1999).

The family plays a role in the cognitive development of children and hence the potential for enhancement of OCD-related beliefs (Pollock and Carter 1999). Salkovskis and colleagues (1999) have identified three possible ways in which the family may influence the cognitive processing of children with OCD. The first possible influence is heightened responsibility as a child. It refers to children who have increased levels of responsibility when young. These children may be given the message that they are responsible for preventing negative outcomes rather than promoting success (Salkovskis *et al.* 1999). The second possible influence is a family environment characterized by high anxiety or worry in which the world is perceived as a threatening or dangerous place. In these families, parental overprotection and criticism for failures is exhibited. Parents may convey a sense that danger is close at hand and that they doubt their child's ability to cope with danger. This parenting style may increase the child's sensitivity to responsibility by limiting their experiences with personal responsibility (Salkovskis *et al.* 1999). Lastly, the child may be exposed to extreme or rigid teachings in the family, school, or religious settings selected by the family. In these contexts children may be taught to follow strict behavioral codes and led to believe that failure to do so may result in blame, guilt, or punishment. This may be a precursor to the development of moral thought–action fusion in which individuals believe that they commit a sin based solely on their thoughts of performing the act (Salkovskis *et al.* 1999).

Predictors of OCD treatment outcome

In order to improve OCD treatment, researchers have tried to identify predictors of treatment response in OCD or, in contrast, predictors of non-response.

An interesting review of literature examined studies published from 1985 to 2007 and focused on predictors of treatment response in pediatric OCD (Ginsburg *et al.* 2008). Both cognitive-behavioral therapy (CBT) and medication studies for pediatric OCD were analyzed. Results suggest that both baseline severity of OCSs and family dysfunction were associated with poorer response to CBT (Table 12.2), whereas comorbid tics and externalizing disorders were associated with poorer response in medication-only studies (Ginsburg *et al.* 2008). The authors suggested that the severity of OBSs at baseline should be taken into consideration when selecting treatment with CBT, developing treatment goals, and determining prognosis.

Concerning family environment, results have mirrored the research on the family role in OCD development. Several studies suggest that parental high expressed emotion (Leonard *et al.* 1993), hostile criticism and emotional overinvolvement (Chambless and Steketee 1999) are associated with greater dropout and/or poor treatment outcome for patients with OCD. Other studies have reported that high family accommodation was associated with a worse response to behavioral therapy in children with OCD (Amir *et al.* 2000). Correspondingly, helping family members disengage from compulsions and resist accommodation during behavioral therapy appeared to improve OCD patient outcomes (Grunes *et al.* 2001; Van Noppen and Steketee 2003; Storch *et al.* 2007). Indeed accommodation has been found to be related to severity of OCD post-treatment (Amir *et al.* 2000) and is associated with poorer outcome at follow-up (Steketee 1993).

Family involvement in treatment

Although more research needs to be carried out, the existing literature suggests that family involvement in treatment can be helpful and it can take many forms. Family involvement is almost universal in the treatment of children with OCD, but there is also research on involving family members and significant others for adults in treatment that suggests it should be used with adults as well.

Treatment of children and adolescents

Parents have long been involved in the treatment of teenagers and children with OCD. The vast majority of case reports, series, and studies of OCD treatment of children and adolescents indicate that parents are involved to some extent. However, there are no studies looking at the impact of parental involvement versus no parental involvement, probably because the need for family involvement in the treatment of children is so accepted and is assumed to be required. It is clear that the treatments involving parents are highly successful and can be recommended; what is unclear is the extent to which the family involvement and other specific elements contribute to the success.

The parents and families are involved in treatment in a variety of important ways. Most often there is psychoeducation about the nature of OCD, its management and CBT treatment specifically (March *et al.* 1994; Piacentini *et al.* 1994, 2002; Scahill *et al.* 1996; Fischer *et al.* 1998; Himle *et al.* 2003). Attention is also focused on the importance of reducing accommodation and how to do it (Piacentini *et al.* 1994, 2002; Scahill *et al.* 1996; Wever and Rey 1997; Waters *et al.* 2001). General parental skills and OCD problem solving are taught (Fischer *et al.* 1998; Waters *et al.* 2001; Himle *et al.* 2003; Barrett *et al.* 2004; Martin and Thienemann 2005). In some cases, parents are used actively as part of the therapy to help with exposures and as co-therapists (Wever and Rey 1997; Benazon *et al.* 2002; Bolton and Perrin 2008).

The intensity of family involvement varies considerably across studies; while there are differences in the planned protocols, family involvement also varies based on the developmental level of the child and other clinical considerations, including family dynamics. Minimally, some protocols offer, but do not require, several sessions for the parents without the patient (Fischer *et al.* 1998). Others report holding a few planned conjoint sessions (often three) with the parents and the patient (March *et al.* 1994; Pediatric OCD Treatment Study Team 2004) with additional family involvement as needed to keep parents apprised of the homework assignments, to get their feedback on the progress of the therapy, and to address any maladaptive family interactions. Some researchers used much more extensive family involvement, with parents attending weekly sessions concurrent with the patient's sessions as well as conjoint sessions as needed (Piacentini *et al.* 1994) or even weekly (Martin and Thienemann 2005). Another strategy is to have the family attend part of every weekly patient session (Wever and Rey 1997) or every other week (Scahill *et al.* 1996); others have parents involved in part of every session and also in some full conjoint sessions (Thienemann *et al.* 2001; Waters *et al.* 2001; Benazon *et al.* 2002; Asbahr *et al.* 2005). Although, as noted, family involvement was often adjusted based on the clinical needs, some researchers held initial sessions with both parent and patient involvement but after that parent involvement varied a great deal according to the clinical needs (Franklin *et al.* 1998; Piacentini *et al.* 2002; Valderhaug *et al.* 2007).

Formal and extensive family involvement has been the focus of two recent studies. In the first, Barrett and her colleagues (2004) conducted a randomized controlled trial of two formats for family CBT for OCD with child and adolescent patients (mean age, 12 years; range, 7–17); the study compared individual family CBT (24 subjects) with group family CBT (29 subjects), and with a wait-list control (24 subjects). Family members included at least one parent for each patient with OCD, as well as siblings if available. The duration of treatment was 14 weeks, with follow-ups at three and six months. The treatment protocol was based on the individual CBT protocol developed by March and colleagues (March et al. 1994; March and Mulle 1998). The family component was addressed in 30 minutes of training in each session and 10 minutes of review of family progress; 50 minutes was focused more directly on the patient. The family component included extensive psychoeducation on OCD and anxiety management, training in appropriate rational responses to OCD, managing behavioral difficulties, problem-solving strategies, and coaching on ways to withdraw accommodation. The therapy protocol was developed into a published manual (Barrett 2007). The results showed that their CBT program involving the family was effective in reducing OCD symptoms in both individual and group formats. At the end of treatment, 88% of the children in the individual family treatment and 76% in the group family treatment were without an OCD diagnosis; all the children on the wait-list retained their OCD diagnosis. Using the diagnostic measure and two symptom severity measures – the Children's Yale–Brown Obsessive Compulsive Scale (CY-BOCS; Scahill et al. 1997) and NIMH Global Obsessive Compulsive Scale (Insel et al. 1983) – there were no differences between the two active groups, but both differed from the control group. A follow-up study of 90% of the original treatment groups found that these gains were maintained at 12 and 18 months, with 70% of those in the individual family CBT and 84% in the group family CBT considered diagnosis free at 18 months (Barrett at al 2005). These treatments also improved family function. There is evidence to suggest that group therapy is somewhat more effective than individual therapy in reducing the young person's anxiety (Barrett et al. 2004).

The second study was conducted by Storch and colleagues (2007) and compared weekly versus intensive individual family CBT. In the intensive condition, 14 sessions were held over three weeks; in the weekly format, the sessions were held over 14 weeks. Treatment was based on the manual developed by Lewin et al. (2005), which was modified to have greater family involvement; at least one parent participated in every session. Although participants were randomly assigned, the weekly group was older and had less-severe OCD than the intensive group. The intensive group showed greater gains at the end of treatment although the two groups were equal at the three-month follow-up.

Treatment of adults

There is some research on family, individual, and group CBT used as the primary therapeutic modality in the treatment of adults with OCD. Unlike the research with OCD in children, these studies did test whether the inclusion of family members was more beneficial than treatment of the individual alone. Unfortunately, the results are not as clear as might be hoped. The inclusion of family members seems to be helpful but in some cases the advantage was not long lasting. It is certainly not a disadvantage to include willing family members, although, understandably, the inclusion of hostile family members can be a problem unless their hostility can be tamed.

Van Noppen and Steketee have developed a successful multifamily behavioral group treatment (Van Noppen et al. 1993, 1997; Steketee and Van Noppen 1998; Van Noppen 2002; Steketee and Van Noppen 2003). In 1997, Van Noppen and her colleagues published a pilot study of group and multifamily group treatment for OCD that showed that the inclusion of families was promising; further research supported the approach, although more research would be valuable to clarify the extent and permanence of the advantage over individual therapy.

The following description of the treatment program is based on three published summaries: Steketee and Van Noppen (1998), Van Noppen (2002), and Van Noppen and Steketee (2003). The groups include five to seven families, resulting in 10 to 16 members per group and are led by two therapists. The intake session(s) for each patient is used to get a detailed history and current OCD status and involve spending time with the patient alone as well as time with the patient and the family member(s) who will participate in the group. The group meets for two hours weekly for 12 weeks and monthly for an additional six months. These sessions are outlined in detail in the publications. They include psychoeducation about OCD (e.g., what is

Table 12.3 Assessment instruments

Title	Variable	Test
Individual	Severity of obsessive-compulsive symptoms	Yale–Brown Obsessive Compulsive Scale (Y-BOCS), child scale (CY-BOCS), self-report (Y-BOCS-SR) (Goodman *et al.* 1989a, 1989b; Scahill *et al.* 1997)
Family	Parental high expressed emotion	Level of Expressed Emotion (LEE) scale (Cole and Kazarian 1988)
	Parental hostile criticism	Perceived criticism measure (Hooley and Teasdale 1989)
	Parental emotional overinvolvement	Influential Relationships Questionnaire (IRQ) (Cole and Kazarian 1988)
	Family accommodation	Family Attitude Scale (FAS) (Calvocoressi *et al.* 1995)

OCD, how is OCD treated, behavior therapy, exposure and response prevention [ERP], neurobiology, medications), family issues (including understanding responses to OCD, guidelines for responding to the OCD patient, communication skills training, contracting), the use of self-help materials, in vivo ERP in and out of session, imaginal ERP.

Summary: the family in OCD treatment

If possible, it seems advisable to integrate the family extensively in the treatment program of children and adolescents and to some extent in the treatment of adults who live with family members (parents or spouses and/or children). In many situations, it may be more feasible to have adjunctive involvement of the family. Some studies have included support groups for family members (Marks *et al.* 1975) or spouses (Hand and Tichatzky 1979), or family psychoeducation without involving the families extensively in the therapy itself (Tynes *et al.* 1990; Krone *et al.* 1991; Black and Blum 1992; Cooper 1993).

Assessment

Moving from the theory and research to plan an efficacious OCD intervention, it is important to assess obsessive-compulsive symptoms, family dysfunction, family accommodation as well as levels of expressed emotion, hostile criticism and emotional over-involvement in significant others. Several instruments have been used to assess these variables

(Table 12.3); these can be used to plan and to assess treatment.

Suggested guidelines for family involvement in treatment

As described above, the treatment of OCD patients can benefit from having their family members or significant others involved in their treatment. While this is common for children, it has not been incorporated into adult treatment on a large scale. Certain treatment centers have developed treatment plans that involve family members in groups but there are many settings, including private practice, where this is not practical. However, what has been learned from research to date can be used to guide family involvement in OCD treatment. Following are suggested topics and interventions that should be considered when treating OCD patients, both children and adults; special considerations for children are included.

Support for family members

Clearly having a family member with OCD is very stressful and it may be valuable in some cases for the family members to receive supportive therapy themselves or, depending on the community, go to meetings for families of OCD patients. Of course, if possible, they can be involved in some sessions with the patients themselves; even if this is not possible, support for the families can be helpful by itself. There are certain family issues that are pertinent to most OCD treatment, but in cases where the family has many additional issues or is highly dysfunctional, it is strongly suggested that their larger issues be addressed in family therapy.

Psychoeducation

In addition to general information about OCD, certain key issues often need to be addressed. Most studies of family involvement in the treatment of OCD have focused some attention on accommodation and hostility, which are critical family problems that can interfere with treatment or lead to relapse. They are best imbedded in the context of general information about OCD itself and OCD treatment.

When working with children, especially young children, special considerations are necessary. It is particularly important to ensure that parents clearly understand the treatment program and rationale before the child is introduced to treatment; this will lay the groundwork because many young children will not fully understand the treatment rationale. Additionally, parents need to be involved more directly in the out of session assignments for young children.

As noted above, psychoeducation can be provided to the patient and family members together or separately. However, in general, it can be valuable for families to have psychoeducation that is comparable to that received by the patients. This would include the following:

- explaining OCD as a medical illness; it can be compared with illnesses such as asthma or diabetes
- correcting erroneous beliefs about OCD
- learning to differentiate OCD from other patient issues
- explaining that anyone can have odd thoughts and the way to deal with them is to ignore them; trying to avoid, suppress or neutralize the thoughts will only cause them to return more strongly than before
- externalizing the OCD by fostering the view of OCD as a medical illness separate from the patient's core identity
- introducing the basics of ERP, including rating anxiety using the Subjective Units of Distress Scale (SUDS; Wolpe 1958) or, for children, a fear thermometer

- covering issues such as confidentiality, attendance, respectful interactions and socializing outside of groups if group therapy is being utilized.

he therapist can help in explaining these points by using techniques such as stories and imagery. For example a story about habits and intrusive thoughts and the effects of control might be where the child is asked to try *not* to picture a white bear in a red landscape. This will show that such an attempt at control might actually increase the frequency of this thought (Bailey 2001). It can also be valuable to create an image of the OCD as an enemy, not just a bad habit. With children, using a disparaging name for OCD can be helpful; for adults, labeling the OCD can serve a similar purpose. The therapist "externalizes" OCD (Epston and White 1990) so that OCD becomes a discrete "enemy" and not a "bad habit," which may have been associated with previous negative experiences or a disliked aspect of the patient's own character. It is important to clarify that both the patient and the family already have some influence on this enemy. In this way, therapist, patient, and family become members of the same team with a unified goal of helping the patient get rid of the OCD.

Change family interactions involving the patient and the OCD

An overarching goal is to have family members disengage from the OCD and develop more normal family functioning and interactions with the affected family member. To accomplish this they need to change their interactions, if the involvement is at all extensive, it needs to be tapered in a planned, slow manner. Guidelines for interacting with the family member include:

Ignore the OCD. The family should find other ways to interact with the patient, reinforcing more positive behaviors not the OCD. Family members can use their attention to change the patient's behavior (Freeman and Garcia 2008). Give attention to behavior they want and withhold attention from the behavior they do not want. Parents, in particular, need to know that children do all sorts of things to get attention. For many children, adult attention is rewarding whether it is positive (i.e., good job!) or negative (I told you to stop doing that!).

Reduce accommodation. Over time, the family should withdraw from accommodating the OCD. In most cases, this is best done in a gradual, planned way that has been negotiated with the patient. Common targets would be to:

- stop offering reassurance
- withdraw from participating in or facilitating rituals (cleaning things for the patient versus buying cleaning supplies)
- stop changing the family activities to help (e.g., going places late because the person needed extra time to perform rituals)
- work on fostering good communication skills, which, in addition to the earlier and ongoing psychoeducation about OCD, will be used to reduce hostility and other aspects of high expressed emotion.

Overinvolvement. Specific attention may need to be paid to overinvolvement, although reducing accommodation will be very helpful with this as well.

Active involvement in therapy

Family members should understand the basics of ERP, how it applies both to classic exposures and to ritual reduction. But as therapy proceeds, they need to understand how it is being applied in the patient's specific therapy and what the weekly therapeutic goals are so that they will understand the therapy and can be guided in how to help the patient. With children, parental involvement will be necessary. With teenage and adult patients, it can be very valuable but care must be taken to involve the patient in negotiating contracts about the ritual changes and in not only agreeing to the specific exposures but agreeing on whether/how the family members would be involved.

The therapist can do parent check-in at the beginning and/or end of each session where the therapist would invite parents to comment on how the child is progressing in the struggle against OCD.

Relaxation training can be used for both the patient and the family members. Parents, in particular, may need to learn to tolerate their own distress in the face of assisting their children with exposure exercises and other homework tasks (Pollack and Carter 1999). Relaxation training could include breathing retraining and progressive muscle relaxation.

Conclusions

Although research is still needed into the role of the family in the development and treatment of OCD, family involvement in the treatment of patients with OCD is established in child treatment and promising in adults. Although the dynamics of individual families certainly differ, certain factors are commonly found to contribute to OCD, interfere with treatment, and predict relapse. These are accommodation to the OCD symptoms and a hostile, critical response. Therefore, it seems wise for therapists to pay attention to the role that family members and significant others play in the life of their patients with OCD and to take steps to work to create a more favorable environment for therapeutic success and the maintenance of gains.

References

Allsopp M, Verduyn C (1990). Adolescents with obsessive–compulsive disorder: a case note review of consecutive patients referred to a provincial regional adolescent psychiatry unit. *J Adolesc* **13**: 157–169.

Alonso P, Menchón J, Mataix-Cols D, *et al.* (2004). Perceived parental rearing style in obsessive–compulsive disorder: relation to symptom dimensions. *Psychiatry Res* **127**: 267–278.

Amir N, Freshman M, Foa E (2000). Family distress and involvement in relatives of obsessive-compulsive disorder patients. *J Anxiety Disord* **14**: 209–217.

Asbahr FR, Castillo AR, Ito LM, *et al.* (2005). Group cognitive–behavioral therapy versus sertraline for the treatment of children and adolescents with obsessive–compulsive disorder. *J Am Acad Child Adolesc Psychiatry* **44**: 1128–1136.

Bailey V (2001). Cognitive–behavioural therapies for children and adolescents. *Adv Psychiatr Treat* **7**: 224–232.

Barrett PM (2007). *FOCUS: Freedom from Obsessions and Compulsions Using Skills (Therapist Manual and Workbooks)*. Brisbane: Pathways Health and Research Centre.

Barrett PM, Rasmussen P, Healy LJ (2001). The effects of obsessive–compulsive disorder on sibling relationships in late childhood and early adolescence: Preliminary findings. *Aust Educ Dev Psychol* **17**: 82–102.

Barrett PM, Shortt A, Healy L (2002). Do parent and child behaviours differentiate families whose children have obsessive-compulsive disorder from other clinic and non-clinic families? *J Child Psychol Psychiatry* **43**: 597–607.

Barrett PM, Healy-Farrell L, March JS (2004). Cognitive-behavioral family treatment of childhood obsessive-compulsive disorder: a controlled trial. *J Am Acad Child Adolesc Psychiatry* **43**: 46–62.

Barrett PM, Farrell LJ, Dadds M, Boulter N (2005). Cognitive–behavioral family treatment of childhood obsessive–compulsive disorder: long-term follow-up and predictors of outcome. *J Am Acad Child Adolesc Psychiatry* **44**: 1005–1014.

Benazon NR, Ager J, Rosenberg DR (2002). Cognitive behavior therapy in treatment-naive children and adolescents with obsessive-compulsive disorder: an open trial. *Behav Res Ther* **40**: 529–39.

Black DW, Blum NS (1992). Obsessive-compulsive disorder support groups: the Iowa model. *Compr Psychiatry* **33**: 65–71.

Bolton D, Perrin S (2008). Evaluation of exposure with response-prevention for obsessive compulsive disorder in childhood and adolescence. *J Behav Ther Exp Psychiatry* **39**: 11–22.

Bolton D, Collins S, Steinberg D (1983). The treatment of obsessive–compulsive disorder in adolescence: a report of 15 cases. *Br J Psychiatry* **142**: 456–464.

Bressi C, Guggeri G (1996). Obsessive-compulsive disorder and the family emotional environment. *New Trend Exp Clin Psychol* **12**: 265–269.

Calvocoressi L, Lewis B, Harris M, *et al.* (1995). Family accommodation in obsessive compulsive disorder. *Am J Psychiatry* **152**: 441–443.

Capps L, Sigman M, Sena R, Henker B, Whalen C (1996). Fear, anxiety and perceived control in children of agoraphobic parents. *J Child Psychol Psychiatry* **37**: 445–452.

Cavedo LC, Parker G (1994). Parental bonding instrument: exploring links between scores and obsessionality. *Social Psychiatry Psychiatr Epidemiol* **29**: 78–82.

Chambless DL, Steketee G (1999). Expressed emotion and behavior therapy outcome: a prospective study with obsessive- compulsive and agoraphobic outpatients. *J Consult Clin Psychol* **67**: 658–665.

Chorpita BF, Barlow DH (1998). The development of anxiety: the role of control in the early environment. *Psychol Bull* **124**: 3–21.

Cole JD, Kazarian SS (1988). The Level of Expressed Emotion Scale: a new measure of expressed emotion. *J Clin Psychol* **44**: 392–397.

Cooper M (1993). A group for families of obsessive-compulsive persons. *Fam Soc* **77**: 301–307.

Cooper M (1996). Obsessive-compulsive disorder: effects on family members. *Am J Orthopsychiatry* **66**: 296–304.

Crisp AH, Gelder MG, Rix S, Meltzer HI, Rowlands OJ (2000). Stigmatisation of people with mental illness. *Br J Psychiatry* **177**: 4–7.

Epston, D, White M (1990). *Narrative Means to Therapeutic Ends*. New York: Norton.

Fischer DJ, Himle JA, Hanna GL (1998). Group behavioral therapy for adolescents with obsessive-compulsive disorder: preliminary outcomes. *Res Social Work Pract* **8**: 629–636.

Franklin ME, Kozak MJ, Cashman LA, *et al.* (1998). Cognitive-behavioral treatment of pediatric obsessive-compulsive disorder: an open clinical trial. *J Am Acad Child Adolesc Psychiatry* **37**: 412–419.

Freeman JB, Garcia AM (2008). *Family Based Treatment for Young Children with OCD: Therapist Guide*. New York: Oxford University Press.

Ginsburg GS, Kingery JN, Drake KL, Grados MA (2008). Predictors of treatment response in pediatric obsessive-compulsive disorder. *J Am Acad Child Adolesc Psychiatry* **47**: 868–878.

Goodman WK, Price LH, Rasmussen SA, *et al.* (1989a). The Yale–Brown obsessive compulsive scale: II validity. *Arch Gen Psychiatry* **46**: 1006–1011.

Goodman WK, Price LH, Rasmussen SA, *et al.* (1989b). The Yale–Brown obsessive compulsive scale: II validity. *Arch Gen Psychiatry* **46**: 1012–1016.

Grunes MS, Neziroglu F, McKay D (2001). Family involvement in the behavioral treatment of obsessive-compulsive disorder: a preliminary investigation. *Behav Ther* **32**: 803–820.

Hand I, Tichatzky M (1979). Behavioral group therapy for obsessions and compulsions: First results of a pilot study. In Sjoden PO, Bates D, Dockens WS (eds.) *Trends in Behavioral Therapy* (pp. 269–297). New York: Academic Press,

Hafner RJ (1998). Obsessive–compulsive disorder: a questionnaire survey of a self-help group. *Int J Soc Psychiatry* **34**: 310–315.

Henin A, Kendall PC (1997). Obsessive-compulsive disorder in childhood and adolescence. *Adv Clin Child Psychol* **19**: 75–131.

Hibbs ED, Hamburger SD, Lenane M, *et al.* (1991). Determinants of expressed emotion in families of disturbed and normal children. *J Child Psychol Psychiatry* **32**: 757–770.

Himle JA, Fischer DJ, Van Etten ML, Janeck AS, Hanna GL (2003). Group behavioral therapy for adolescents with tic-related and non-tic-related obsessive-compulsive disorder. *Depress Anxiety* **17**: 73–77.

Hollander E, Kwon K, Stein DJ, *et al.* (1996). Obsessive-compulsive and spectrum disorders: Overview and quality of life issues. *J Clin Psychiatry* **57**(Suppl 8): 3–6.

Hooley JM, Teasdale JD (1989). Predictors of relapse in unipolar depressives: expressed emotion, marital distress, and perceived criticism. *J Abnorm Psychol* **98**: 229–235.

Insel TR, Murphy DL, Cohen RM, *et al.* (1983). Obsessive-compulsive disorder: a double-blind trial of clomipramine and clorgyline. *Arch Gen Psychiatry* **40**: 605–612.

Kalra H, Kamath P, Trivedi JK, Janca A (2008). Caregiver burden in anxiety disorders. *Curr Opin Psychiatry* **21**: 70–3.

Kohlmann CW, Schumacher A, Streit R (1988). Trait anxiety and parental child-rearing behavior: support as a moderator variable. *Anxiety Res* **1**: 53–64.

Koran L (2000). Quality of life in obsessive-compulsive disorder. *Psychiatr Clin N Am* **23**: 509–517.

Krone KP, Himle JA, Nesse RM (1991). A standardized behavioral group treatment program for obsessive-compulsive disorder: preliminary outcomes. *Behav Res Ther* **29**: 627–632.

Leonard H, Swedo SE, Lenane MC, *et al.* (1993). A 2- to 7-year follow-up study of 54 obsessive-compulsive children and adolescents. *Arch Gen Psychiatry* **50**: 429–439.

Lewin AB, Storch EA, Merlo LJ, *et al.* (2005), Intensive cognitive behavioral therapy for pediatric obsessive compulsive disorder: a treatment protocol for mental health providers. *Psychol Serv* **2**: 91Y104.

Livingston-Van Noppen B, Rasmussen SA, Eisen J, McCarthey L (1990). Family function and treatment in obsessive-compulsive disorder. In Jenike MA, Baer L, Minichiello WE (eds.) *Obsessive Compulsive Disorders: Theory and Management* (pp. 325–340). Chicago, IL: Yearbook Medical.

Magliano L, Tosini P, Guarneri M, Marasco C, Catapano F (1996). Burden on the families of patients with obsessive-compulsive disorder: a pilot study. *Eur Psychiatry* **11**: 192–197.

March J, Mulle K (1998). *OCD in Children and Adolescents: A Cognitive-Behavioral Treatment Manual*. New York: Guilford Press.

March JS, Mulle K, Herbel B (1994). Behavioral psychotherapy for children and adolescents with obsessive–compulsive disorder: an open trial of a new protocol driven treatment package. *J Am Acad Child Adolesc Psychiatry* **33**: 333–341.

Marks IM, Hodgson R, Rachman S (1975). Treatment of chronic obsessive-compulsive neurosis by in-vivo exposure: a two-year follow-up and issues in treatment. *Br J Psychiatry* **527**: 349–364.

Martin JL, Thienemann M (2005). Group cognitive-behavior therapy with family involvement for middle-school-age

children with obsessive-compulsive disorder: a pilot study. *Child Psychiatry Hum Dev* **36**: 113–127.

Pediatric OCD Treatment Study Team (2004). Cognitive–behavioral therapy, sertraline, and their combination for children and adolescents with obsessive–compulsive disorder: The Pediatric OCD Treatment Study (POTS) randomized controlled trial. *JAMA* **292**: 1969–1976.

Phelan JC, Link BG (1998). The growing belief that people with mental illnesses are violent: the role of the dangerousness criterion for civil commitment. *Social Psychiatry Psychiatr Epidemiol* **33**(Suppl 1): S7–S12.

Phelan JC, Bromet EJ, Link BG (1998). Psychiatric illness and family stigma. *Schizophr Bull* **24**: 115–126.

Piacentini J, Gitow A, Jaffer M, Graae F, Whitaker A (1994). Outpatient behavioral treatment of child and adolescent obsessive-compulsive disorder. *J Anxiety Disord* **8**: 277–289.

Piacentini J, Bergman RL, Jacobs C, McCracken JT, Kretchman J (2002). Open trial of cognitive behavior therapy for childhood obsessive-compulsive disorder. *J Anxiety Disord* **16**: 207–219.

Pollock RA, Carter AS (1999). The familial and developmental context of obsessive-compulsive disorder. *Child Adolesc Psychiatr Clin N Am* **8**: 461–479.

Rachman S (1993). Obsessions, responsibility, and guilt. *Behav Res Ther* **31**: 149–154.

Rachman S (1997). A cognitive theory of obsessions. *Behav Res Ther* **36**: 385–401.

Rachman S (1998). A cognitive theory of obsessions: elaborations. *Behav Res Ther* **35**: 793–802.

Rachman SJ, Hodgson RJ (1980). *Obsessions and Compulsions* (pp. 57–68). Englewood Cliffs, NJ: Prentice-Hall.

Renshaw KD, Chambless DL, Rodebaugh TL, Steketee G (2000). Living with severe anxietydisorders: relatives' distress and reactions to patient behaviours. *Clin Psychol Psychother* **7**: 190–200.

Renshaw KD, Chambless DL, Steketee G (2003). Perceived criticism predicts severity of anxiety symptoms after behavioral treatment in patients with obsessive-compulsive disorder and panic disorder with agoraphobia. *J Clin Psychol* **59**: 411–421.

Salkovskis PM (1985). Obsessional compulsive problems: a cognitive behavioral analysis. *Behav Res Ther* **23**: 571–583.

Salkovskis PM (1998). Cognitive behavioral approach to understanding obsessional thinking. *Br J Psychiatry* **173** (Suppl 35): 53–63.

Salkovskis PM, Richards CH, Forrester E (1995). The relationship between obsessional problems and intrusive thoughts. *Behav Cogn Psychother* **23**: 281–299.

Salkovskis P, Shafran R, Rachman S, Freeston MH (1999). Multiple pathways to inflated responsibility beliefs in obsessional problems: possible origins and implications for therapy and research. *Behav Res Ther* 37: 1055–1072.

Scahill L, Vitulano LA, Brenner EM, Lynch KA, King RA (1996). Behavioral therapy in children and adolescents with obsessive-compulsive disorder: a pilot study. *J Child Adolesc Psychopharmacol* 6: 191–202.

Scahill L, Riddle M, McSwiggin-Hardin M, *et al.* (1997). Children's Yale–Brown Obsessive Compulsive Scale: reliability and validity. *J Am Acad Child Adolesc Psychiatry* 36: 844–852.

Shafran R, Ralph J, Tallis F (1995). Obsessive-compulsive symptoms and the family. *Bull Menninger Clin* 59: 472–479.

Stein DJ, Roberts M, Hollander E, Rowland C, Serebro P (1996). Quality of life and pharmaco-economic aspects of obsessive-compulsive disorder. *S Afr Med J* 36: 1579–1585.

Steketee G (1993). Social support and treatment outcome of obsessive compulsive disorder at 9-month follow-up. *Behav Psychother* 21: 81–95.

Steketee G (1997). Disability and family burden in obsessive-compulsive disorder. *Can J Psychiatry* 42: 919–928.

Steketee G, Van Noppen B (1998). Group and family treatment for obsessive-compulsive disorder. In Jenike MA, Baer L, Minichiello WE (eds.) *Obsessive-Compulsive Disorders: Practical Management*, 3rd edn (pp. 443–468). St Louis, MO: Mosby.

Steketee G, Van Noppen B (2003). Family approaches to treatment for obsessive-compulsive disorder. *Rev Bras Psiquiatr* 25: 43–50.

Stengler-Wenzke K, Trosbach J, Dietrich S, Angermeyer MC (2004). Experience of stigmatization by relatives of patients with obsessive compulsive disorder. *Arch Psychiatr Nurs* 18: 88–96.

Stengler-Wenzke K, Kroll M, Matschinger H, Angermeyer MC (2006). Quality of life of relatives of patients with obsessive compulsive disorder. *Compr Psychiatry* 47: 523–527.

Stewart SE, Beresin C, Haddad S, *et al.* (2008). Predictors of family accommodation in obsessive-compulsive disorder. *Ann Clin Psychiatry* 20: 65–70.

Storch EA, Geffken GR, Merlo LJ, *et al.* (2007). Family-based cognitive-behavioral therapy for pediatric obsessive-compulsive disorder: comparison of intensive and weekly approaches. *J Am Acad Child Adolesc Psychiatry* 46: 469–478.

Thienemann M, Martin J, Cregger B, Thompson HB, Dyer-Friedman J (2001). Manual-driven group cognitive-behavioral therapy for adolescents with obsessive-compulsive disorder: a pilot study. *J Am Acad Child Adolesc Psychiatry* 11: 1254–1260.

Tynes L, Salins C, Winstead D (1990). Obsessive-compulsive patients: familial frustration and criticism. *J Louisiana State Med Soc* 142: 24–26, 28–29.

Valderhaug R, Larsson B, Götestam KG, Piacentini J (2007). An open clinical trial of cognitive–behavior therapy in children and adolescents with obsessive–compulsive disorder administered in regular outpatient clinics. *Behav Res Ther* 45: 577–589.

Valleni-Basile LA, Garrison CZ, Jackson KL, *et al.* (1995). Family and psychosocial predictors of obsessive compulsive disorder in a community sample of young adolescents. *J Child Fam Stud* 4: 193–206.

Van Noppen B (2002). Multifamily behavioral treatment (MFBT) for obsessive-compulsive disorder: a step by step model. *Brief Treat Crisis Interv* 2: 107–122.

Van Noppen B, Steketee G (2003). Family responses and multifamily behavioral treatment for obsessive-compulsive disorder. *Brief Treat Crisis Interv* 3: 231–247.

Van Noppen B, Pato M, Rasmussen S (1993). *Learning to Live with OCD*. Milfor, MA: Obsessive Compulsive Foundation.

Van Noppen B, Steketee G, McCorkle BH, Pato M (1997). Group and multifamily behavioral treatment for obsessive-compulsive disorder. *J Anxiety Disord* 11: 431–46.

Wahl OF, Harman CR (1989). Family views of stigma. *Schizophr Bull* 15: 131–139.

Waters TL, Barrett PM (2000). The role of the family in childhood obsessive–compulsive disorder. *Clin Child Fam Psychol Rev* 3: 173–184.

Waters TL, Barrett PM, March JS (2001). Cognitive-behavioral family treatment of childhood obsessive-compulsive disorder: preliminary findings. *Am J Psychother* 55: 372–387.

Wever C, Rey JM (1997). Juvenile obsessive-compulsive disorder. *Aust N Z J Psychiatry* 31: 105–113.

WHOQOL Group (1998). Development of the World Health Organization WHOQOL–BREF quality of life assessment. *Social Sci Med* 28: 551–558.

Wolpe J (1958). *Psychotherapy by Reciprocal Inhibition*. Stanford, CA: Stanford University Press.

Providing treatment for patients with obsessive-compulsive disorder

Terri Laterza, Kalie D. Pierce, and Robert Hudak

Introduction

The purpose of this chapter is to provide an overview of the data concerning the intensity of exposure with response prevention (ERP) and its effect on the treatment of obsessive-compulsive disorder (OCD). The different levels of intensity will be discussed, as well as the factors that clinicians need to consider when determining the proper level of care for their patients. Case examples will be provided to illustrate how decision making was utilized in determining which type of care would lead to the best outcome. Finally, a list of programs which provide intensive treatment for OCD will be provided.

The ERP approach is a specific type of cognitive-behavioral therapy (CBT) that is used in the treatment of OCD. It has been shown to be the most effective psychotherapy for the treatment of OCD (Chs. 8 and 10) and is superior to other psychotherapies, such as relaxation therapy (Griest *et al.* 2002). However, even with the efficacy of ERP well studied, only 18% of patients with OCD have been offered an adequate trial of ERP (Blanco *et al.* 2006). Since ERP is considered a first-line treatment for OCD (March *et al.* 1997), it should be offered to more individuals. While simply obtaining adequate ERP is important, determining the specific design of the treatment protocol that should be implemented is equally important in setting up a treatment plan for patients. There are different levels of ERP treatment available, such as regular outpatient visits (typically one or more hours per week), intensive outpatient therapy (IOP; typically three hours per day at least three days per week), intensive residential treatment (IRT), or inpatient hospital treatment. There has been limited research regarding the appropriate setting and level of care of ERP, and some guidelines do not address appropriate levels of care

(American Academy of Child Adolescent Psychiatry 1998). Additional data are needed in areas such as the optimal length of a psychotherapy session, frequency of sessions, and in the number of sessions (American Psychiatric Association 2007). Other ways to design therapy sessions such as individual versus group therapy and therapies that include family members are also not adequately studied as of this time. The different levels of care available can be summarized as follows:

Outpatient treatment. This consists of visits with a therapist trained in the treatment of OCD by utilizing ERP, as well as other psychotherapeutic interventions such as additional cognitive techniques as appropriate. Treatment may be individual or in a group. Since ERP is generally not taught in any of the advanced graduate programs for mental health professionals, a therapist must learn ERP in other ways. Typically, a qualified therapist has either trained in a specialized OCD treatment center or has taken a weekend long seminar dedicated to teaching ERP. The Behavioral Therapy Institute, run in conjunction with the International Obsessive Compulsive Disorder Foundation, has trained many therapists in this manner. Their course also provides telephone supervision after the seminar has concluded. Self-assisted therapy using workbooks along with a voice-activated telephone system are available and the efficacy of these programs has been studied (Marks *et al.* 1998).

Intensive outpatient therapy. Such intensive therapy is provided in multi-hour sessions performed several days per week. There is no single standard regarding the construction of an IOP program for OCD. Different formats

---

Clinical Obsessive-Compulsive Disorders in Adults and Children, ed. Robert Hudak and Darin D. Dougherty.
Published by Cambridge University Press. Copyright © Cambridge University Press 2011.

exist in different treatment centers, and it may consist of individual and/or group sessions.

Partial hospitalization. This approach has been used successfully in the treatment of OCD (Bystritsky *et al.* 1996) and is useful in providing transition from the structure of an inpatient setting to the patient's normal environment. Reducing symptoms to a level consistent with less-intensive therapeutic settings is a primary goal. It typically runs approximately six hours a day and occurs five days per week. Nursing care, ERP, pharmacotherapy, and illness education is typically offered in individual and group formats. Partial hospitalization treatment settings have become less common in the USA as IOP as become more popular. Reimbursement by insurance companies was a major influence in this trend.

Intensive residential treatment. A very limited number of sites in the USA provide IRT. It is a specialized approach in which patients stay at the treatment center, thus enabling close monitoring. Participants will typically receive two to four hours of psychotherapy daily in a highly structured environment, as well as weekly sessions with a psychopharmacologist. Patients also meet with social work staff, nurses, behavioral therapists, and participate in both individual sessions and group psychotherapy (Stewart *et al.* 2005).

Inpatient hospital treatment. The use of specialized OCD units is currently not available in the USA but is available in the UK. This is reserved for patients who cannot be managed as outpatients owing to the nature or extent of their condition and the need for 24-hour nursing care (Drummond *et al.* 2007). Reasons for inpatient care include being a danger to self, either through suicide risk or self-neglect, or having complicating comorbid conditions (Boschen *et al.* 2008).

In order to obtain the maximum benefit from outpatient psychotherapy, ERP sessions should be scheduled at least on a once a week basis (March *et al.* 1997) and between 13–20 sessions are recommended for the majority of patients although Van Noppen *et al.* (1997) noted improvement with as few as 10 sessions in a group format. In that study, the first session was educational in nature, with the remaining sessions focusing on treatment. Advantages to the group format included reducing the stigma of OCD, allowing patients to imitate and learn positive techniques from each other, and the competitive nature of groups, which enabled people to feel comfortable taking more risks. Patients whose illness is more severe or who have required more intensive therapy in the past should be considered for more intensive treatment. A study involving therapy on two days a week versus five days a week showed that there was no significant difference with the more intensive regimen, although there was a trend towards greater improvement in that group (Abramowitz *et al.* 2003). Severe, treatment-resistant OCD has been shown to respond to inpatient treatment, with the majority of participants obtaining a significant reduction in the severity of their symptoms (Drummond 1993; Drummond *et al.* 2007). Additionally, these individuals have maintained their progress as assessed in follow-up evaluations 18 months following discharge (Boschen *et al.* 2008). Patients can be treated with group therapy as well and individual treatment.

According to the Expert Consensus Guidelines (March *et al.* 1997), patients with mild OCD symptoms can be offered ERP as a first-line treatment, medication in conjunction with ERP being reserved for moderate and severe symptoms. While traditional outpatient ERP is recommended at initial presentation, IRT can also be offered as first-line treatment for any OCD regardless of symptoms or severity if the patient desires greater than one hour per week of treatment.

The IRT approach was developed to treat patients with severe OCD who had failed other standard outpatient treatment modalities (Stewart *et al.* 2005) and as an alternative to other approaches for refractory illness such as neurosurgery or intravenous medications. More intensive treatment has been shown to be successful even when less-intensive interventions have not worked. The predictors of positive outcomes in IRT include factors such as the presence of contamination obsessions, overt rituals, absence of depression, living with family, being employed during treatment, never having been treated previously (Buchanan *et al.* 1996), female gender, lower initial OCD severity, and higher psychosocial functioning (Stewart *et al.* 2006). The greater response is likely a gender effect rather than other confounding factors, and females have been found to be more compliant with CBT in general. The reason for the response to IRT in treatment-refractory patients is hypothesized to be at least partially caused by a "last chance" mentality, as patients usually have failed all other prior treatment modalities (Stewart *et al.* 2009). The finding that living alone after IRT predicts a worse outcome is significant. This may be because of such factors as a decrease in social supports, and so recommending that patients live with family after IRT may improve outcomes (Stewart *et al.* 2009).

Considerations for intensive treatments

There are various factors to consider when determining if a patient with OCD may need a higher level of care than traditional outpatient ERP therapy. While overall severity of the illness (as measured by a scale such as the Yale–Brown Obsessive Compulsive Scale [Y-BOCS]) is an important consideration, an individual's psychosocial functioning is not always directly correlated to the severity of symptoms. Among psychiatric illnesses, OCD is unusual in that patients can have marked differences in their level of impairment in different facets of their lives. It is common for patients to report that they function at work reasonably well, but "save up" their rituals for when they go home at night. If their rituals are severe enough, they may spend most of their non-work time involved with compulsions, with little time left over for socializing, family, and even eating and sleeping. As a result, someone may function well at work but perform very poorly in other spheres of their life. Therefore, a good psychosocial assessment is needed to fully evaluate not only the severity of patient's symptom but all of the areas of their life that the illness may be impacting. Regardless of the patient's impairment, most clinicians will agree that patients with moderate/severe level of symptoms should be offered intensive therapy, and that even patients with mild symptoms can be given intensive outpatient therapy if the patient requests it (March *et al.* 1997).

A partial but inadequate treatment response to lower levels of care is a reason to consider a referral to a higher level of care. This may be indicative of treatment effectiveness and need for greater frequency of sessions. A patient may be appropriate for a higher level of care if they are unable to resist rituals without environmental interventions or if their functioning has been significantly impaired in several aspects. For example, a patient who has washing rituals and is unable to resist engaging in these rituals unless the water in the house has been turned off, or a patient whose symptoms have rendered him confined to his home or strict geographical area, is likely to benefit from a higher level of care. A significant comorbid illness such as major depressive disorder and difficulty tolerating anxiety or discomfort may also be reasons to refer a client to a higher level of care. Maintaining the safety and increasing an individual's general coping skills (e.g., sleep hygiene, healthful eating, and managing other factors that increase emotional vulnerability) may also suggest a more concentrated treatment protocol. A patient may have difficulty tolerating the anxiety of an exposure without a therapist, whose mere presence creates a level of /safety. This situation will often necessitate longer and more frequent sessions, with the goal of increasing independence as the patient builds confidence in the treatment. Patients who have difficulty interpreting their obsessions as irrational may do well with higher levels of care. For example, a patient may hold the beliefs that having an intrusive thought means they are very likely to act on it: having the thought is just as bad as having done the action (thought–fusion action) and indicative of their "true nature." A patient with such belief (e.g., involving harming obsessions) initially may do better in a more structured and, to the patient, a "safer" environment to ensure them that they and others are safe. With slightly reduced anxiety from being in safe place (an intensive treatment setting with trained professionals who may stop the patient from acting on thoughts), the patient may be willing to explore and address these obsessions with the eventual goal of successfully completing similar work in lower levels of care.

Another factor to consider is the impact the OCD exerts on the individual's general health. Rituals may have progressed to the point where they have a negative impact on the patient's and/or family's health and well-being. Examples include using industrial grade chemicals to decontaminate the house, threatening his or her and the family's health; using chemicals on the skin to the point where integrity of skin has been compromised; and rituals that significantly interfere with activities of daily living including sleep cycle, patient's ability to eat/drink, and the ability to care for children.

A lack of social/family support as well as additional life stressors may indicate a need for a higher level of care. Patients may be unable to engage in family and social activities, unable to complete activities of daily living/household chores, unable to work, and/or laid off from work. The lack of daily structure that these activities provide is likely to create an opportunity for the patient to engage in obsessions and compulsions for longer amounts of time. Higher levels of care often provide a helpful structure to a patient's day. In addition, it creates a framework in which patients are given more support; are held accountable for homework exposures, and helps them to engage in exposures in different environments and with different people in order to generalize treatment gains.

When deciding what level of care is appropriate, it is also important to consider such practical factors as time constraints, patient willingness and motivation, family willingness and motivation, availability of treatment, and financial aspects including insurance coverage. Some patients will choose to participate in higher levels of care because of time constraints (e.g., college students on a break hoping to return when classes resume and people on time-limited leave from work). Some patients may not have a flexible enough schedule to participate in higher levels of care (may not have time off from work/school or adequate childcare), requiring them to participate in a lower level of care. Also, a patient's motivation to engage in treatment of any kind, including higher levels of care, may increase when approaching a life transition or particular circumstance (e.g., partner threatens to leave if patient does not get treatment, new romantic relationship, new job, pregnancy, starting college, etc.). Given the limited number of IOP, partial hospitalization, and IRT programs, if a patient is not fortunate enough to live near a facility offering intensive treatment and does not have financial means to travel to one of these programs, then a lower level of care will be their only option. Health insurance is another factor to consider when determining level of care. Not all insurances cover all levels of care. It is important to consider coverage as well as co-payments and the financial impact this will have on the patient.

Case example 1

Ms. M is a 22-year-old woman who lived at home with her father and presented to the clinic with severe (Y-BOCS 27) OCD symptoms focused mainly on her fear of harming others; she was diagnosed with comorbid depression. She was initially referred to IOP treatment instead of regular outpatient treatment because of the severe decrease in functioning she was having from

symptoms. She was not able to attend school or work because of her preoccupation with the symptoms, which took up most of her day. In addition, the nature of her symptoms (fear of harm to others) made her isolate herself from others, causing significant psychosocial dysfunction. Her habituation during exposure therapy took longer than the typical length of an outpatient session and she had difficulty finishing the exposure sessions on her own. Ms. M began treatment in the IOP program but was soon transferred to a higher level of care when it became clear that she had extreme fears resulting in the belief that the only way she could guarantee she would not act on her intrusive thoughts to harm others was to end her life. She did not respond to CBT while in the OCD IOP to challenge this belief. Ms. M had difficulty seeing her intrusive thoughts as "just thoughts" without carrying special meaning about her "true character" and her "true desire." While in IOP, her distress tolerance was low: she was unable to sit through any level of exposures long enough to habituate. Her depression contributed to this situation, as she would cry during exposure work and start to experience suicidal ideations. Ms. M's father was unsupportive and even counter-productive to treatment, despite several family contacts and attempts to educate him. He kept telling the patient to simply "snap out of it" and would yell at the patient whenever she verbalized any symptoms. Because of these multiple factors, the decision was made to transfer her to a different level of care, partial hospitalization. Ms. M was referred to a general adult partial hospitalization program where she was seen five days a week for five hours a day. The OCD IOP staff remained closely involved in her treatment to ensure that the patient continued to receive education about her illness. While in the partial hospital program, she received CBT, including illness education. Her psychosocial stressors were likewise addressed with more intensive family meetings and education. Treatment focused on increasing her coping skills utilizing Linehan's skills training workbook (Linehan 1993). While in the partial hospitalization program, Ms. M moved into a more supportive living environment with her mother and a friend, who were supportive and willing to be involved in her treatment. Contact with father was stopped. Her depression improved; suicidal ideation stopped, and she began to challenge her interpretations of her intrusive thoughts. Once the patient demonstrated an ability to tolerate stress and participate in exposure therapy, she was transferred back to the specialty OCD program at the IOP level of care. She was better able to participate in ERP and had the experience of full habituation which increased her motivation to engage in more difficult exposures. Once patient developed a significant level of clinical improvement (greater than 50% decrease in Y-BOCS) and demonstrated the ability to do self-guided exposures without the constant presence of a therapist, she was referred to and successfully treated as an outpatient.

Case example 2

Mr. A is a very bright 18-year-old single male who lives with his family and recently graduated from high school. Mr. A was resigned to not being able to start college in the fall because of his significant symptoms. His OCD was severe (Y-BOCS 24) with harming and aggressive contamination obsessions. Mr. A's family relationships and friendships were suffering significantly as a result of his rituals of seeking reassurance and checking. He stopped engaging in hobbies as obsessions and rituals took up the majority of his time. He had difficulty academically at the end of his senior year in high school. Mr. A also had concentration and attention problems, in part as a result of a traumatic brain injury that he had suffered approximately five months earlier. This made it difficult for him to remember to do homework outside of regular therapy sessions, which stalled his improvement. The family and therapist felt that more frequent sessions would be required to reduce the severity of symptoms. Initially in IOP, Mr. A had much difficulty following through on homework assignments despite a clear understanding of the rationale for the treatment as well as the family's understanding of the treatment and supportive involvement. He had the ability to engage in ERP if he had the close supervision of a therapist to help him to stay focused. His ability to perform homework was still poor, and intensive treatment made it obvious that his lack of follow through was because of poor concentration. It was decided that he needed a more intensive level of care than IOP, so a referral to an IRT program was made. During IRT assessment, Mr. A revealed that the fear of not starting college in the fall with his peers was a factor in his motivation to participate in and focus on treatment. He related that he received a great deal of self-esteem and sense of accomplishment through his academic work, which was stellar. Once his family agreed that he could start college with his peers on time if his symptoms reduced, Mr. A began to fully participate in the treatment while at the IRT. The close supervision ensured that he completed homework assignments. Soon after, Mr. A began to design and complete his own exposures above and beyond what the treatment team had assigned. His symptoms reduced significantly (Y-BOCS 15) and he was discharged to an outpatient level of care. Use of IRT was the key to his improvement because he needed round-the-clock monitoring to help him to follow through on assignments. The motivation of more rapid improvement from intensive therapy enabled him to meet the goal of getting better in order to attend school with his peers.

Intensive programs

What follows are a list of programs that offer treatment for OCD in intensive settings. Information on these programs was obtained via internet searches, personal communications, and/or listings from various OCD advocacy groups. When protocols advertised differ from standard templates as noted above, the specific protocols used in that program are listed if known.

ANXIETY DISORDERS PROGRAM AT REMUDA RANCH (*inpatient*) One East Apache St., Wickenburg, AZ 85390 www.remudaranch.com

THE ANXIETY TREATMENT CENTER (*IOP*) 8980 Alderson Ave, Sacramento, CA 95864 www.anxietytreatmentexperts.com

THE COGNITIVE BEHAVIOR THERAPY CENTER FOR OCD AND ANXIETY (*IOP*) 990 A St., Suite 401, San Rafael, CA 94901–3000 www.cbtmarin.com

STANFORD UNIVERSITY DEPARTMENT OF PSYCHIATRY AND BEHAVIORAL SCIENCES, OCD RESEARCH PROGRAM (*IOP*) 401 Quarry Rd., Stanford, CA 94305–5721 www.ocd.stanford.edu

UCLA OBSESSIVE COMPULSIVE DISORDER INTENSIVE TREATMENT PROGRAM (*1 h/day, 5 days/week*) 300 UCLA Medical Plaza, Los Angeles, CA 90095–6968 www.semel.ucla.edu/adc/about/ocd

NEUROBEHAVIORAL INSTITUTE (*IOP*) 2233 North Commerce Parkway, Suite 3, Weston, FL 33326 www.NBIWeston.com

OCD AND ANXIETY TREATMENT CENTER (*IOP*) 3030 Starkey Blvd., Suite 128, New Port Richey, FL 34655 www.ocdandanxietytreatment.com

OCD RESOURCE CENTER OF FLORIDA (*2 h/day, 5–6 days/week*) 3475 Sheridan St. 310, Hollywood, FL 33021 www.ocdhope.com

UNIVERSITY OF FLORIDA OCD PROGRAM (*IOP*) PO Box 100234, Gainesville, FL 32610 www.psychiatry.ufl.edu/UFOCD

UNIVERSITY OF SOUTH FLORIDA OCD PROGRAM (*1.5 h/day, 5 days/week*) 800 6th St. South, 4th Floor North, Box 7523, St. Petersburg, FL 33701 health.usf.edu/medicine/pediatrics/rothman/index.htm

CENTER FOR ANXIETY AND OBSESSIVE COMPULSIVE DISORDER AT ALEXIAN BROTHERS BEHAVIORAL HEALTH HOSPITAL (*IOP, partial hospitalization*) 1650 Moon Lake Blvd., Hoffman Estates, IL 60169 www.abbhh.org

KANSAS CITY CENTER FOR ANXIETY TREATMENT 10540 Marty, Suite 200, Overland Park, Kansas 66212 www.kcanxiety.com

THE LINDNER CENTER OF HOPE (*residential, IOP*) 4075 Old Western Row Rd., Mason, OH 45040 www.lindnercenterofhope.org

ADULT OCD INTENSIVE OUTPATIENT PROGRAM AT WESTERN PSYCHIATRIC INSTITUTE AND CLINIC Bellefield Towers, 100 North Bellefield Ave, 4th Floor, Pittsburgh, PA 15213 www.upmc.com/HospitalsFacilities/Hospitals/wpic

ANXIETY AND AGORAPHOBIA TREATMENT CENTER (*IOP*) 112 Bala Ave., Bala Cynwyd, PA 19004 www.aatcphila.com

CENTER FOR THE TREATMENT AND STUDY OF ANXIETY, UNIVERSITY OF PENNSYLVANIA (*IOP*) 3535 Market St., 6th Floor, Philadelphia, PA 19104 www.med.upenn.edu/ctsa

CHILD OCD INTENSIVE OUTPATIENT PROGRAM AT WESTERN PSYCHIATRIC INSTITUTE AND CLINIC 1011 Bingham St., Pittsburgh, PA 15203www.upmc.com/HospitalsFacilities/Hospitals/wpic

UNIVERSITY OF PENNSYLVANIA CHILD/ADOLESCENT OCD, TICS, TRICHOTILLOMANIA AND ANXIETY GROUP 3535 Market St., 6th Floor, Philadelphia, PA 19104 www.med.upenn.edu/cottage

THE AUSTIN CENTER FOR THE TREATMENT OF OCD 6633 Highway 290 East, Suite 300, Austin, TX 78723 www.austinocd.com

UCLA CHILD/ADOLESCENT OBSESSIVE COMPULSIVE DISORDER INTENSIVE TREATMENT PROGRAM

(*IOP*) 300 UCLA Medical Plaza, Suite 1315, Los Angeles, CA 90095 www.semel.ucla.edu/caap/ocd-intensive-treatment

WESTWOOD INSTITUTE FOR ANXIETY DISORDERS (*IOP*) 921 Westwood Blvd., Suite 223, Los Angeles, CA 90024 www.hope4ocd.com

ANXIETY DISORDERS CENTER AT THE INSTITUTE OF LIVING (*15sessions of 1.5–2 h over 3 weeks*) 200 Retreat Ave., Hartford, CT 06106 www.instituteofliving.org/adc

YALE OCD RESEARCH CLINIC (*inpatient*) 34 Park St.; 3rd Floor, CNRU, New Haven, CT 06508 http://info.med.yale.edu/psych/clinics/OCD%20Research%20Clinic/OCDindex.htm

ANXIETY SOLUTIONS OF NORTHERN NEW ENGLAND, PLLC (*IOP*) PO Box 70, Raymond, ME 04071 www.anxietysolutions.net

OCD INSTITUTE (*residential*) McLean Hospital, 115 Mill St., Belmont, MA 02478 www.mclean.harvard.edu/patient/adult/ocd.php

DEPARTMENT OF PSYCHIATRY AND PSYCHOLOGY, MAYO CLINIC (*2 sessions/day for 1 week*) West 11, 200 First St., SW Rochester, MN 55905 http://www.mayoresearch.mayo.edu/mayo/research/whiteside_lab

ANXIETY DISORDERS CENTER AT THE SAINT LOUIS BEHAVIORAL MEDICINE INSTITUTE 1129 Macklind Ave., St. Louis, MO 63110 info@slbmi.com

BIO BEHAVIORAL INSTITUTE (*IOP*) 935 Northern Blvd., Suite 102, Great Neck, New York, NY 11021 www.biobehavioralinstitute.com

ANXIETY DISORDERS TREATMENT CENTER (*weekend treatment session*) 3011 Jones Ferry Rd., Chapel Hill, NC 27516 www.anxieties.com/weekend.php

UNC ANXIETY AND STRESS DISORDERS CLINIC Department of Psychology, University of North Carolina at Chapel Hill, CB 3270, Davie Hall, Chapel Hill, NC 27599 www.uncanxietyclinic.com

THE HOUSTON OCD PROGRAM (*residential, IOP*) 1401 Castle Court, Houston, TX 77006 www.HoustonOCDProgram.org

OCD CENTER AND COGNITIVE-BEHAVIORAL THERAPY SERVICES, ROGERS MEMORIAL HOSPITAL (*residential, partial hospitalization*) 34700 Valley Road, Oconomowoc, WI 53066 www.rogershospital.org

MCMASTER UNIVERSITY MEDICAL CENTRE, HHS Box 2000 Hamilton, Ontario L8N 3Z5 Canada www.hhsc.ca/body.cfm?ID=232

OCD CENTRE (*IOP*) 9 Eccleston St., London www.ocdcentre.com

MAUDSLEY HOSPITAL (*residential, 1 week intensive outpatient*) Denmark Hill, London www.slam.nhs.uk/services/sitelist.aspx?site=Maudsley+Hospital

THE PRIORY HOSPITAL Priory Road, Edgbaston, Birmingham, UK www.bmihealthcare.co.uk/priory

OCD CLINIC NATIONAL INSTITUTE OF MENTAL HEALTH AND NEURO SCIENCES Deemed University Bangalore 560 029 India www.nimhans.kar.nic.in

ANXIETY DISORDERS PROGRAM ST. PATRICK'S UNIVERSITY HOSPITAL (*IOP*) James St. Dublin 8, Ireland www.stpatrickshosp.ie/index.php/the-programmes/anxiety-disorder

NEUROSCIENCES INSTITUTE FLORENCE ITALY (*IOP*) www.istitutodineuroscienze.it

References

Abramowitz JS, Foa EB, Franklin ME (2003). Exposure and ritual prevention for obsessive-compulsive disorder: effects of intensive versus twice-weekly sessions. *J Consult Clin Psychol* **71**: 394–398.

American Academy of Child Adolescent Psychiatry (1998). Official action summary of the practice parameters for the assessment and treatment of children and adolescents with obsessive-compulsive disorder. *J Am Acad Child Adolesc Psychiatry* **37**(Suppl 10): S27–45.

American Psychiatric Association (2007). *Practice Guidelines for the Treatment of Patients with Obsessive Compulsive Disorder*. Washington, DC: American Psychiatric Press.

Blanco C, Olfson M, Stein DJ, et al. (2006). Treatment of obsessive-compulsive disorder by US psychiatrists. *J Clin Psychiatry* **67**: 946–951.

Boschen MJ, Drummond LM, Pillay A (2008). Treatment of severe, treatment refractory obsessive-compulsive disorder: a study of inpatient and community treatment. *CNS Spectr* **13**: 1056–1085.

Buchanan AW, Meng KS, Marks IM (1996). What predicts improvement and compliance during the behavioral treatment of obsessive compulsive disorder? *Anxiety* **2**: 22–27.

Bystritsky A, Munford PR, Rosen RM, et al. (1996). A preliminary study of partial hospital management of severe obsessive-compulsive disorder. *Psychiatr Serv* **47**: 170–174.

Drummond LM (1993). The treatment of severe, chronic, resistant obsessive-compulsive disorder. an evaluation of an in-patient programme using behavioral psychotherapy in combination with other treatments. *Br J Psychiatry* **163**: 223–229.

Drummond LM, Pillay A, Kolb P, Rani S (2007). Specialised in-patient treatment for severe, chronic, resistant obsessive-compulsive disorder. *Psychiatr Bull* **31**: 49–52.

Griest JH, Marks IM, Baer L, et al. (2002). Behavior therapy for obsessive-compulsive disorder guided by a computer or by a clinician compared with relaxation as a control. *J Clin Psychiatry* **63**: 138–145.

Linehan MM (1993). *Skills Training Manual for Treating Borderline Personality Disorder*. New York: Guilford Press.

March JS, Frances A, Carpenter D, et al. (1997). The Expert Consensus Guidelines Series: treatment of obsessive-compulsive disorder. *J Clin Psychiatry* **58** (Suppl 4): 1–72.

Marks IM, Baer L, Greist JH, et al. (1998). Home self-assessment of obsessive-compulsive disorder. Use of a manual and a computer-conducted telephone interview: two UK–US studies. *Br J Psychiatry* **172**: 406–412.

Stewart SE, Stack DE, Farrell C, Pauls DL, Jenike MA (2005). Effectiveness of intensive residential treatment (IRT) for severe, refractory obsessive-compulsive disorder. *J Psychiatr Res* **39**: 603–609.

Stewart SE, Yen CH, Stack DE, Jenike MA (2006). Outcome predictors for severe obsessive-compulsive patients in intensive residential treatment. *J Psychiatr Res* **40**: 511–519.

Stewart SE, Stack DE, Tsilker S, et al. (2009). Long-term outcome following intensive residential treatment of obsessive-compulsive disorder. *J Psychiatr Res* **43**: 1118–1123.

Van Noppen BL, McCorkle BH, Pato MT (1997). Group and multifamily behavioral treatment for obsessive compulsive disorder: a pilot study. *J Anxiety Disord* **11**: 431–446.

Body dysmorphic disorder

Katharine A. Phillips

Introduction

Body dysmorphic disorder (BDD) is a relatively common disorder that is often considered to be related to obsessive-compulsive disorder (OCD) (e.g., Cohen and Hollander 1997; Castle and Phillips 2006; Mataix-Cols *et al.* 2007). It is associated with high levels of distress, markedly impaired psychosocial functioning, very poor quality of life, and high rates of suicidality. Despite its severity and prevalence, BDD is under-recognized in a variety of clinical settings.

The *Diagnostic and Statistical Manual of Mental Disorders,* 4th edition (DSM-IV; American Psychiatric Association 1994) defines BDD as a preoccupation with an imagined or slight defect in appearance. In other words, individuals with BDD are preoccupied with the belief that they look abnormal, whereas in reality the physical appearance defects they perceive are slight or non-existent. The preoccupation must cause clinically significant distress or impairment in social, occupational/academic, or role functioning, and it must not be better accounted for by another psychiatric disorder (e.g., anorexia nervosa).

History

There is a long historical tradition for BDD, having been consistently described around the world for more than a century (Phillips 1991). The original term for this disorder, "dysmorphophobia," was coined by Enrico Morselli in the 1880s (Morselli 1891). This term is derived from *dysmorphia,* a Greek word meaning ugliness, specifically the face, which first appeared in the *Histories of Herodotus* (Phillips 1991). Morselli noted that patients with BDD have prominent obsessions and compulsive behaviors, similar to patients with OCD. He also emphasized the suffering that these patients experience, writing that

dysmorphophobic patients are "really miserable" and that their "fear of deformity ... may reach a very painful intensity, even to the point of weeping and desperation" (Morselli 1891).

Kraepelin (1909–1915) and Janet (1903) subsequently described BDD at the turn of the twentieth century. Janet emphasized the extreme shame that patients with BDD feel, and he classified BDD within a group of syndromes similar to OCD, referring to BDD as "obsession with shame of the body." Janet underscored the morbidity that BDD can cause in his description of a young woman who worried that she would never be loved because she was "ugly and ridiculous," and who for five years confined herself to a tiny apartment that she rarely left.

"Dermatologic hypochondriasis," "beauty hypochondria" (*Schönheitshypochondrie*), and "one who is worried about being ugly" (*Hässlichkeitskümmerer*) are other terms used to describe BDD over the years (Phillips 1991). In DSM-III, BDD was listed as an example of an atypical somatoform disorder, but it did not have diagnostic criteria. It was first accorded separate diagnostic status, as a somatoform disorder, in DSM-IIIR. Sustained research over the past 15 years has greatly advanced understanding of this intriguing disorder.

Prevalence

Available data indicate that BDD is relatively common. The point prevalence in community and population-based studies is 0.7–2.4% (Faravelli *et al.* 1997; Bienvenu *et al.* 2000; Otto *et al.* 2001; Rief *et al.* 2006; Koran *et al.* 2008), making it somewhat more common than schizophrenia or anorexia nervosa. It appears that BDD is even more common than this among patients with other psychiatric disorders. It

---

Clinical Obsessive-Compulsive Disorders in Adults and Children, ed. Robert Hudak and Darin D. Dougherty.
Published by Cambridge University Press. Copyright © Cambridge University Press 2011.

Box 14.1   Case example 1

Ms. A, an attractive 28-year-old single Hispanic teacher, presented with a chief complaint of: "I'm obsessed with my appearance, and my plastic surgeon has been trying to get me to see a psychiatrist for four years." Since early adolescence, Ms. A had disliked "everything" about her appearance, including her supposedly "scarred" and "discolored" skin, "flat" hair, "big and bumpy" nose, "receding" chin, "thin" lips, "high" forehead, "flabby" thighs, "fat" stomach, and "stumpy" legs. She thought about these supposed flaws for more than eight hours a day. Because she believed she looked "hideous and revolting," she did not date and avoided most social situations unless she first became intoxicated with alcohol to diminish her anxiety. Her appearance preoccupations and frequent mirror checking diminished her concentration and productivity at work. She missed work several times a month and was underemployed because she felt too ugly to be seen and too distressed to try a more challenging job. Ms. A had had 15 cosmetic surgeries, which had cost nearly $100 000 and drained her family's finances. These procedures had not alleviated her body image concerns; as she stated, "After each surgery I just started hating something else."

---

has been reported in 8–37% of patients with OCD (Hollander *et al.* 1993; Brawman-Mintzer *et al.* 1995; Wilhelm *et al.* 1997), 11–13% of patients with social phobia (Brawman-Mintzer *et al.* 1995; Wilhelm *et al.* 1997), 26% of patients with trichotillomania (Soriano *et al.* 1996), and 39% of patients with anorexia nervosa (Grant *et al.* 2002).

Among patients with atypical major depressive disorder, a prevalence of 14% (Phillips *et al.* 1996), 16% (Nierenberg *et al.* 2002), and 42% (Perugi *et al.* 1998) has been reported. In a study of 122 general psychiatric inpatients, 13% had BDD, a prevalence that was higher than for many other disorders in the study, including schizophrenia, OCD, post-traumatic stress disorder, and eating disorders (Grant *et al.* 2001). In that study, 81% of BDD subjects said that BDD was their major or biggest problem. A more recent study of 100 general psychiatric inpatients found that 16.0% (95% confidence interval [CI], 8.7–23.3) had BDD (Conroy *et al.* 2008). Box 14.1 gives a case example of BDD.

Clinical features of body dysmorphic disorder

The clinical features have been consistently described in a variety of studies and settings (Hollander *et al.* 1993; Phillips *et al.* 1993, 2005a; Veale *et al.* 1996a; Perugi *et al.* 1997a). The disorder occurs in all age groups and most often begins during early adolescence. Although the gender ratio has varied in different studies, the female to male ratio appears to be in the range of 1:1 to 3:2 (Phillips and Diaz 1997; Phillips *et al.* 2005a; Rief *et al.* 2006; Koran *et al.*

2008). The clinical features appear to be generally similar in men and women, although some gender differences have been found (Perugi *et al.* 1997b; Phillips and Diaz 1997; Phillips *et al.* 2006a). There also appears to be more similarities than differences in BDD in different cultures, although this important issue has received very little investigation (Phillips 2005a).

Obsessional preoccupation with perceived appearance "defects"

Individuals with BDD are obsessed with the belief that there is something wrong with how they look (Hollander *et al.* 1993; Phillips *et al.* 1993, 2005a; Veale *et al.* 1996a; Perugi *et al.* 1997a; Phillips 2005a). They may describe themselves as looking ugly, unattractive, "not right," deformed, or abnormal. Some patients use more extreme terms to describe their perceived appearance flaws, such as "hideous," "freak," or "monster." The preoccupation most often focuses on the face or head, typically the skin (e.g., acne, scarring, skin color), hair (e.g., hair thinning or excessive body hair), or nose (e.g., size or shape). However, any body area can be the focus of concern. A common misconception about BDD is that the appearance concerns must focus on only one specific body area; in fact, most patients are preoccupied with numerous body areas, and some dislike virtually every body area, saying that they look generally ugly. On average, the appearance preoccupations occur for three to eight hours a day, and they are often difficult to resist or control.

Insight is usually absent or poor

A clinically important aspect of BDD is that insight is usually poor or absent. Most patients are convinced or fairly certain that they look abnormal (Phillips *et al.* 1994; Phillips 2004). Very few patients, prior to treatment, realize that the perceived appearance defects are actually slight or non-existent. In addition, many patients do not realize that their appearance concerns are because of a psychiatric disorder. This is one of the reasons so many patients with BDD pursue surgery, dermatologic treatment, and other cosmetic treatment.

Ideas and delusions of reference are also common, with a majority of patients believing that other people take special notice of their "defects" in a negative way, for example, mocking them, laughing at them, or recoiling in horror because of how they look (Phillips 2004). Patients with BDD worry more about being mocked or rejected than about being harmed, differentiating them from patients with classic paranoia.

Compulsive behaviors

Although compulsive behaviors are not part of BDD's definition, nearly all patients perform some of these behaviors in an attempt to diminish the anxiety caused by their appearance preoccupations (Neziroglu and Yaryura-Tobias 1993; Phillips *et al.* 1993, 2005a; Veale *et al.* 1996a; Perugi *et al.* 1997a; Phillips 2005a). The purpose of these behaviors is generally to check, hide, or fix the perceived appearance defects. These behaviors are usually time consuming and, like the preoccupations, are typically difficult to resist or control.

Common behaviors include compulsively comparing the disliked body areas with the same body areas of other people, examining the perceived defects in mirrors and other reflecting surfaces (Veale and Riley 2001), excessively grooming (e.g., hair combing or styling, hair plucking or pulling, or shaving), touching the body areas to check them, seeking reassurance from other people about the perceived flaws, frequently changing clothes to find a more flattering outfit, and compulsively buying clothes, makeup, or beauty products. About one quarter of patients with BDD compulsively tan – sometimes to the point of causing severe skin damage – in an effort to darken "pale" skin or cover perceived acne scarring or facial marks (Phillips *et al.* 2006b).

Nearly all patients with BDD attempt to camouflage their perceived defects. For example, they may try to hide "love handles" by wearing loose shirts, cover perceived facial scarring with makeup, hide perceived hair loss by wearing a hat or toupee, conceal "freakish" eyes with sunglasses, or hide the "bad" side of their face by turning it away from people.

About one third to one half of BDD patients compulsively pick their skin (Phillips and Diaz 1997; Phillips *et al.* 2005a; Grant *et al.* 2006). The intent of this behavior is to improve the skin's appearance (e.g., "smooth out" or remove blemishes) (Phillips and Taub 1995). However, because skin picking can occur for hours a day and may involve use of sharp implements such as pins, needles, razor blades, or knives, it can cause considerable skin damage. Consequentlys, some individuals with BDD who pick their skin are an exception to the rule that people with BDD look normal. Skin picking may even be life threatening, for example, when picking ruptures, or nearly ruptures, major blood vessels (O'Sullivan *et al.* 1999).

Comorbidity

Comorbidity is common (Gunstad and Phillips 2003; Phillips *et al.* 2005a). Major depressive disorder is the most frequently co-occurring disorder, with a lifetime prevalence of approximately 75% (Gunstad and Phillips 2003; Phillips *et al.* 2005a). The melancholic subtype is most common, and a majority of patients have recurrent depressive episodes (Phillips *et al.* 2007). About one third of patients have comorbid lifetime OCD, and nearly 40% have comorbid lifetime social phobia (Gunstad and Phillips 2003; Phillips *et al.* 2005a).

While rates of substance use disorders have varied across studies (Hollander *et al.* 1993; Veale *et al.* 1996a; Zimmerman and Mattia 1998), in the largest studies, which used the Structured Clinical Interview for DSM-IV (SCID), 30% of 175 participants in a phenomenology series had a lifetime substance use disorder (Gunstad and Phillips 2003) and 48% of a more broadly ascertained sample of 200 subjects had a lifetime substance use disorder (Phillips *et al.* 2005a). In the latter study, 68% of individuals with a comorbid substance use disorder reported that BDD symptoms contributed to their substance use (Grant *et al.* 2005). Conversely, in a study of 34 adult psychiatric inpatients with a current substance use disorder, a notably high proportion, 26.5%, had BDD (Grant *et al.* 2001).

Other clinical features

Individuals with BDD tend to have poor self-esteem and high levels of depressive symptoms (Rosen and Ramirez 1998; Phillips *et al.* 2004a, 2004b). Core BDD beliefs often focus on being unlovable, inadequate, and generally defective (Veale *et al.* 1996a; Phillips 2005a). Levels of social anxiety tend to be high and in the range seen in anxiety disorders (Pinto and Phillips 2005). High levels of anxiety, neuroticism, and anger/hostility, as well as very low levels of extroversion, have also been reported (Phillips and McElroy 2000; Phillips *et al.* 2004b).

Morbidity

Functioning and quality of life

People with BDD experience significant distress and impairment in social, occupational, and academic functioning (Phillips *et al.* 1993, 2005b; Perugi *et al.* 1997b). While level of functioning varies, it is typically very poor. In the author's series of 507 individuals with BDD (Gunstad and Phillips 2003; Phillips *et al.* 2005a), 43% had a history of psychiatric hospitalization; 31% had been completely housebound for at least one week because of BDD; 36% were currently not working because of psychopathology; and 32% were currently unable to be in school or do schoolwork because of psychopathology. Compared with subjects who worked in the past month, those who were not currently working because of psychopathology had more severe and chronic BDD (Didie *et al.* 2008).

Two studies of quality of life, one with 62 participants and one with 176, indicated markedly poor mental health-related quality of life (Phillips 2000; Phillips *et al.* 2005b). For example, on the 36-Item Short Form Health Survey, individuals with BDD scored notably worse in all mental health domains than norms for the general US population or for patients with clinical depression (major depressive disorder and/or dysthymia), type II diabetes, or a recent myocardial infarction (Phillips 2000; Phillips *et al.* 2005b). More severe BDD symptoms were associated with poorer mental health-related quality of life on the 36-Item Short Form Health Survey and other quality of life measures. On another measure, quality of life was even poorer than has been reported for many other severe psychiatric disorders, including chronic depression and post-traumatic stress disorder (Rapaport *et al.* 2005).

Suicidality

Case reports from psychiatry, dermatology, and surgery settings underscore the suicidal ideation, suicide attempts, and completed suicide that can occur in BDD (Phillips 1991). Studies have reported high lifetime rates of suicidal ideation (78–81%) and suicide attempts (24–28%) (Veale *et al.* 1996a; Phillips and Diaz 1997; Phillips *et al.* 2005c). In a study of 200 broadly ascertained individuals with BDD, 78% of subjects reported lifetime suicidal ideation and 28% had attempted suicide (Phillips *et al.* 2005c). The BDD was the primary reason for suicidal ideation in 71% of those with a history of ideation and nearly 50% of subjects with a past attempt. In logistic regression analyses, suicidal ideation was significantly predicted by comorbid major depression and greater lifetime impairment through BDD. Suicide attempts were significantly predicted by post-traumatic stress disorder, a substance use disorder, and greater lifetime impairment by BDD. Therefore, more severe BDD and certain comorbid disorders appear to increase the risk of suicidality.

Regarding completed suicide, a retrospective study of patients in two dermatology practices known to have committed suicide over 20 years found that most of the patients who committed suicide had acne or BDD (Cotterill and Cunliffe 1997). In the only prospective study of the course of BDD, the annual rate of completed suicide was 0.3% per year (Phillips and Menard 2006). This rate translates into a standardized mortality ratio that is higher than that reported for nearly any other mental illness (Harris and Barraclough 1997). While these data are very preliminary and require confirmation, they underscore the importance of carefully monitoring BDD patients for suicidality and instituting appropriate treatment that focuses specifically on BDD symptoms and the comorbid disorders noted above.

Body dysmorphic disorder in youth

The disorder usually begins during early adolescence (mode of age 13 and mean of age 16–17). Only two studies have examined a broad range of clinical features in youth with BDD, and only one of these studies directly compared adolescents (36) with adults (164) (Albertini and Phillips 1999; Phillips *et al.* 2006c). These studies suggest that BDD's clinical features in youth are generally similar to those seen in adults. Youth appear to have similar preoccupations, compulsions, body areas of concern, comorbidity, and other clinical features. They also have high levels of distress and impairment in psychosocial functioning. In these two series, approximately 20% of youth had dropped out of school primarily because of BDD symptoms.

In the adolescent–adult comparison study, the two groups were comparable on many variables. However, several differences raise the possibility that adolescents may be more severely ill than adults (Phillips *et al.* 2006c). A higher proportion of adolescents than adults reported a lifetime suicide attempt (44.4% vs. 23.8%; *p* =0.012). Adolescents also had more delusional BDD beliefs (*p* < 0.001). In addition, lifetime rates of comorbidity and functional impairment were similar in adolescents and adults, despite the adolescents having had fewer years in which to develop these problems. While severe illness and impaired functioning are problematic at any age, they have particular salience and importance during adolescence, given this period's critical developmental tasks.

Treatment strategies for body dysmorphic disorder

Establishing an alliance and providing psychoeducation

It is important to take patients' appearance concerns seriously rather than dismissing them or simply reassuring patients that they look normal. Most patients do not believe reassurance and may interpret it as trivializing their concerns. However, it is also important not to agree with the patient's view that there is something wrong with their appearance, as this may be devastating and may even trigger suicidal thinking.

It is important to provide psychoeducation by telling patients that they have the diagnosis of BDD, and explaining what BDD is and that it is a relatively common and treatable body image disorder. It can be helpful to note that people with BDD view their appearance differently to other people, for reasons that are unclear. It can also be helpful to emphasize that people with BDD are preoccupied with their appearance and as a result experience significant distress and difficulty functioning, because most patients can readily agree with this. For patients who resist the diagnosis and treatment, insisting that they truly are ugly, it is best to avoid arguments over how they actually look.

Instead, focus on the potential for psychiatric treatment to diminish their excessive preoccupation, suffering, and impaired functioning. Clinical experience suggests that motivational interviewing techniques (Miller and Rollnick 2002) that are adapted for BDD (Wilhelm *et al.* 2010) may encourage reluctant patients to try psychiatric treatment.

Research suggests that serotonin reuptake inhibitors and cognitive-behavioral therapy (CBT) are often efficacious for BDD. No study has directly compared the efficacy of these two treatments or examined whether their combination is more efficacious than either treatment when used alone. Clinical judgment and other factors must be weighed when deciding which treatment to use or whether to use them together (this is discussed more extensively by Phillips [2009]). In the author's clinical experience, patients who are too severely ill and depressed to engage in CBT may benefit from first trying an SRI, which may diminish symptoms and increase motivation to the point where CBT can be successfully implemented. The author recommends that both treatments be used in combination for more highly suicidal patients.

Discouraging surgery and other cosmetic treatment

Many patients with BDD receive surgical, dermatologic, dental, or other cosmetic treatment for their perceived defects. In a study of 250 subjects with BDD, 190 (76%) had sought such treatment, and 165 (66%) had received a total of 484 treatments (Phillips *et al.* 2001a). A study of 200 broadly ascertained individuals with BDD similarly found that 142 (71%) had sought such treatment, and 128 (64%) had received it (Crerand *et al.* 2005). Both studies found that dermatologic treatment was most frequently sought and received (most often, topical acne agents), followed by surgery (most often, rhinoplasty). Some patients with BDD even perform their own surgery, – for example attempting to replace their nose cartilage with chicken cartilage in the desired shape (Phillips 2005a) or attempting a facelift with a staple gun (Veale 2000).

The surgery and dermatology literature describe BDD as very difficult to treat (Koblenzer 1985; Cotterill 1996). As one dermatologist wrote, "The author knows of no more difficult patients to treat than those with body dysmorphic disorder" (Cotterill

1996). A 2001 survey of plastic surgeons found that BDD patients tend to have a poor surgical outcome, and 40% said a BDD patient had threatened them legally and/or physically (Sarwer 2002). Occasional patients have committed suicide or murdered the physician (Phillips 1991; Phillips *et al.* 1992; Cotterill 1996; Ladee 1966). Such reports underscore the critical importance of recognizing BDD and implementing appropriate psychiatric treatment.

Although it appears that most individuals who do not have BDD are satisfied with the outcome of cosmetic surgery (Honigman *et al.* 2004), those with BDD appear to respond poorly to surgery and other types of cosmetic treatment. In the study described above of 250 patients, only 7% of retrospectively assessed treatments led to overall improvement in BDD over the longer term (i.e., decreased preoccupation, distress, and impairment related to all BDD concerns) (Phillips *et al.* 2001a). In the other study of 200 participants, only 4% of all procedures improved overall BDD symptoms over the longer term (Crerand *et al.* 2005). In a study of 50 subjects with BDD, 41 (81%) reported being dissatisfied with past medical consultation or surgery (Veale *et al.* 1996a). In a prospective study of the course of BDD, receipt of cosmetic treatment for BDD concerns was not associated with a higher probability of remission from BDD over one year of follow-up (Phillips *et al.* 2005d). Most treatment outcome data are retrospective, and additional prospective studies are needed to further examine treatment outcomes.

A challenge for clinicians, however, is that many patients pursue such treatment, some ardently. In fact, patients with BDD have been referred to as "polysurgery addicts" (Fukuda 1977). Research has not examined how to successfully dissuade patients from obtaining such treatment. In the author's clinical experience, the following approach may be helpful. First, explain to the patient that they have BDD, a body image disorder, and discuss the reasons this diagnosis applies to them. Second, provide psychoeducation about BDD. Third, explain that as best anyone knows, surgery, dermatologic treatment, and other cosmetic treatments do not appear to help BDD. In fact, the vast majority of patients do not improve, and some develop increased appearance concerns, depression, and anxiety following such treatment, and they regret having had the procedure. Fourth, acknowledge that while the patient can probably obtain such treatment if they wish (if you or the doctor they are requesting it from deny it, the patient will likely find it elsewhere), emphasize that you cannot recommend the treatment because they are not likely to improve, and after receiving it they may dislike their appearance even more. Fifth, if the patient will not agree to forgo such treatment, encourage them to at least delay it and first try psychiatric treatment, which is much more likely to help. Sixth, explain that effective treatments are available for BDD (see below) and strongly encourage the patient to try them. Finally, recommend reading about these treatments (e.g., Phillips 2005a, 2009).

Pharmacotherapy

The following strategies are based on evidence from controlled studies, open-label trials, and the author's clinical experience. More detailed pharmacotherapy reviews and recommendations are available elsewhere (Phillips 2005a; National Collaborating Center for Mental Health 2006; Phillips and Hollander 2008). No medications currently have FDA approval for BDD because insufficient studies designed to receive such approval have been carried out for BDD.

Serotonin uptake inhibitors

Controlled studies, open-label studies, and clinical series consistently indicate that SRIs are often efficacious for BDD (Phillips 2005a; Phillips and Hollander 2008). These medications usually improve BDD-related appearance preoccupations, distress, and insight as well as compulsive BDD behaviors. Functioning and associated symptoms such as depression and suicidality often improve as well. In a double-blind crossover trial, clomipramine was more efficacious than desipramine for BDD symptoms and functional disability (Hollander *et al.* 1999). In a placebo-controlled study, fluoxetine was significantly more efficacious than placebo for BDD symptoms and functional disability (Phillips *et al.* 2002). Four systematic open-label SRI studies have been published (with 15–30 subjects), two with fluvoxamine, one with citalopram, and one with escitalopram (Perugi *et al.* 1996; Phillips *et al.* 1998a; Phillips and Najjar 2003; Phillips 2006;). In intention-to-treat analyses, BDD response rates in these studies ranged from 63% to 83%. Available data, while limited, suggest that a substantial proportion of patients who fail an initial SRI trial will respond to a subsequent SRI (Phillips *et al.* 2001b). A recent open-label study of venlafaxine in 17 patients suggested that this medication may be efficacious (Allen *et al.* 2008), although serotonin–norepinephrine reuptake inhibotors are not currently considered a first-line treatment for BDD.

Of note, studies have shown that delusional patients (i.e., those who are completely convinced that they look abnormal) are as likely as non-delusional patients to respond to an SRI (Hollander *et al.* 1999; Phillips *et al.* 1994, 2002). In contrast, antipsychotic drugs as monotherapy do not appear efficacious for delusional BDD (Phillips *et al.* 1994), although data are very limited. A small case series suggests that pimozide as monotherapy is unlikely to be efficacious for BDD (Phillips 2005a), although systematic studies are needed on this important question.

Dosage of serotonin uptake inhibitors

Methodologically rigorous studies have not compared different SRI doses; however, BDD appears to often require higher SRI doses than those typically used for depression (Phillips 2005a, 2006d). Some patients benefit from doses that exceed the maximum recommended dose (this approach is not advised for clomipramine). Most patients with BDD, however, appear to receive relatively low SRI doses, which a retrospective study found to be associated with a poorer treatment response than higher doses (Phillips *et al.* 2006d). In the author's clinical practice, the mean daily selective SRI (SSRI) doses used are (Phillips 2005a):

- fluoxetine: 67 ± 24 mg
- clomipramine: 203 ± 53 mg
- fluvoxamine: 308 ± 49 mg
- sertraline: 202 ± 46 mg
- paroxetine: 55 ± 13 mg
- citalopram: 66 ± 36 mg
- escitalopram: 29 ± 12 mg.

The average time to response has varied in different studies, from four to five weeks to as much as nine weeks (Phillips and Hollander 2008). However, some patients will not respond until the tenth or twelfth week of SRI treatment, even with fairly rapid dose titration. If SRI response is inadequate after 12–16 weeks of treatment, and the highest dose recommended by the manufacturer or tolerated by the patient has been tried for two to three weeks, it is recommended that the medication be changed.

Augmentation strategies

In the only placebo-controlled SRI augmentation study, pimozide was not more efficacious than placebo, regardless of whether the appearance beliefs were delusional or non-delusional (Phillips 2005b). In a small case series, olanzapine augmentation of SRIs was not efficacious for BDD symptoms (Phillips 2005c), but clinical experience suggests that augmentation of an SRI with an atypical antipsychotic is sometimes helpful, especially for symptoms of anxiety and agitation. Buspirone may be a helpful SRI augmentation for BDD symptoms, and adjunctive benzodiazepines should be considered for coexisting anxiety, agitation, or insomnia, especially when these symptoms are severe (Phillips 2005a; Phillips and Hollander 2008).

Cognitive-behavioral therapy

Although psychotherapy research is limited, data from clinical series and studies using waiting-list controls indicate that CBT provided individually or in a group format is often efficacious for BDD (Neziroglu and Khemlani-Patel 2002; Phillips 2005a; National Collaborating Center for Mental Health 2006). The psychotherapy of choice for BDD is currently CBT, although studies of other types of psychotherapy are needed.

In a case series of 17 patients treated with 20 daily sessions of 90 minutes CBT over one month, 12 patients had a 50% or greater reduction in BDD symptom severity (Neziroglu 1996). In a randomized study of 19 subjects who received 12 one-hour weekly individual CBT sessions, the patients receiving CBT improved significantly more than those on a waiting list (Veale *et al.* 1996b). In a study of six weeks of intensive treatment with 30 sessions of 90 minutes each of exposure and response prevention (without cognitive therapy), BDD symptoms improved significantly and remained stable at follow-up (McKay *et al.* 1997a).

Several studies have examined the efficacy of CBT provided in a group setting. In one randomized study of group treatment, 54 women were assigned to eight sessions of two hours in group CBT or a waiting list; subjects who received CBT had significantly greater improvement in BDD symptoms, self-esteem, and depression than those on the waiting list (Rosen *et al.* 1995). In another study of group CBT in 13 adults, BDD and depression severity significantly improved with 12 sessions of 90 minutes each (Wilhelm *et al.* 1999). The severity scores for BDD decreased from the severe to the moderate range; the authors noted that further improvement might have occurred with a longer treatment.

Core elements of cognitive-behavioral therapy

When CBT is used for BDD (Rosen *et al.* 1995; Veale *et al.* 1996b; Wilhelm *et al.* 1999, 2010; Neziroglu and Khemlani-Patel 2002; Phillips 2005a), the following core elements are usually involved:

1. Cognitive restructuring, which focuses on identifying inaccurate beliefs and cognitive errors and developing more accurate and helpful new beliefs;
2. Exposure, which helps patients enter feared and avoided situations (typically, social situations) without ritualizing. Exposure is usually combined with behavioral experiments, in which patients empirically test inaccurate and dysfunctional beliefs;
3. Response (ritual) prevention, which teaches patients how to resist repetitive behaviors such as mirror checking and excessive grooming.

Additional techniques include the following (Wilhelm *et al.* 2010):

- cognitive restructuring and other techniques: to address core beliefs, which usually involve negative beliefs about oneself as a person (e.g., I'm unlovable; I'm inadequate)
- perceptual retraining: helps patients to learn to see themselves more holistically and less negatively
- activity scheduling: for more severely depressed patients
- mindfulness approaches
- habit reversal for compulsive skin picking and hair pulling or plucking.

Clinical experience suggests that effective CBT for BDD differs in some ways from CBT for "near-neighbor" disorders, because of differences between BDD and these disorders. These differences include the content of the preoccupation (appearance), the presence of prominent compulsive behaviors (unlike social phobia or depression), and the poorer insight in BDD than in OCD. Problematic behaviors that are not characteristic of other similar disorders – such as pursuit of cosmetic treatment and abuse of anabolic steroids to build muscle mass

(Pope *et al.* 2005) – need to be specifically targeted in treatment.

Frequency and duration of cognitive-behavioral therapy

The optimal session frequency and treatment duration for CBT are unclear. Treatment provided in studies has ranged from eight weekly two-hour sessions to 12 weeks of daily CBT (60 sessions). Most experts would recommend weekly or more frequent sessions for at least five to six months, plus daily homework. More severely ill patients may need longer or more intensive treatment. Maintenance/booster sessions following treatment should be considered, especially for more severely ill patients, to reduce the risk of relapse.

Relationship of body dysmorphic disorder to OCD

While BDD is currently classified as a somatoform disorder, it is widely considered to be an OCD spectrum disorder (Cohen and Hollander 1997; Castle and Phillips 2006a; Mataix-Cols *et al.* 2007). In fact, a close relationship between these two disorders was proposed more than a century ago (Morselli 1891). Solyom *et al.* (1985) suggested that BDD may even be a type of "obsessive psychosis," which he defined as an atypical and more malignant form of OCD.

A number of studies have directly compared BDD with OCD, finding many similarities between the disorders across a variety of domains as well as some clinically relevant differences (McKay *et al.* 1997b; Phillips *et al.* 1998a, 2006e; Saxena *et al.* 2001; Eisen *et al.* 2004; Frare *et al.* 2004). (More extensive reviews of this topic are available elsewhere [Phillips and Kaye 2007].) Phenomenologic similarities between BDD and OCD are notable. The preoccupations in BDD have many similarities to OCD obsessions, for example, their unwanted nature, and their intrusiveness, repetitiveness, and persistence. In one study, scores for 53 subjects with BDD or 53 with OCD did not significantly differ on any individual obsession item on the Yale–Brown Obsessive Compulsive Scale (Y-BOCS; Phillips *et al.* 1998b). Furthermore, some BDD preoccupations have some content similarities with OCD obsessions, for example those focusing on symmetry, "just right" concerns, or a desire for perfection.

However, the BDD obsessions differ from OCD obsessions in that, by definition, they focus on physical appearance. In addition, feelings of embarrassment and shame appear nearly universal in BDD, and the core beliefs underlying obsessions appear to focus more on being unacceptable as a person (e.g., believing oneself to be inadequate or unlovable). Another important difference is that BDD obsessions are characterized by poorer insight (greater delusionality) than OCD obsessions (McKay *et al.* 1997b; Phillips *et al.* 1998b, 2006e; Eisen *et al.* 2004). Studies have found that 27–39% of BDD patients have currently delusional beliefs compared with only 2% of patients with OCD (Eisen *et al.* 2004; Phillips *et al.* 2006e). Regarding specific components of delusionality, BDD patients are usually more convinced than patients with OCD that their underlying belief (e.g., "I am ugly and deformed") is accurate, more likely to think that other people agree with their belief, less willing to consider the possibility that their belief is inaccurate, and less likely to recognize that their belief has a psychiatric/psychological cause (Eisen *et al.* 2004).

Like patients with OCD, nearly all patients with BDD engage in repetitive, time-consuming compulsive behaviors that are performed intentionally, in response to an obsession, and which aim to reduce anxiety or distress and prevent an unwanted event (e.g., being rejected by others or looking "ugly"). Carrying out the act is not pleasurable (Phillips 2005a). One study found that scores for patients with BDD or OCD did not significantly differ on any individual Y-BOCS compulsion item (Phillips *et al.* 1998b). Furthermore, some OCD and BDD compulsions (e.g., checking and reassurance seeking) overlap to some extent in content/phenomenology. Other compulsions differ, however (see above). Furthermore, some BDD compulsions (e.g., mirror checking) do not appear to follow a simple model of anxiety reduction that occurs with OCD compulsions (Veale and Riley 2001).

Both BDD and OCD appear to be generally similar in terms of gender ratio and age of onset (Phillips *et al.* 1998b, 2006e; Frare *et al.* 2004), although one study found an earlier age of onset for BDD (Frare *et al.* 2004), and several studies found that individuals with BDD are less likely to be married (Phillips *et al.* 1998b; Frare *et al.* 2004). Both disorders often appear to be chronic (Eisen *et al.* 1999; Phillips *et al.* 2005d). A recent longitudinal study of BDD found that BDD and comorbid OCD tended to similarly vary together over time, suggesting that BDD and OCD symptoms may be related and linked for some people (Phillips

and Stout 2006). However, full-criteria BDD persisted in approximately half of subjects after their OCD remitted, suggesting that BDD is not simply a symptom of OCD.

Three studies that used the SCID found that 32–38% of patients ascertained for BDD had lifetime comorbid OCD, suggesting that BDD and OCD are related disorders (Gunstad and Phillips 2003; Phillips *et al.* 2005a). Studies that examined the converse have yielded rates of BDD among patients with OCD that ranged from 3% to 37%, with an average of approximately 15% (e.g., Hollander *et al.* 1993; Brawman-Mintzer *et al.* 1995; Simeon *et al.* 1995; Wilhelm *et al.* 1997; Phillips *et al.* 1998b; Jaisoorya *et al.* 2003; Diniz *et al.* 2004). Patterns of comorbidity with other disorders vary somewhat across studies, but BDD appears to have more comorbidity than OCD does, in particular with major depressive disorder, dysthymia, substance use disorders, paranoid personality disorder, and possibly social phobia (Phillips and Kaye 2007).

Several studies suggest that functioning and quality of life are similarly very poor in both disorders or even somewhat poorer in BDD than in OCD (Frare *et al.* 2004; Didie *et al.* 2007). In addition, BDD may also be associated with higher rates of suicidal ideation and suicide attempts than OCD (Phillips *et al.* 1998b, 2006e; Frare *et al.* 2004).

A controlled and blinded family study (80 case probands and 73 control probands) found that BDD occurred significantly more frequently in first-degree relatives of OCD probands than control probands, suggesting that BDD and OCD may be related disorders (Bienvenu *et al.* 2000). While data on BDD's pathophysiology are still very limited, they offer some (although somewhat mixed) support for a relationship between BDD and OCD; these data also suggest that these disorders are not identical. A small, preliminary morphometric magnetic resonance imaging study of 16 subjects with BDD found that the caudate nucleus differed in subjects and controls, consistent with conceptualization of BDD as an OCD spectrum disorder (Rauch *et al.* 2003). However, the BDD group had a relative leftward shift in caudate nucleus asymmetry, whereas OCD studies that have implicated lateralized abnormalities have suggested a rightward shift in striatal asymmetry (Jenike *et al.* 1996). Whereas some previous OCD studies have shown reduced white matter volume (Breiter *et al.* 1994; Jenike *et al.* 1996), BDD subjects in this study had greater total white matter volume. A small uncontrolled BDD single-photon emission computed tomography study of six subjects yielded a broad range of discrepant findings that did not support a close relationship between BDD and OCD (Carey *et al.* 2004).

In a neuropsychological study of 35 subjects, those with BDD had impaired verbal and non-verbal memory compared with healthy controls (Deckersbach *et al.* 2000), similar to findings for an OCD group in the same laboratory (although BDD and OCD subjects were not directly compared). In an information processing study, BDD subjects were more likely than healthy controls to interpret a range of ambiguous situations (appearance related, social, and general) as threatening; OCD patients exhibited this negative interpretive bias only for general situations (not for appearance-related or social situations) (Buhlmann *et al.* 2002). In another study, both BDD patients and OCD patients were less accurate than a healthy control group in identifying facial expressions of emotion. However, relative to the control and OCD groups, the BDD group more often misidentified emotional expressions as angry (Buhlmann *et al.* 2004).

Like OCD, BDD appears to respond preferentially to SRIs (although studies of non-SRI medications in BDD are still very limited). However, BDD and OCD do not always respond to the same SRI concurrently, suggesting that they are not identical disorders (Phillips *et al.* 1998a). In addition, while some CBT techniques for BDD are quite similar to those used for OCD (namely, exposure and response prevention), some aspects of CBT differ for the two disorders. For example, in BDD there is a greater focus on cognitive approaches and behavioral experiments; perceptual retraining exercises are often used, and certain symptoms are treated with habit reversal.

Taken together, the above findings indicate many similarities but also some clinically important differences between BDD and OCD. Occurrence of BDD may also be related to major depression, social phobia, and eating disorders (Phillips 2005a, 2009). In fact, in the longitudinal study discussed above, BDD appeared to be more closely related to major depressive disorder than to OCD (Phillips and Stout 2006). In Asian cultures, BDD is conceptualized as a type of social phobia (*taijin-kyofusho*) (Kleinknecht *et al.* 1997). To the author's knowledge, however, no direct comparison studies with these other disorders have been carried out, and such studies are needed.

Recognizing and diagnosing body dysmorphic disorder

The importance of detecting BDD in clinical settings has been emphasized (Thompson and Durrani 2007). However, BDD is under-recognized and underdiagnosed, despite its prevalence, severity, and the availability of effective treatments. Five studies have found that mental health clinicians fail to diagnose BDD, even when BDD is a major problem or the primary diagnosis (Phillips *et al.* 1993, 1996; Zimmerman and Mattia 1998; Grant *et al.* 2001; Conroy *et al.* 2008). Common reasons for this include patients being embarrassed about their symptoms, fearing that their healthcare provider will judge them negatively, believing that the provider will not understand their concerns, and not knowing that the problem is treatable (Conroy *et al.* 2008). Instead, patients may reveal only symptoms of depression, anxiety, social anxiety, or substance use, which may lead to misdiagnosis of BDD or to diagnosis of comorbid disorders but not BDD. As a result, treatment may not target BDD or be appropriate for this disorder. A study in a psychiatric inpatient setting found that no patient with BDD revealed their appearance concerns to their clinician, even though all patients considered their appearance concerns a major problem or their biggest problem, because they were too embarrassed to reveal them (Grant *et al.* 2001). However, all of the patients in this study wanted their clinician to know about their BDD symptoms. Consequently, it is often up to the clinician to recognize clues to BDD's presence and to screen patients for BDD.

Diagnosis of BDD can be relatively straightforward using questions such as those in Box 14.2 (Phillips 2005a). Useful screening questions are: "Are you very worried about your appearance in any way?" "Are you unhappy with how you look?" If the patient replies affirmatively, the clinician can then ask more about the appearance concerns, such as what body areas the patient worries about, and then ascertain that DSM-IV criteria for BDD are met. It is important to be aware that, because patients with BDD usually have poor or absent insight, they should *not* be asked whether they are preoccupied with an imagined defect. The word "imagined" is usually off-putting to patients. Even more important, most patients have poor or absent insight, considering their perceived defects to be real rather than imagined.

Box 14.2 Questions to ask patients to diagnose body dysmorphic disorder (BDD)

Criterion A Preoccupation with an imagined or slight defect in appearance

1. Are you very worried about your appearance in any way? *or* Are you unhappy with how you look?
   Note: Do not ask the patient if they are concerned about an imagined defect in their appearance.
2. Invite the patient to describe their concern by asking "What don't you like about how you look?" *or* "Can you tell me about your concern?"
3. Ask if there are other disliked body areas to ensure none are missed; for example, "Are you unhappy with any other aspects of your appearance, such as your face, skin, hair, nose, or the shape or size of any other body area?"
4. Ascertain that the patient is preoccupied with these perceived flaws by asking "Does this concern preoccupy you? That is, do you think about it a lot and wish you could worry about it less? If you add up all the time you spend each day thinking about your appearance, how much time would you estimate you spend?"

Criterion B Clinically significant distress or impairment in functioning

1. Ask "How much distress do these concerns cause you?" Ask specifically about resulting anxiety, social anxiety, depression, feelings of panic, and suicidal thinking.
2. Ask about effects of the appearance preoccupations on the patient's life, for example: "Do these concerns interfere with your life or cause problems for you in any way?" Ask specifically about effects on:
   - work, school, other aspects of role functioning (e.g., caring for children)
   - relationships, intimacy, family and social activities
   - household tasks
   - leisure activities
   - effects on family or friends
   - other types of interference.

Criterion C Preoccupation is not better accounted for by another mental disorder (e.g., dissatisfaction with body shape and size in anorexia nervosa)

For patients with problematic weight concerns, clinicians need to ascertain that weight concerns are not better accounted for by an eating disorder.

Some clues to the presence of BDD

1. While compulsive behaviors are not required for the diagnosis, most patients perform at least one of them (usually many). Ask about the most common ones: camouflaging, comparing, mirror checking, excessive grooming, reassurance seeking, touching the disliked body areas, clothes changing, skin picking, tanning, dieting, excessive exercise, and excessive weightlifting.
2. Screen carefully for BDD in patients with major depressive disorder, OCD, social phobia, or a substance use disorder.
3. Screen for BDD in patients who have unnecessary cosmetic procedures, especially if they have them repeatedly, with persistence of appearance concerns.

Clues to BDD's presence include the behaviors described above, such as excessive mirror checking, camouflaging (e.g., covering one's face with a hat or hair), skin picking, excessive tanning, or seeking reassurance about how one looks (Phillips 2005a). Other clues include the frequently comorbid disorders noted above, ideas or delusions of reference, depression or anxiety, social avoidance, being housebound, and unnecessary cosmetic treatment.

One diagnostic complexity is that, according to DSM-IV-TR, patients whose appearance beliefs are non-delusional are diagnosed with the somatoform disorder BDD, whereas those with delusional beliefs are diagnosed with delusional disorder, somatic type. However, delusional disorder may be double coded with BDD – in other words, delusional patients may receive diagnoses of both BDD and delusional disorder. Giving both diagnoses reflects the likelihood that

BDD's delusional and non-delusional variants are actually one and the same disorder, characterized by a range of insight (Phillips 2004; Phillips *et al.* 1994). Indeed, BDD's delusional and non-delusional variants appear to have far more similarities than differences and, of note, appear to respond to the same treatments (Phillips *et al.* 1994; Phillips 2004).

The ICD-10 (World Health Organization 1994) classifies BDD as a type of hypochondriasis, although there is no research or clinical support for this. Unlike patients with hypochondriasis, somatic complaints and fear of having a serious disease are not the primary concern of patients with BDD. In addition, their scores on measures of somatization appear no higher than those of patients with other psychiatric disorders (Phillips *et al.* 2004b). Furthermore, many patients do not seek medical evaluation and reassurance for their perceived appearance defect, as required by the diagnostic criteria for hypochondriasis. Requiring these symptoms and behaviors is likely to lead to underdiagnosis of BDD. Indeed, the literature offers more support for a relationship between BDD and OCD or possibly social phobia or major depressive disorder (Phillips 2005a; Phillips and Kaye 2007).

Another challenging issue is how to diagnose BDD in surgical and medical settings. Diagnosing BDD in these settings can be complex because many patients in these settings seek such treatments for minimal deformities, and, by definition, they have some appearance concerns. This important issue has not been well studied. However, in the author's experience, the DSM-IV-TR diagnostic criteria for BDD can be applied in these settings. Although patients who seek cosmetic surgery have some appearance concerns, most of them are not preoccupied with these concerns, and most do not experience clinically significant distress or impairment as a result of their appearance concerns.

Future trends

As recently the mid 1990s, BDD was largely unknown in the field of psychiatry, despite having been described for more than a century. Even now, BDD has received much less empirical investigation than most other serious mental illnesses, and it remains an under-recognized and understudied disorder. Therefore, there is a great need for research on virtually all aspects of BDD. Additional research on

psychiatric treatments is particularly needed, for example, placebo-controlled studies of SRIs and other medications; studies of augmentation of SRIs with pharmacotherapy or CBT; and continuation, maintenance, and relapse prevention studies. Use of CBT for BDD needs to be more rigorously tested, and studies are needed that compare CBT with an SRI and with combined CBT/SRI treatment. Alternative types of psychotherapy need to be developed. Phenomenology and treatment studies are especially needed in adolescents, as this is the age when BDD usually begins. More research is needed on how to best screen for and identify BDD in surgical and non-psychiatric medical settings, and how to persuade patients with BDD to forgo cosmetic procedures and try psychiatric treatment instead. Finally, research is needed to elucidate BDD's etiology and pathophysiology, which are likely complex. Such investigation will clarify BDD's relationship to other disorders and may provide fruitful new leads for BDD's treatment and prevention.

Acknowledgements

This chapter was adapted with permission from Phillips KA (2006). Body dysmorphic disorder: clinical features and treatment of an underrecognized somatoform disorder. In Blumenfeld M, Strain JJ (eds.) *Psychosomatic Medicine in the 21st Century*. Baltimore, MD: Lippincott, Williams & Wilkins.

This work was supported by a grant from the National Institute of Mental Health (K24-MH63975).

References

Albertini RS, Phillips KA (1999). 33 cases of body dysmorphic disorder in children and adolescents. *J Am Acad Child Adolesc Psychiatry* **38**: 453–459.

Allen A, Hadley SJ, Kaplan A, *et al.* (2008). An open-label trial of venlafaxine in body dysmorphic disorder. *CNS Spectr* **13**: 138–144.

American Psychiatric Association (1994). *Diagnostic and Statistical Manual of Mental Disorders*, 4th edn. Washington, DC: American Psychiatric Press.

Bienvenu OJ, Samuels JF, Riddle MA, *et al.* (2000). The relationship of obsessive-compulsive disorder to possible spectrum disorders: results from a family study. *Biol Psychiatry* **48**: 287–293.

Brawman-Mintzer O, Lydiard RB, Phillips KA, *et al.* (1995). Body dysmorphic disorder in patients with anxiety disorders and major depression: a comorbidity study. *Am J Psychiatry* **152**: 1665–1667.

Breiter HC, Filipek PA, Kennedy DN, *et al.* (1994). Retrocallosal white matter abnormalities in patients with obsessive-compulsive disorder. *Arch Gen Psychiatry* **51**: 663–664.

Buhlmann U, Wilhelm S, McNally RJ, *et al.* (2002). Interpretive biases for ambiguous information in body dysmorphic disorder. *CNS Spectr* **7**: 435–443.

Buhlmann U, McNally RJ, Etcoff NL, *et al.* (2004). Emotion recognition deficits in body dysmorphic disorder. *J Psychiatr Res* **38**: 201–206.

Carey P, Seedat S, Warwick J, *et al.* (2004). SPECT imaging of body dysmorphic disorder. *J Neuropsychiat Clin Neurosci* **16**: 357–335.

Castle D, Phillips KA (2006). The OCD spectrum of disorders: a defensible construct?. *Aust N Z J Psychiatry* **40**: 114–120.

Cohen LR, Hollander E (1997). Obsessive-compulsive spectrum disorders. In Hollander E, Stein DJ (ed.) *Obsessive-Compulsive Disorders* (pp. 47–74). New York: Marcel Dekker.

Conroy M, Menard W, Fleming-Ives K, *et al.* (2008). Prevalence and clinical characteristics of body dysmorphic disorder in an adult inpatient setting. *Gen Hosp Psychiatry* **30**: 67–72.

Cotterill JA (1996). Body dysmorphic disorder. *Dermatol Clin* **14**: 457–463.

Cotterill JA, Cunliffe WJ (1997). Suicide in dermatological patients. *Br J Dermatol* **137**: 246–250.

Crerand CE, Phillips KA, Menard W, *et al.* (2005). Nonpsychiatric medical treatment of body dysmorphic disorder. *Psychosomatics* **46**: 549–555.

Deckersbach T, Savage CR, Phillips KA, *et al.* (2000). Characteristics of memory dysfunction in body dysmorphic disorder. *J Int Neuropsychol Soc* **6**: 673–681.

Didie ER, Walters MM, Pinto A, *et al.* (2007). Comparison of quality of life and psychosocial functioning in obsessive-compulsive disorder versus body dysmorphic disorder. *Ann Clin Psychiatry* **19**: 181–186.

Didie ER, Menard W, Stern AP, Phillips KA (2008). Occupational functioning and impairment in adults with body dysmorphic disorder. *Compr Psychiatry* **49**: 561–569.

Diniz JB, Rosario-Campos MC, Shavitt RG, *et al.* (2004). Impact of age at onset and duration of illness on the expression of comorbidities in obsessive-compulsive disorder. *J Clin Psychiatry* **65**: 22–27.

Eisen JL, Goodman WK, Keller MB, *et al.* (1999). Patterns of remission and relapse in obsessive-compulsive disorder: a 2-year prospective study. *J Clin Psychiatry* **60**: 346–351.

Eisen JL, Phillips KA, Coles ME, *et al.* (2004). Insight in obsessive compulsive disorder and body dysmorphic disorder. *Compr Psychiatry* **45**: 10–15.

Faravelli C, Salvatori S, Galassi F, *et al.* (1997). Epidemiology of somatoform disorders: a community survey in Florence. *Soc Psychiatry Psychiatr Epidemiol* **32**: 24–29.

Frare F, Perugi G, Ruffolo G, *et al.* (2004). Obsessive-compulsive disorder and body dysmorphic disorder: a comparison of clinical features. *Eur Psychiatry* **19**: 292–298.

Fukuda O (1977). Statistical analysis of dysmorphophobia in out-patient clinic. *Jpn J Plast Reconstruct Surg* **20**: 569–577.

Grant JE, Kim SW, Crow SJ (2001). Prevalence and clinical features of body dysmorphic disorder in adolescent and adult psychiatric inpatients. *J Clin Psychiatry* **62**: 517–522.

Grant JE, Kim SW, Eckert ED (2002). Body dysmorphic disorder in patients with anorexia nervosa: prevalence, clinical features, and delusionality of body image. *Int J Eat Disord* **32**: 291–300.

Grant JE, Menard W, Pagano ME, *et al.* (2005). Substance use disorders in individuals with body dysmorphic disorder. *J Clin Psychiatry* **66**: 309–316.

Grant JE, Menard W, Phillips KA (2006). Pathological skin picking in individuals with body dysmorphic disorder. *Gen Hosp Psychiatry* **28**: 487–493.

Gunstad J, Phillips KA (2003). Axis I comorbidity in body dysmorphic disorder. *Compr Psychiatry* **44**: 270–276.

Harris EC, Barraclough B (1997). Suicide as an outcome for mental disorders: a meta-analysis. *Br J Psychiatry* **170**: 205–228.

Hollander E, Cohen LJ, Simeon D (1993). Body dysmorphic disorder. *Psychiatr Ann* **23**: 359–364.

Hollander E, Allen A, Kwon J, *et al.* (1999). Clomipramine vs desipramine crossover trial in body dysmorphic disorder: selective efficacy of a serotonin reuptake inhibitor in imagined ugliness. *Arch Gen Psychiatry* **56**: 1033–1039.

Honigman RJ, Phillips KA, Castle DJ (2004). Psychosocial outcomes for patients seeking cosmetic surgery: oppurtunities and risks. *Plast Reconstr Surg* **113**: 1229–1237.

Jaisoorya TS, Reddy YC, Srinath S (2003). The relationship of obsessive-compulsive disorder to putative spectrum disorders: results from an Indian study. *Compr Psychiatry* **44**: 317–23.

Janet P (1903). *Les Obsessions et la Psychasthenie*. Paris: Felix Alcan.

Jenike MA, Breiter HC, Baer L, *et al.* (1996). Cerebral structural abnormalities in obsessive-compulsive disorder: a quantitative morphometric magnetic resonance imaging study. *Arch Gen Psychiatry* 53: 625–632.

Kleinknecht RA, Dinnel DL, Kleinknecht EE, *et al.* (1997). Cultural factors in social anxiety: a comparison of social phobia symptoms and Taijin kyofusho. *J Anxiety Disord* 11: 157–177.

Koblenzer CS (1985). The dysmorphic syndrome. *Arch Dermatol* 121: 780–784.

Koran LM, Abujaoude E, Large MD, *et al.* (2008). The prevalence of body dysmorphic disorder in the United States adult population. *CNS Spectr* 13: 316–322.

Kraepelin E (1909–1915). *Psychiatrie*, 8th edn. Leipzig: JA Barth.

Ladee GA (1966). *Hypochondriacal Syndromes.* Amsterdam: Elsevier.

Mataix-Cols D, Pertusa A, Leckman JF (2007). Issues for DSM-V: how should obsessive-compulsive and related disorders be classified? *Am J Psychiatry* 164: 1313–1314.

McKay D, Todaro J, Neziroglu F, *et al.* (1997a). Body dysmorphic disorder: a preliminary evaluation of treatment and maintenance using exposure with response prevention. *Behav Res Ther* 35: 67–70.

McKay D, Neziroglu F, Yaryura-Tobias JA (1997b). Comparison of clinical characteristics in obsessive-compulsive disorder and body dysmorphic disorder. *J Anxiety Disord* 11: 447–454.

Miller WR, Rollnick S (2002). *Motivational Interviewing.* New York: Guilford Press.

Morselli E (1891). Sulla dismorfofobia e sulla tafefobia. *Boll R Accad Genova* 6: 110–119.

National Collaborating Center for Mental Health (2006). *NICE Clinical Guidance CG31: Core Interventions in the Treatment of Obsessive Compulsive Disorder and Body Dysmorphic Disorder.* London: British Psychiatric Society and Royal College of Psychiatrists.

Neziroglu F (1996). Effect of cognitive behavior therapy on persons with body dysmorphic disorder and comorbid axis II disorders. *Behav Ther* 27: 67–77.

Neziroglu F, Khemlani-Patel S (2002). A review of cognitive and behavioral treatment for body dysmorphic disorder. *CNS Spectr* 7: 464–471.

Neziroglu F, Yaryura-Tobias JA (1993). Exposure, response prevention, and cognitive therapy in the treatment of body dysmorphic disorder. *Behav Ther* 24: 431–438.

Nierenberg AA, Phillips KA, Petersen TJ, *et al.* (2002). Body dysmorphic disorder in outpatients with major depression. *J Affect Disord* 69: 141–148.

O'Sullivan RL, Phillips KA, Keuthen NJ, *et al.* (1999). Near-fatal skin picking from delusional body dysmorphic disorder responsive to fluvoxamine. *Psychosomatics* 40: 79–81.

Otto MW, Wilhelm S, Cohen LS, *et al.* (2001). Prevalence of body dysmorphic disorder in a community sample of women. *Am J Psychiatry* 158: 2061–2063.

Perugi G, Giannotti D, Di Vaio S, *et al.* (1996). Fluvoxamine in the treatment of body dysmorphic disorder (dysmorphophobia). *Int Clin Psychopharmacol* 11: 247–254.

Perugi G, Giannotti D, Frare F, *et al.* (1997a). Prevalence, phenomenology and comorbidity of body dysmorphic disorder (dysmorphophobia) in a clinical population. *Int J Psych Clin Pract* 1: 77–82.

Perugi G, Akiskal HS, Giannotti D, *et al.* (1997b). Gender-related differences in body dysmorphic disorder (dysmorphophobia). *J Nerv Ment Dis* 185: 578–582.

Perugi G, Akiskal HS, Lattanzi L, *et al.* (1998). The high prevalence of "soft" bipolar (II) features in atypical depression. *Compr Psychiatry* 39: 63–71.

Phillips KA (1991). Body dysmorphic disorder: the distress of imagined ugliness. *Am J Psychiatry* 148: 1138–1149.

Phillips KA (2000). Quality of life for patients with body dysmorphic disorder. *J Nerv Ment Dis* 188: 170–175.

Phillips KA (2004). Psychosis in body dysmorphic disorder. *J Psychiatr Res* 38: 63–72.

Phillips KA (2005a). *The Broken Mirror: Understanding and Treating Body Dysmorphic Disorder*, revised edn. New York: Oxford University Press.

Phillips KA (2005b). Placebo-controlled study of pimozide augmentation of fluoxetine in body dysmorphic disorder. *Am J Psychiatry* 162: 377–379.

Phillips KA (2005c). Olanzapine augmentation of fluoxetine in body dysmorphic disorder. *Am J Psychiatry* 162: 1022–1023.

Phillips KA (2006). An open-label study of escitalopram in body dysmorphic disorder. *Int Clin Psychopharmacol* 21: 177–179.

Phillips KA (2009). *Understanding Body Dysmorphic Disorder: An Essential Guide.* New York: Oxford University Press.

Phillips KA, Diaz SF (1997). Gender differences in body dysmorphic disorder. *J Nerv Ment Dis* 185: 570–577.

Phillips KA, Hollander (2008). Treating body dysmorphic disorder with medication: evidence, misconceptions and a suggested approach. *Body Image* 5: 13–27.

Phillips KA, Kaye WH (2007). The relationship of body dysmorphic disorder and eating disorders to obsessive-compulsive disorder. *CNS Spectr* 12: 347–358.

Phillips KA, McElroy SL (2000). Personality disorders and traits in patients with body dysmorphic disorder. *Compr Psychiatry* **41**: 229–236.

Phillips KA, Menard W (2006). Suicidality in body dysmorphic disorder: a prospective study. *Am J Psychiatry* **163**: 1280–1282.

Phillips KA, Najjar F (2003). An open-label study of citalopram in body dysmorphic disorder. *J Clin Psychiatry* **64**: 715–720.

Phillips KA, Stout RL (2006). Associations in the longitudinal course of body dysmorphic disorder with major depression, obsessive compulsive disorder, and social phobia. *J Psychiatr Res* **40**: 360–369.

Phillips KA, Taub SL (1995). Skin picking as a symptom of body dysmorphic disorder. *Psychopharmacol Bull* **31**: 279–288.

Phillips KA, McElroy SL, Lion JR (1992). Body dysmorphic disorder in cosmetic surgery patients. *J Plast Reconst Surg* **90**: 333–334.

Phillips KA, McElroy SL, Keck PE, Jr., *et al.* (1993). Body dysmorphic disorder: 30 cases of imagined ugliness. *Am J Psychiatry* **150**: 302–308.

Phillips KA, McElroy SL, Keck PE, Jr., *et al.* (1994). A comparison of delusional and nondelusional body dysmorphic disorder in 100 cases. *Psychopharmacol Bull* **30**: 179–186.

Phillips KA, Nierenberg AA, Brendel G, *et al.* (1996). Prevalence and clinical features of body dysmorphic disorder in atypical major depression. *J Nerv Ment Dis* **184**: 125–129.

Phillips KA, Dwight MM, McElroy SL (1998a). Efficacy and safety of fluvoxamine in body dysmorphic disorder. *J Clin Psychiatry* **59**: 165–171.

Phillips KA, Gunderson CG, Mallya G, *et al.* (1998b). A comparison study of body dysmorphic disorder and obsessive-compulsive disorder. *J Clin Psychiatry* **59**: 568–575.

Phillips KA, Grant J, Siniscalchi J, *et al.* (2001a). Surgical and non-psychiatric medical treatment of patients with body dysmorphic disorder. *Psychosomatics* **42**: 504–510.

Phillips KA, Albertini RS, Siniscalchi JM, *et al.* (2001b). Effectiveness of pharmacotherapy for body dysmorphic disorder: a chart-review study. *J Clin Psychiatry* **62**: 721–727.

Phillips KA, Albertini RS, Rasmussen SA (2002). A randomized placebo-controlled trial of fluoxetine in body dysmorphic disorder. *Arch Gen Psychiatry* **59**: 381–388.

Phillips KA, Pinto A, Jain S (2004a). Self-esteem in body dysmorphic disorder. *Body Image* **1**: 385–390.

Phillips KA, Siniscalchi JM, McElroy SL (2004b). Depression, anxiety, anger, and somatic symptoms in patients with body dysmorphic disorder. *Psychiatr Q* **75**: 309–320.

Phillips KA, Menard W, Fay C, *et al.* (2005a). Demographic characteristics, phenomenology, comorbidity, and family history in 200 individuals with body dysmorphic disorder. *Psychosomatics* **46**: 317–25.

Phillips KA, Menard W, Fay C, *et al.* (2005b). Psychosocial functioning and quality of life in body dysmorphic disorder. *Compr Psychiatry* **46**: 254–260.

Phillips KA, Coles ME, Menard W, *et al.* (2005c). Suicidal ideation and suicide attempts in body dysmorphic disorder. *J Clin Psychiatry* **66**: 717–725.

Phillips KA, Pagano ME, Menard W, *et al.* (2005d). Predictors of remission from body dysmorphic disorder: a prospective study. *J Nerv Ment Dis* **193**: 564–567.

Phillips KA, Menard W, Fay C, *et al.* (2006a). Gender similarities and differences in 200 individuals with body dysmorphic disorder. *Compr Psychiatry* **47**: 77–87.

Phillips KA, Conroy M, Dufresne RG, *et al.* (2006b). Tanning in body dysmorphic disorder. *Psychiatr Q* **77**: 129–138.

Phillips KA, Didie ER, Menard W, *et al.* (2006c). Clinical features of body dysmorphic disorder in adolescents and adults. *Psychiatry Res* **141**: 305–314.

Phillips KA, Pagano ME, Menard W (2006d). Pharmacotherapy for body dysmorphic disorder: treatment received and illness severity. *Ann Clin Psychiatry* **18**: 251–257.

Phillips KA, Pinto A, Menard W, *et al.* (2006e). Obsessive-compulsive disorder versus body dysmorphic disorder: a comparison study of two possibly related disorders. *Depress Anxiety* **24**: 399–409.

Phillips KA, Didie ER, Menard W (2007). Clinical features and correlates of major depressive disorder in individuals with body dysmorphic disorder. *J Affect Disord* **97**: 129–135.

Pinto A, Phillips KA (2005). Social anxiety in body dysmorphic disorder. *Body Image* **2**: 401–405.

Pope CG, Pope HG, Menard W, *et al.* (2005). Clinical features of muscle dysmorphia among males with body dysmorphic disorder. *Body Image* **2**: 395–400.

Rapaport MH, Clary C, Faayed R, *et al.* (2005). Quality-of-life impairment in depressive and anxiety disorders. *Am J Psychiatry* **162**: 1171–1178.

Rauch SL, Phillips KA, Segal E, *et al.* (2003). A preliminary morphometric magnetic resonance imaging study of regional brain volumes in body dysmorphic disorder. *Psychiatry Res* **122**: 13–19.

Rief W, Buhlmann U, Wilhelm S, *et al.* (2006). The prevalence of body dysmorphic disorder: a population-based survey. *Psychol Med* **36**: 877–885.

Rosen JC, Ramirez E (1998). A comparison of eating disorders and body dysmorphic disorder on body image and psychological adjustment. *J Psychosom Res* **44**: 441–449.

Rosen JC, Reiter J, Orosan P (1995). Cognitive-behavioral body image therapy for body dysmorphic disorder. *J Consult Clin Psychol* **63**: 263–269.

Sarwer DB (2002). Awareness and identification of body dysmorphic disorder by aesthetic surgeons: results of a survey of American Society for Aesthetic Plastic Surgery members. *Aesth Surg J* **22**: 531–535.

Saxena S, Winograd A, Dunkin JJ, *et al.* (2001). A retrospective review of clinical characteristics and treatment response in body dysmorphic disorder versus obsessive-compulsive disorder. *J Clin Psychiatry* **62**: 67–72.

Simeon D, Hollander E, Stein DJ, *et al.* (1995). Body dysmorphic disorder in the DSM-IV field trial for obsessive-compulsive disorder. *Am J Psychiatry* **152**: 1207–1209.

Solyom L, DiNicola VF, Phil M, *et al.* (1985). Is there an obsessive psychosis? Aetiological and prognostic factors of an atypical form of obsessive-compulsive neurosis. *Can J Psychiatry* **30**: 372–380.

Soriano JL, O'Sullivan RL, Baer L, *et al.* (1996). Trichotillomania and self-esteem: a survey of 62 female hair pullers. *J Clin Psychiatry* **57**: 77–82.

Thompson CM, Durrani AJ (2007). An increasing need for early detection of body dysmorphic disorder by all specialties. *J R Soc Med* **100**: 61–62.

Veale D (2000). Outcome of cosmetic surgery and "DIY" surgery in patients with body dysmorphic disorder. *Psychiatric Bull* **24**: 218–221.

Veale D, Riley S (2001). Mirror, mirror on the wall, who is the ugliest of them all? The psychopathology of mirror gazing in body dysmorphic disorder. *Behav Res Ther* **39**: 1381–1393.

Veale D, Boocock A, Gournay K, *et al.* (1996a). Body dysmorphic disorder. A survey of fifty cases. *Br J Psychiatry* **169**: 196–201.

Veale D, Gournay K, Dryden W, *et al.* (1996b). Body dysmorphic disorder: a cognitive behavioural model and pilot randomised controlled trial. *Behav Res Ther* **34**: 717–729.

Wilhelm S, Otto MW, Zucker BG, *et al.* (1997). Prevalence of body dysmorphic disorder in patients with anxiety disorders. *J Anxiety Disord* **11**: 499–502.

Wilhelm S, Otto MW, Lohr B, *et al.* (1999). Cognitive behavior group therapy for body dysmorphic disorder: a case series. *Behav Res Ther* **37**: 71–75.

Wilhelm S, Phillips KA, Steketee G (2010). *A Cognitive Behavioral Treatment Manual for Body Dysmorphic Disorder*. New York: Guilford Press, in press.

World Health Organization (1994). *International Statistical Classification of Diseases and Related Health Problems*, 10th revision. Geneva: World Health Organization.

Zimmerman M, Mattia JI (1998). Body dysmorphic disorder in psychiatric outpatients: recognition, prevalence, comorbidity, demographic, and clinical correlates. *Compr Psychiatry* **39**: 265–270.

Trichotillomania and other impulse control disorders

Michael H. Bloch

Introduction

Trichotillomania is classified as an impulse-control disorder in the *Diagnostic and Statistical Manual of Mental Disorders*, 4th edition revised (DSM-IVR; American Psychiatric Association, 2000). Trichotillomania is characterized by recurrent hair pulling that causes noticeable hair loss and significant distress or impairment (DSM-IVR). Additionally, according to DSM-IVR, trichotillomania requires that an individual sometimes experiences urges prior to pulling and a sense of pleasure, gratification, or relief after pulling. These two diagnostic criteria for trichotillomania remain controversial as a substantial proportion of adults and a majority of children with chronic hair pulling that causes impairment do not report experiencing urges prior to pulling or gratification/relief after pulling. The DSM-IVR criteria for trichotillomania are depicted in Box 15.1.

Trichotillomania is currently classified in DSM-IV as an impulse control disorder, alongside kleptomania, pyromania, pathological gambling, and intermittent explosive disorder. Impulse control disorders are characterized by an inability to resist the impulse to perform an action that is harmful to oneself or others. Trichotillomania, however, has long been hypothesized to belong to group of disorders closely related to obsessive-compulsive disorder (OCD) termed the obsessive-compulsive spectrum disorders (Swedo and Leonard 1992). Obsessive-compulsive spectrum disorders are characterized by repetitive thoughts and actions akin to OCD. Evidence supporting trichotillomania's inclusion as an obsessive-compulsive spectrum disorder include initial evidence suggesting that trichotillomania responded to the same medications, (this has been largely disproven in later studies), and the high comorbidity between OCD and

trichotillomania (Swedo *et al.* 1989; Stewart *et al.* 2005). Other spectrum disorders include OCD, Tourette's syndrome, body dysmorphic disorder, eating disorders, hypochondrias, and compulsive skin picking. In terms of conceptualization, it may be more fruitful to envision trichotillomania as closely related to Tourette's syndrome rather than OCD. Trichotillomania is characterized by premonitory urges and responds to similar behavioral interventions and possibly similar medications as Tourette's syndrome. Furthermore, as in Tourette's syndrome, neuroimaging studies have suggested basal ganglis abnormalities in trichotillomania (O'Sullivan *et al.* 1997). Additionally, Tourette's syndrome and trichotillomania tend to cluster together as comorbidities in individuals with OCD.

Epidemiology and natural history

Trichotillomania has an estimated lifetime prevalence of roughly 0.6%, based on an epidemiologic survey of college students (Christenson *et al.* 1991a). However, the estimated lifetime prevalence increases to roughly 3% when preceding urges and pleasure/relief afterwards are removed from the diagnostic criteria (Christenson *et al.* 1991a). Trichotillomania has a range of comorbidities, with approximately 82% of adults presenting for treatment experiencing at least one other axis I psychiatric disorder (Christenson *et al.* 1991a). Common comorbidities include depression, anxiety disorders, OCD, substance use disorders, post-traumatic stress disorder and other body-focused impulse control disorders.

In adults with trichotillomania, the average age of onset is around 13 years of age (Mansueto *et al.* 1997). Trichotillomania in adults has a strong female predominance and has a chronic waxing and waning

Clinical Obsessive-Compulsive Disorders in Adults and Children, ed. Robert Hudak and Darin D. Dougherty.
Published by Cambridge University Press. Copyright © Cambridge University Press 2011.

Box 15.1 Diagnostic criteria for trichotillomania

A. Recurrent pulling out of one's hair resulting in noticeable hair loss.

B. An increasing sense of tension immediately before pulling out the hair or when attempting to resist the behavior.

C. Pleasure, gratification, or relief when pulling out the hair.

D. The disturbance is not better accounted for by another mental disorder and is not caused by a general medical condition (e.g., a dermatological condition).

E. The disturbance causes clinically significant distress or impairment in social, occupational, or other important areas of functioning.

Source: adapted with permission from American Psychiatric Association 2000.

---

course. Longitudinal studies of adults with trichotillomania have demonstrated little improvement in symptoms over time (Keuthen *et al.* 2001). However, most outcome studies were conducted prior to the availability of effective behavioral techniques for trichotillomania

By contrast, it is important to distinguish trichotillomania from chronic hair pulling in young children. In children under one year of age, it is common to pull a parent's hair and this is considered a behavior consistent with developmentally appropriate environment exploration (Tay *et al.* 2004). Additionally, many preschool children engage in chronic, habitual hair pulling; this behavior is often associated with bedtime and tiredness and may be a self-limiting condition like nail biting or thumb sucking (Tay *et al.* 2004). Trichotillomania also exists in teenagers. This developmental stage of trichotillomania more closely mimics the form of trichotillomania in adults but is likely more responsive to behavioral techniques and has a better clinical outcome as it is earlier in the disease course.

Genetics

Trichotillomania appears to have a hereditary component as trichotillomania is more common in first-degree relatives of trichotillomania patients than in the general population. Genetic studies in trichotillomania have been exceedingly sparse. One recent study demonstrated a mutation in the gene *SLITRK1* in 2 of 44 individuals with trichotillomania and absent in 2192 control samples (Zuchner *et al.* 2006). This gene encodes a dendritic growth factor (SLIT and NTRK-like protein 1) expressed in the striatum, globus pallidus, thalamus, and cortical plate (Abelson *et al.* 2005). Mutations of *SLITRK1* have also been

implicated in the pathogenesis of Tourette's syndrome (Abelson *et al.* 2005).

Neuropsychological deficits

Trichotillomania patients have demonstrated deficits in the ability to inhibit motor behaviors compared with healthy controls (Chamberlain *et al.* 2006; Bohne *et al.* 2008). These deficits have been shown to be in excess compared with other disorders with impaired motor inhibition such as OCD (Chamberlain *et al.* 2006; Bohne *et al.* 2008). These motor inhibition deficits have been demonstrated on two separate tasks of motor inhibition, the Stop-Signal Task and a Go-No-Go task, by two separate groups (Chamberlain *et al.* 2006; Bohne *et al.* 2008). Motor inhibition is a neuropsychological measure of impulsivity and these tasks have been used extensively to study neuropsychological deficits in attention-deficit hyperactivity disorder. Trichotillomania patients have also demonstrated deficits in spatial working memory and in divided attention when compared with healthy controls in some, but not all studies (Keuthen *et al.* 1996; Stanley *et al.* 1997; Chamberlain *et al.* 2006; Bohne *et al.* 2008).

Neuroimaging

Few neuroimaging studies exist in trichotillomania. Small, pilot structural magnetic resonance imaging (MRI) studies have demonstrated reductions in putamen (O'Sullivan *et al.* 1997) and cerbellar volumes (Keuthen *et al.* 2007) in trichotillomania subjects compared with healthy controls. However, the results of structural neuroimaging studies have never been replicated across multiple samples.

Functional neuroimaging (fMRI) has demonstrated reduced resting glucose metabolism in the cerebellum of adult females with trichotillomania compared with healthy controls (Leonard *et al.* 1991). A recent fMRI study examined brain activation patterns during the Serial Reaction Time (SRT) task. The SRT task is an implicit learning task designed to cortico-striatal function. This study failed to demonstrate any evidence for cortico-striatal dysfunction in trichotillomania patients: the patients performed similarly to healthy controls on the SRT and did not show any differences on striatal or cortical brain activation (Rauch *et al.* 2007). Further neuroimaging studies that involve larger samples and probe neuropsychological deficits specific to trichotillomania are needed to further elucidate the neuroanatomy of trichotillomania.

Assessment

A proper assessment in a patient with trichotillomania involves getting a detailed history of their hair pulling. This involves having the patient recount the first instance in which they pulled as well as their current pulling behaviors. When discussing hair pulling behaviors, it is important to discuss antecedent cognitions, behaviors, and feelings prior to pulling (Swedo and Leonard 1992); the settings in which pulling occurs (Swedo *et al.* 1989); the body locations from which pulling occurs (Stewart *et al.* 2005); and behavior after pulling. Trichotillomania patients commonly experience emotions such as boredom, tension, and anxiety prior to hair pulling episodes and/or a physical urge to pull. Commonly experienced cognitions prior to hair pulling include beliefs about the inappropriate appearance of certain hairs (gray, course, etc.), that hairlines or lengths of hair need to be symmetrical or that she or he is unattractive or unlovable because of appearance. Trichotillomania patients also usually have specific places where they pull (e.g., the bedroom or the bathroom). Common post-pulling behaviors involve biting, rubbing, or eating the hair. Also, discarding the hairs in fairly stereotyped ways is the norm. In patients who ingest their own hair, trichobezoars (conglomerations of hair and food that form in the gastrointestinal tract) are of particular concern as they can lead to weight loss, iron-deficiency anemia, malabsorption, and even gastrointestinal tract obstructions.

A detailed history of which body locations a patient pulls from is important. The most common sites of hair pulling are the scalp (73%), eyebrows (56%), eyelashes (53%), pubic region (46%), and legs (15%)

(Woods *et al.* 2006a). A physical examination of areas of hair pulling can uncover areas of irritation, follicle damage, and atypical regrowth of hair, which are common in patients with trichotillomania.

Distinguishing between automatic and focused hair pulling can be important for behavioral treatments. Focused pulling describes pulling with awareness – in response to an urge or an emotion. Automatic pulling describes subconscious pulling that occurs outside of awareness. Often individuals will be well into an automatic pulling episode before they become aware that they are doing it. In clinical samples, automatic pulling behaviors form a slight majority, although most individuals practice both focused and automatic pulling behaviors. Rating scales exist for both adults and children that are designed to distinguish automatic and focused pulling behaviors in individual patients (Woods *et al.* 2006a; Flessner *et al.* 2008). Rating scales such as the Massachusetts General Hospital Hairpulling Scale, a patient self-report form, and the National Institute of Health Trichotillomania Severity Scale, a clinician-rated form, are useful in tracking changes in symptom severity over time (Swedo *et al.* 1989; Keuthen *et al.* 1995; O'Sullivan *et al.* 1995). These scales, as well as the Milwaukee Inventory of Styles of Trichotillomania (Flessner *et al.* 2007), are freely available through the cited references or via internet links.

Since the vast majority of trichotillomania patients suffer from comorbid conditions such as depression, anxiety disorders, OCD, substance use disorders, and other repetitive grooming disorders such as compulsive skin picking, it is important to screen and treat these conditions. Perhaps most important in a clinical evaluation of trichotillomania is to learn how the disorder is impacting an individual's life. Individuals with trichotillomania frequently avoid intimate encounters, social relationships, or certain occupations because of embarrassment about their condition. Trichotillomania can also have a serious negative impact on studying behaviors. Other activities such as swimming or leaving the house on hot or windy days are eschewed because of fears of their hair loss being discovered.

Behavioral treatments

Habit reversal therapy (HRT) is a behavioral therapy designed for the treatment of trichotillomania and tics (Azrin *et al.* 1980). The therapy is covered by a manual

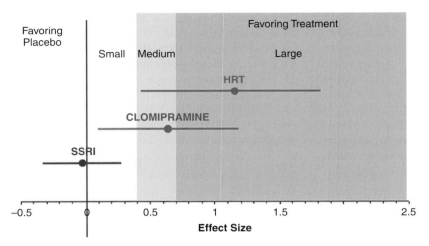

Fig. 15.1 Relative efficacy of treatments in trichotillomania. Effect sizes of habit reversal therapy (HRT), clomipramine, and serotonin reuptake inhibitors (SSRI). Circles represent the point estimate (and lines the 95% confidence intervals) for effect sizes for each of these interventions from the comparison of this intervention with respect to placebo in a meta-analysis of treatments for trichotillomania. (Adapted with permission from Bloch *et al.* 2007.)

and is a behavioral technique that is administered over a period of two to three months with a maintanence period for relapse prevention. The therapy has several components: self-monitoring, awareness training, stimulus control and competing response training. The self-monitoring component of HRT requires patients to keep records of their hair pulling. Awareness training works to increase patient awareness of hair pulling behaviors and of high-risk situations that increase the risk of hair pulling. Stimulus control employs interventions designed to decrease the opportunities to pull and to intervene or prevent pulling behaviors. Competing response training involves teaching a patient to engage in a physical behavior that is incompatible with pulling for a set period of time when they feel the urge to pull. In HRT, patients are only permitted to pull after they have engaged in the competing response behaviors (Woods *et al.* 2006b).

In three randomized, parallel-group studies, HRT demonstrated superior efficacy compared with wait-list or placebo controls (Ninan *et al.* 2000; van Minnen *et al.* 2003; Woods *et al.* 2006a). It also demonstrated superiority to pharmacotherapy with fluoxetine or clomipramine in two of these randomized trials (Ninan *et al.* 2000; van Minnen *et al.* 2003). A recent meta-analysis of randomized, controlled trials of trichotillomania showed that HRT had superior effect sizes compared with pharmacological agents for trichotillomania (Bloch *et al.* 2007) (Fig. 15.1). Further trials are needed to demonstrate that HRT will maintain efficacy when compared with control conditions that account for the non-specific aspects of therapy

(i.e., supportive psychotherapy and psychoeducation). Additionally, a major challenge to HRT is one of access. Given the relative rarity with which trichotillomania patients reach psychiatric attention and the novelty of HRT, few clinicians are currently trained in this invention and most of them are clustered around a few academic centers.

Pharmacological treatments

Selective serotonin reuptake inhibitors

Selective serotonin reuptake inhibitors (SSRI) are currently the most commonly utilized intervention to treat trichotillomania (Woods *et al.* 2006a). Initial open-label trials showed improvement over time in trichotillomania patients taking an SSRI. However, in two blinded, placebo-controlled crossover trials and two randomized, blinded, placebo-controlled parallel group studies, SSRIs have failed to separate out from placebo (Christenson *et al.* 1991b; Streichenwein and Thornby 1995; van Minnen *et al.* 2003; Dougherty *et al.* 2006). A recent meta-analysis that combined the results of these four trials failed to show any evidence of an improvement compared with placebo treatment (Bloch *et al.* 2006). Although there were substantial issues with trial design in early SSRI trials in trichotillomania – small sample size (Christenson *et al.* 1991b; Streichenwein and Thornby 1995; van Minnen *et al.* 2003), crossover design (Christenson *et al.* 1991b; Streichenwein and Thornby 1995), and inadequate treatment duration (Christensen *et al.* 1991b) – even later trials without these design issues have failed to demonstrate even a trend towards efficacy with treatment (Dougherty *et al.* 2006).

Although there is substantial evidence that pharmacological treatment with SSRI is no more effective than placebo in the treatment of primary hair pulling, these medications still may be quite effective in treating comorbid illness in these patients. Depression, anxiety disorders, and post-traumatic stress disorder are all common comorbidities in trichotillomania patients and there is substantial evidence demonstrating improvements in these with SSRI pharmacotherapy. Consequently, when SSRI pharmacotherapy is initiated in a trichotillomania patient, the goal of therapy should be to specifically target comorbid illness that is impairing to the patient, as SSRI pharmacotherapy for primary trichotillomania has little evidence of effecicacy.

Tricyclic antidepressants

Clomipramine is the only tricyclic antidepressant that has been extensively studied in the treatment of trichotillomania. Initial results from a 10 week, randomized, double-blind, crossover study of 13 women that compared clomipramine, a serotonergically selective tricyclic antidepressant, with desipramine, a non-selective tricyclic antidepressant, demonstrated substantial improvement in trichotillomania patients treated with clomipramine (Swedo *et al.* 1989). However, most of the patients in this trial experienced a relapse in their symptoms after longer-term treatment with clomipramine (Swedo *et al.* 1993). Another small, nine-week, randomized, placebo-controlled parallel group study showed some increased improvement of trichotillomania symptoms with clomipramine compared with placebo but not to the level of statistical significance (Ninan *et al.* 2000). Clomipramine treatment was very poorly tolerated in this trial, with 4 of 10 subjects treated with clomipramine dropping out early (Ninan *et al.* 2000). Common side effects associated with clomipramine include weight gain, anticholinergic symptoms, and sedation.

There is some evidence to suggest that clomipramine may be modestly effective in the treatment of trichotillomania although this benefit may be short lived. Clomipramine has also been demonstrated to be effective in common comorbid disorders in trichotillomania such as depression, OCD, and anxiety disorders. Therefore, based on currently available

evidence, clomipramine may be viewed as the pharmacological treatment of choice by default. It should be noted that in head-to-head trials (Ninan *et al.* 2000) and the meta-analysis of randomized, controlled clinical trials behavioral therapy with HRT appears to be a superior intervention where available (Bloch *et al.* 2006).

Emerging treatments

A substantial number of case reports and uncontrolled trials have suggested the possible efficacy of both typical and atypical antipsychotics (Stein and Hollander 1992; Stein *et al.* 1997; Potenza *et al.* 1998; Epperson *et al.* 1999; Van Ameringen *et al.* 1999; Gabriel 2001; Senturk and Tanriverdi 2002; Stewart and Nejtek 2003; Pathak *et al.* 2004; Srivastava *et al.* 2005). Individual case reports have reported improvement with both haloperidol and pimozide in individual trichotillomania patients (Stein *et al.* 1997; Van Ameringen *et al.* 1999). Larger case series have suggested that a large proportion of trichotillomania patients may improve with treatment with atypical antipsychotics such as olanzapine, risperidone, aripiprazole, and quetiapine (Stein *et al.* 1997; Potenza *et al.* 1998; Epperson *et al.* 1999; Gabriel 2001; Senturk and Tanriverdi 2002; Stewart and Nejtek 2003; Pathak *et al.* 2004; Srivastava *et al.* 2005). These anecdotal reports have suggested improvement with antipsychotic treatment alone and as an augmentation agent to SSRI. A 12-week, double-blind, placebo-controlled study of olanzapine for trichotillomania demonstrated significant improvement in the olanzapine-treated group based on clinician-rated global improvement compared with placebo (Van Ameringen *et al.* 2006). Differences in improvement between the groups on rating scales of trichotillomania were much less robust (Van Ameringen *et al.* 2006). Significant side effects of antipsychotics such as weight gain, sedation, and tardive dyskinesia often limit patient acceptance or long-term use of these agents in trichotillomania.

Clinical observations and knowledge of psychopharmacology also support the possible efficacy of dopamine-blocking agents such as antipsychotics in the treatment of trichotillomania. The de novo onset or exacerbation of trichotillomania symptoms in children has been observed to occur with the introduction of psychostimulants (Martin *et al.* 1998). Psychostimulants are known to increase striatal dopamine release. Furthermore, the urges to pull experienced by trichotillomania patients are very similar in character to the premonitory urges many patients with Tourette's syndrome experience prior to tics. Antipsychotic agents are currently the most effective medication of the treatment of tics (Scahill et al. 2000).

A few lines of evidence point to the potential efficacy of glutamate-modulating compounds in the treatment of trichotillomania. Riluzole is an FDA-approved agent for the treatment of amyotrophic lateral sclerosis. Riluzole is thought to be neuroprotective and acts via inhibition of certain voltage-gated sodium channels, which can lead to reduced neurotransmitter release and enhanced astrocytic uptake of extracellular glutamate (Pittenger et al. 2006). Open-label case series have suggested that riluzole may be effective in the treatment of depression, OCD, bipolar depression, and generalized anxiety disorder (Coric et al. 2003, 2005; Zarate et al. 2004). Case report data suggest the possible efficacy of this agent in trichotillomania (Bloch et al. 2007). Similarly, topiramate, an FDA-approved agent for epilepsy that also has glutamate modulating activity, has been studied in trichotillomania. Topiramate acts by modulating voltage-gated sodium and calcium channels, by enhancing gamma-aminobutyrate (GABA) activity at the non-benzodiazepine site of the $GABA_A$ receptor, and by blocking kainite/AMPA (α-amino-3-hydroxyl-5-methyl-4-isoxazole-propionate) glutamate receptors (Shank et al. 2000). Topiramate has also shown efficacy in the treatment of other impulse-control disorders such as binge eating and pathological gambling in randomized, blinded trials. An open-label case series of 14 adults with trichotillomania reported six responders to treatment after 16 weeks of treatment (Lochner et al. 2006). There was also significant improvement with time across the cohort on standard ratings of trichotillomania severity.

N-Acetylcysteine is a hepatoprotective antioxidant that stimulates inhibitory metabotropic glutamate receptors, reducing the synaptic release of glutamate (Grant et al. 2009). A 12-week double-blind placebo-controlled study showed a statistically significant decrease in hair pulling symptoms in the treated group: 56% of the treatment group reported improvements while only 16% of the group taking placebo showed improvement. This is the first double-blind placebo-controlled study of a glutamatergic agent in the treatment of trichotillomania (Grant et al. 2009).

Naltexone is an opioid antagonist used to treat urge-related disorders such as alcoholism and pathological gambling (Volpicelli et al. 1992; Kim et al. 2001). Multiple case reports of adults with trichotillomania and a large open-label uncontrolled trial of children with trichotillomania have suggested the possible efficacy of naltrexone in the treatment of trichotillomania (Carrion 1995; De Sousa 2008).

Skepticism is warranted when viewing the likely efficacy of any treatment of trichotillomania studied in an unblinded, uncontrolled fashion. Many patients with trichotillomania improve over the short-term regardless of treatment after presenting for initial treatment. Greater familiarity and psychoeducation about the disorder, meeting other individuals with the disorder, supportive clinicians, and engaging in any active intervention against the disorder are all powerful forces towards patient improvement. These aspects of treatment along with the waxing and waning course of trichotillomania make it difficult to assess efficacy in uncontrolled trials. There is currently a great need for effective pharmacological treatments for trichotillomania as behavioral treatments are not widely available. However, properly conducted, well-powered, blinded, controlled clinical trials are needed to truly evaluate the efficacy of new treatments for trichotillomania.

Support groups

The Trichotillomania Learning Center based in Santa Cruz, California can be quite helpful in providing treatment referrals and support to individuals experiencing trichotillomania. Often, hearing other individuals' stories, coping mechanisms, and strategies for trichotillomania can be quite helpful in living with and overcoming this illness.

Conclusions

Trichotillomania can be a source of substantial impairment for the individual. There have been great advancements in recent years in the development of HRT to treat trichotillomania. A major challenge to the widespread implementation of this treatment is one of access. Currently, expert HRT treatment is available at only a few academic centers. The relative rarity with which trichotillomania reaches psychiatric attention makes this a particularly daunting challenge. However, treatment manuals of HRT that are of high-quality and are relatively easy to administer are currently available. Research into effective pharmacological treatment for trichotillomania is currently lagging behind that of behavioral therapies. No pharmacological agent has convincingly demonstrated long-term efficacy in the treatment of trichotillomania. Novel pharmacological treatments are urgently needed given the access problem to effective behavioral treatments and the substantial proportion of patients who still do not experience adequate symptom relief despite committing to currently available treatments.

References

Abelson JF, Kwan KY, O'Roak BJ, *et al*. (2005). Sequence variants in SLITRK1 are associated with Tourette's syndrome. *Science* **310**: 317–320.

American Psychiatric Association (2000). *Diagnostic and Statistical Manual*, 4th edn, revised. Washington, DC: American Psychiatric Press.

Azrin NH, Nunn RG, Frantz SE (1980). Treatment of hair pulling (trichotillomania): a comparative study of habit reversal and negative practice training. *Behav Ther Exp Psychiatry* **11**: 13–20.

Bloch MH, Landeros-Weisenberger A, Kelmendi B, *et al*. (2006). A systematic review: antipsychotic augmentation with treatment refractory obsessive-compulsive disorder. *Mol Psychiatry* **11**: 622–632.

Bloch MH, Landeros-Weisenberger A, Dombrowski P, *et al*. (2007). Systematic review: pharmacological and behavioral treatment for trichotillomania. *Biol Psychiatry* **62**: 839–846.

Bohne A, Savage CR, Deckersbach T, Keuthen NJ, Wilhelm S (2008). Motor inhibition in trichotillomania and obsessive-compulsive disorder. *J Psychiatry Res* **42**: 141–150.

Carrion VG (1995). Naltrexone for the treatment of trichotillomania: a case report. *J Clin Psychopharmacol* **15**: 444–445.

Chamberlain SR, Fineberg NA, Blackwell AD, Robbins TW, Sahakian BJ (2006). Motor inhibition and cognitive flexibility in obsessive-compulsive disorder and trichotillomania. *Am J Psychiatry* **163**: 1282–1284.

Chamberlain SR, Fineberg NA, Blackwell AD, *et al*. (2007). A neuropsychological comparison of obsessive-compulsive disorder and trichotillomania. *Neuropsychologia* **45**: 654–662.

Christenson GA, Pyle RL, Mitchell JE (1991a). Estimated lifetime prevalence of trichotillomania in college students. *J Clin Psychiatry* **52**: 415–417.

Christenson GA, Mackenzie TB, Mitchell JE, Callies AL (1991b). A placebo-controlled, double-blind crossover study of fluoxetine in trichotillomania. *Am J Psychiatry* **148**: 1566–1571.

Coric V, Milanovic S, Wasylink S, *et al*. (2003). Beneficial effects of the antiglutamatergic agent riluzole in a patient diagnosed with obsessive-compulsive disorder and major depressive disorder. *Psychopharmacology (Berl)* **167**: 219–220.

Coric V, Taskiran S, Pittenger C, *et al*. (2005). Riluzole augmentation in treatment-resistant obsessive-compulsive disorder: an open-label trial. *Biol Psychiatry* **58**: 424–428.

De Sousa A (2008). An open-label pilot study of naltrexone in childhood-onset trichotillomania. *J Child Adolesc Psychopharmacol* **18**: 30–33.

Dougherty DD, Loh R, Jenike MA, Keuthen NJ (2006). Single modality versus dual modality treatment for trichotillomania: sertraline, behavioral therapy, or both? *J Clin Psychiatry* **67**: 1086–1092.

Epperson CN, Fasula D, Wasylink S, Price LH, McDougle CJ (1999). Risperidone addition in serotonin reuptake inhibitor-resistant trichotillomania: three cases. *J Child Adolesc Psychopharmacol* **9**: 43–49.

Flessner CA, Woods DW, Franklin ME, *et al*. (2007). The Milwaukee Inventory for Styles of Trichotillomania-Child Version (MIST-C): initial development and psychometric properties. *Behav Modif* **31**: 896–918.

Flessner CA, Conelea CA, Woods DW (2008). Styles of pulling in trichotillomania: exploring differences in symptom severity, phenomenology, and functional impact. *Behav Res Ther* **46**: 345–357.

Gabriel A (2001). A case of resistant trichotillomania treated with risperidone-augmented fluvoxamine. *Can J Psychiatry* **46**: 285–286.

Grant JE, Odlaug BL, Kim SW (2009). *N*-Acetylcysteine, a glutamate modulator, in the treatment of trichotillomania: a double-blind, placebo controlled study. *Arch Gen Psychiatry* **66**: 756–763.

Keuthen NJ, O'Sullivan RL, Ricciardi JN, *et al*. (1995). The Massachusetts General Hospital (MGH) Hairpulling Scale: 1. development and factor analyses. *Psychother Psychosom* **64**: 141–145.

Keuthen NJ, Savage CR, O'Sullivan RL, *et al*. (1996). Neuropsychological functioning in trichotillomania. *Biol Psychiatry* **39**: 747–749.

Keuthen NJ, Fraim C, Deckersbach T, *et al*. (2001). Longitudinal follow-up of naturalistic treatment outcome in patients with trichotillomania. *J Clin Psychiatry* **62**: 101–107.

Keuthen NJ, Makris N, Schlerf JE, *et al*. (2007). Evidence for reduced cerebellar volumes in trichotillomania. *Biol Psychiatry* **61**: 374–381.

Kim SW, Grant JE, Adson DE, Shin YC (2001). Double-blind naltrexone and placebo comparison study in the treatment of pathological gambling. *Biol Psychiatry* **49**: 914–921.

Leonard HL, Lenane MC, Swedo SE, Rettew DC, Rapoport JL (1991). A double-blind comparison of clomipramine and desipramine treatment of severe onychophagia (nail biting). *Arch Gen Psychiatry* **48**: 821–827.

Lochner C, Seedat S, Niehaus DJ, Stein DJ (2006). Topiramate in the treatment of trichotillomania: an open-label pilot study. *Int Clin Psychopharmacol* **21**: 255–259.

Mansueto CS, Stemberger RM, Thomas AM, Golomb RG (1997). Trichotillomania: a comprehensive behavioral model. *Clin Psychol Rev* **17**: 567–577.

Martin A, Scahill L, Vitulano L, King RA (1998). Stimulant use and trichotillomania. *J Am Acad Child Adolesc Psychiatry* **37**: 349–350.

Ninan PT, Rothbaum BO, Marsteller FA, Knight BT, Eccard MB (2000). A placebo-controlled trial of cognitive-behavioral therapy and clomipramine in trichotillomania. *J Clin Psychiatry* **61**: 47–50.

O'Sullivan RL, Keuthen NJ, Hayday CF, *et al.* (1995). The Massachusetts General Hospital (MGH) Hairpulling Scale: 2. reliability and validity. *Psychother Psychosom* **64**: 146–148.

O'Sullivan RL, Rauch SL, Breiter HC, *et al.* (1997). Reduced basal ganglia volumes in trichotillomania measured via morphometric magnetic resonance imaging. *Biol Psychiatry* **42**: 39–45.

Pathak S, Danielyan A, Kowatch RA (2004). Successful treatment of trichotillomania with olanzapine augmentation in an adolescent. *J Child Adolesc Psychopharmacol* **14**: 153–154.

Pittenger C, Krystal JH, Coric V (2006). Glutamate-modulating drugs as novel pharmacotherapeutic agents in the treatment of obsessive-compulsive disorder. *Neurotherapeutics* **3**: 69–81.

Potenza MN, Wasylink S, Epperson CN, McDougle CJ (1998). Olanzapine augmentation of fluoxetine in the treatment of trichotillomania. *Am J Psychiatry* **155**: 1299–1300.

Rauch SL, Wright CI, Savage CR, *et al.* (2007). Brain activation during implicit sequence learning in individuals with trichotillomania. *Psychiatry Res* **154**: 233–240.

Scahill L, Chappell PB, King RA, Leckman JF (2000). Pharmacologic treatment of tic disorders. *Child Adolesc Psychiatr Clin N Am* **9**: 99–117.

Senturk V, Tanriverdi N (2002). Resistant trichotillomania and risperidone. *Psychosomatics* **43**: 429–430.

Shank RP, Gardocki JF, Streeter AJ, Maryanoff BE (2000). An overview of the preclinical aspects of topiramate: pharmacology, pharmacokinetics, and mechanism of action. *Epilepsia* **41**(Suppl 1): S3–S9.

Srivastava RK, Sharma S, Tiwari N, Saluja B (2005). Olanzapine augmentation of fluoxetine in trichotillomania: two cases. *Aust N Z J Psychiatry* **39**: 112–113.

Stanley MA, Hannay HJ, Breckenridge JK (1997). The neuropsychology of trichotillomania. *J Anxiety Disord* **11**: 473–488.

Stein DJ, Hollander E (1992). Low-dose pimozide augmentation of serotonin reuptake blockers in the treatment of trichotillomania. *J Clin Psychiatry* **53**: 123–126.

Stein DJ, Bouwer C, Hawkridge S, Emsley RA (1997). Risperidone augmentation of serotonin reuptake inhibitors in obsessive-compulsive and related disorders. *J Clin Psychiatry* **58**: 119–122.

Stewart RS, Nejtek VA (2003). An open-label, flexible-dose study of olanzapine in the treatment of trichotillomania. *J Clin Psychiatry* **64**: 49–52.

Stewart SE, Jenike MA, Keuthen NJ (2005). Severe obsessive-compulsive disorder with and without comorbid hair pulling: comparisons and clinical implications. *J Clin Psychiatry* **66**: 864–869.

Streichenwein SM, Thornby JI (1995). A long-term, double-blind, placebo-controlled crossover trial of the efficacy of fluoxetine for trichotillomania. *Am J Psychiatry* **152**: 1192–1196.

Swedo SE, Leonard HL (1992). Trichotillomania. An obsessive compulsive spectrum disorder? *Psychiatr Clin N Am* **15**: 777–790.

Swedo SE, Leonard HL, Rapoport JL, *et al.* (1989). A double-blind comparison of clomipramine and desipramine in the treatment of trichotillomania (hair pulling). *N Engl J Med* **321**: 497–501.

Swedo SE, Lenane MC, Leonard HL (1993). Long-term treatment of trichotillomania (hair pulling). *N Engl J Med* **329**: 141–142.

Tay YK, Levy ML, Metry DW (2004). Trichotillomania in childhood: case series and review. *Pediatrics* **113**: e494–e498.

Van Ameringen M, Mancini C, Oakman JM, Farvolden P (1999). The potential role of haloperidol in the treatment of trichotillomania. *J Affect Disord* **56**: 219–226.

Van Ameringen MA, Mancini CL, Patterson B, Bennett M, Oakman J (2010). A randomized, double-blind, placebo-controlled trial of olanzapine in the treatment of trichotillomania. *J Clin Psychiatry* Apr 20 [Epub ahead of print].

van Minnen A, Hoogduin KA, Keijsers GP, Hellenbrand I, Hendriks GJ (2003). Treatment of trichotillomania with behavioral therapy or fluoxetine: a randomized, waiting-list controlled study. *Arch Gen Psychiatry* **60**: 517–522.

Volpicelli JR, Alterman AI, Hayashida M, O'Brien CP (1992). Naltrexone in the treatment of alcohol dependence. *Arch Gen Psychiatry* **49**: 876–880.

Woods DW, Flessner CA, Franklin ME, *et al.* (2006a). The Trichotillomania Impact Project (TIP): exploring phenomenology, functional impairment, and treatment utilization. *J Clin Psychiatry* **67**: 1877–1888.

Woods DW, Wetterneck CT, Flessner CA (2006b). A controlled evaluation of acceptance and commitment therapy plus habit reversal for trichotillomania. *Behav Res Ther* **44**: 639–656.

Zarate CA, Jr., Payne JL, Quiroz J, *et al.* (2004). An open-label trial of riluzole in patients with treatment-resistant major depression. *Am J Psychiatry* **161**: 171–174.

Zuchner S, Cuccaro ML, Tran-Viet KN, *et al.* (2006). *SLITRK1* mutations in trichotillomania. *Mol Psychiatry* **11**: 887–889.

Resources

OCD Ireland www.ocdireland.org/

OCD Organizations and Support Groups http://www.geonius.com/ocd/organizations.html

Tricotillomania Learning Center 207 McPherson St, Suite H, Santa Cruz, CA 95060-5863 http://www.trich.org/

Index